The Men'sHealth Guide to Peak Conditioning

The Men'sHealth Guide to
Peak Conditioning

By **Richard Laliberte, Stephen C. George**

and the Editors of Men'sHealth Books

Rodale Press, Inc.

Emmaus, Pennsylvania

Notice

The information in this book is meant to supplement, not replace, proper exercise training. All forms of exercise pose some inherent risks. The editors and publisher advise readers to take full responsibility for their safety and know their limits. Before practicing the exercises in this book, be sure that your equipment is well-maintained, and do not take risks beyond your level of experience, aptitude, training and fitness. The programs in this book are not intended as a substitute for any exercise routine or treatment that may have been prescribed by your doctor.

Library of Congress Cataloging-in-Publication Data

Laliberte, Richard.
    The men's health guide to peak conditioning / by Richard Laliberte, Stephen C. George and the editors of Men's Health Books.
        p.   cm.
    Includes index.
    ISBN 0–87596–323–4 paperback
    1. Physical fitness for men. 2. Exercise for men. I. George, Stephen C.
II. Men's Health Books. III. Title.
GV482.5.L35   1997
613.7'0449—dc20   96–34087

Distributed in the book trade by St. Martin's Press

12 14 16 18 20 19 17 15 13   paperback

── OUR PURPOSE ──

"We inspire and enable people to improve their lives and the world around them."

The Men's Health Guide to Peak Conditioning Editorial Staff

Senior Managing Editor: Neil Wertheimer

Writers: Richard Laliberte, Stephen C. George

Contributing Writer: K. Winston Caine

Lead Researchers: Jan Eickmeier, Deborah Pedron

Researchers and Fact Checkers: Susan E. Burdick, Carol J. Gilmore, Jane Unger Hahn, Sandra Salera-Lloyd, Kathryn Piff

Copy Editor: Amy K. Kovalski

Art Director: Jane Colby Knutila

Cover and Book Designer: Charles Beasley

Illustrators: Charles Beasley (pages 328, 331), J. Andrew Brubaker (pages 54, 325)

Studio Manager: Stefano Carbini

Layout Artist: Eugenie S. Delaney

Photo Editor: Susan Pollack

Photographer: Mitch Mandel

Manufacturing Coordinator: Patrick T. Smith

Office Staff: Roberta Mulliner, Julie Kehs, Bernadette Sauerwine, Mary Lou Stephen

Men's Health Books

Vice-President and Editorial Director: Debora T. Yost

Research Manager: Ann Gossy Yermish

Copy Manager: Lisa D. Andruscavage

Book Manufacturing Director: Helen Clogston

Contents

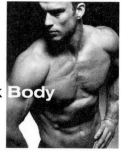

Part Three
Achieving a Peak Body

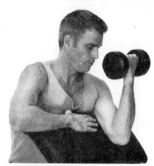

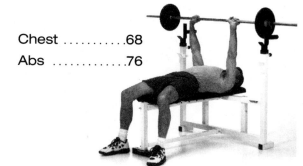

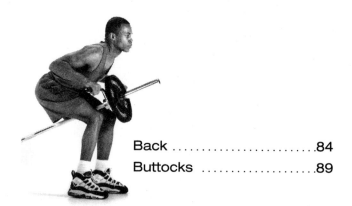

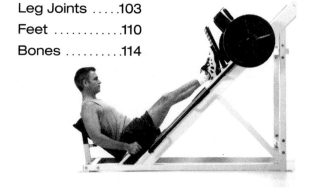

Part Four
Workouts for Every Scenario

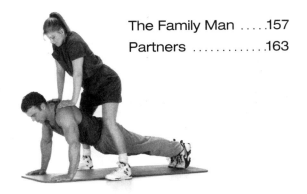

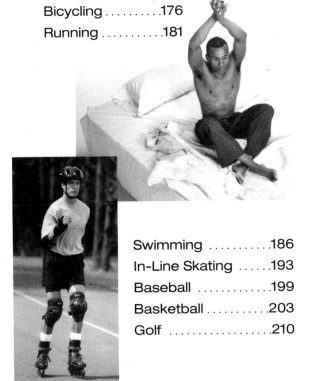

Part Five
Body Maintenance

Part Six
Getting Equipped

Illustrated Exercises

Introduction

The men of America come in a hundred million different sizes, colors, ages, backgrounds. But most of us share one thing: the ability to tell scary stories about our grade-school gym teachers.

Remember the time the entire class watched as your teacher forced you to wrestle a guy 150 pounds bigger than you? Or when you loudly split your gym shorts on your 53rd consecutive sit-up, just as the gym was getting quiet with exertion, and how your teacher called you Rip for the rest of the year? Or the time you fell on your head while your teacher stood three feet away, grade book in hand, watching to see if you could do something—*anything*—on the parallel bars? We have no proof to back this up, but we suspect millions of men have avoided the gym their entire adult lives because of flashback fears.

Gymteacherphobia—as good a reason as any for why men don't work out. Which is to say, there's *no* good reason to blow off exercise. Sure, as a whole, we are working long hours. We have families, communities, friends who need us. We have no time to exercise, and frankly, it's not a priority.

And yet, three hours of exercise per week—that's 1.8 percent of your time—is all you need to be healthy and strong. Compare that with the 20-plus hours of television you watch in a week (yes, the U.S. TV-consumption average now exceeds 3 hours a day). And so, year after year goes by, and the men of America get fatter and lazier.

But we're starting to sound like your old gym teacher. We know we can't scare you, or guilt you, or paddle your butt into exercising more. That you're holding this book suggests you are one of the brilliant who know the benefits and joys of being fit and strong. If so, you're going to love all this book has to offer. But if you're new to this, here's why being fit makes so much sense.

First and foremost, realize that exercise, done right, is pleasure, not pain. Particularly if you do things you enjoy. Running, bicycling, bowling, rowing, throwing a baseball. This is the stuff of life, of laughter, of good times.

Second, the feeling you get after exercise is exquisite. Your body has this calm euphoria about it. Blood is flowing, your breathing is deep, your mind is sharp. It's hard to explain this post-workout aura, but if you exercise, you know.

Third, exercise lets you eat more. And not just to make up what you burned off during workouts. Toned muscles need more fuel even when they are idling. That means you'll need more food merely to get through a night of sleep.

Fourth, exercise gives you energy. To stay up late. To play longer. To love better.

Fifth, exercise makes you look great. Your belly flattens, you gain definition, your posture straightens, your demeanor gets confident.

Pretty good list, no? And that doesn't even include the stuff the doctor will tell you. Like how exercise can help prevent heart disease. Strokes. Cancer. Impotence. Bone degeneration. And on and on.

All for a few hours a week.

The Training Gap

The thing is that most men don't really know how to exercise. The only training many of us got came from the gym teachers and coaches of our youth. You're an adult now. You can't succeed very well in business with an eighth-grade education; how can you succeed at fitness with that level of schooling?

Sure, men have an instinctive knowledge of how to pound a baseball mitt or ride a bike. But a true understanding of what fitness is and how to get it? We men are surprisingly naive. Which is one of the biggest reasons why we wrote *The Men's Health Guide to Peak Conditioning*. Men need better information about how to reach their peak fitness levels. Gut instinct won't do it—no matter how big our guts have become.

For example, it is astounding how many myths and half-truths are widely considered as fact, we discovered in our research. That weight lifting is just for bodybuilders. That stretching isn't very important. That being sore is good. That you need to consume more salt when you exercise.

We were also struck at how so much instruction presented by books and magazines is "one size fits all," as if a single exercise program will work for most every guy in America. This, too, isn't right. We all know that every man is different: different goals, preferences, body types, lifestyles, time constraints.

So we set goals for our book. First, to tell the complete, practical truth about exercise—how much time to allot for it, the right way to do it, how much money you should spend on it. And we set out to tell you in as easy, entertaining and actionable a format as possible. Hey, that's our stock and trade here at *Men's Health*.

We also decided to write *Peak Conditioning* in a way that truly *does* offer fitness tips for every guy in America. To do this, we sat in a room and brainstormed all the different exercise challenges our readers might encounter. Like living in the country. Or living in the inner city. Or approaching middle age. Or having kids. Or working at a job that takes 50 intense hours of your week. Then we pondered all the goals our readers might have. Like getting better at golf. Recovering from an illness. Improving sexual stamina. Losing weight. Bulking up.

Armed with these lists, we came up with our approach: Offer exercise routines and solutions for roughly three dozen different goals, lifestyles or activities. That way, readers could dip into each situation that is relevant to them and build their own program. Say a guy loves tennis, is 43 years old and needs to lose 25 pounds. He would go to the "Racquet Sports," "The Forties" and "Ridding Fat" chapters to learn the stretches, exercises and strategies to be the best at all three.

Finally, as we pondered all the books and magazines out there that deal with exercise, we came to the conclusion that they were written in a vacuum, as if a guy has unlimited time and resources to achieve a state of peak fitness. So we tried to put exercise in context with the full gamut of modern life. We teach you how to buy equipment. How to make time for exercise. How to stay motivated. How to give a massage. How to eat. How to work out at lunch without changing your clothes. How to teach your kids about exercise. How not to get arrested when riding a mountain bike through city streets. And on and on.

How We Organized the Book

As we said, jumping blindly into an exercise routine just doesn't work: You need some education first. And that's what we provide. Part 1, "The Peak Lifestyle," teaches how to make exercise a part of your life with as little effort as possible. Part 2, "Achieving Peak Conditioning," gets into the art and science of exercise—the what, how and why of it all. It's fascinating reading.

Of course, what good is a workout book without great exercises? In part 3, "Achieving a Peak Body," we go muscle group by muscle group, offering the best exercises for each. These exercises are the ingredients for part 4, "Workouts for Every Scenario," where we go through the nearly three dozen goal- and lifestyle-specific workouts.

Part 5, "Body Maintenance," discusses how to keep your body healthy and sound. In it, we teach how to give a massage, how to avoid injury and how to treat one if one indeed occurs.

We wrap things up with part 6, "Getting Equipped," in which we discuss all the gear you'll need to achieve your goals.

A word regarding photography: Our approach was to provide instructional photographs each time we introduce a new exercise. If a chapter mentions an exercise previously discussed and you do not know how to do it, take at look at the Reference Points box that accompanies the chapter. It will list where every exercise in that chapter is first detailed.

In all, *Peak Conditioning* provides nearly 500 photos showing how to stretch, pump and otherwise strengthen your body. Our hope is that you will take this book with you to the gym, the basement, wherever you exercise. If this book stays on your night table, we will consider ourselves failures.

Your First Lesson

In the course of writing *Peak Conditioning*, we interviewed hundreds of fitness experts, read dozens of books, digested untold number of research papers and studies. We also tested out virtually every exercise on our own to make sure it felt right and was easy to do. We learned a lot of things, one of which is that there is not much consensus about the proper methods or amounts of exercise. For all the research into health and fitness, in many ways, exercise is as much art as science.

Yet we still needed a foundation on which to build the book. And so we established some underlying assumptions and approaches, based on experts' opinions. Each of these are discussed at length in the pages that follow. But knowing them up front will help you considerably in your quest for success. So consider this roundup of assorted facts and assumptions as your first lesson for achieving peak conditioning.

• The elements of fitness. Every exercise regimen should blend stretching, aerobic activity and strength training. While specific goals—running a marathon or sculpting your body, for example—might emphasize one of the three, it's still necessary to work in all three aspects to truly be at your peak.

• The way to weight lift. Resistance training benefits everything you do. There's not a guy in America who shouldn't be doing it. The trick is to find the right method for you. There's no such thing as "just doing" bench presses—the outcome of the exercise will vary incredibly based solely on how much weight you use, how many repetitions you do and how much you rest between sets. We'll be offering five different approaches.

1. Weight lifting for brute strength
2. Weight lifting for general fitness
3. Weight lifting for stamina
4. Weight lifting for body shaping
5. Weight lifting that blends the best of each using what's known as a periodization program

It's your job to decide your personal goals. From there, we'll teach you what you need to know.

• Machines versus free weights. We are biased toward free weights over machines. One obvious reason is practicality: Many men don't have access to a gym and would prefer to work out in their basements. For these guys, there is no choice but to buy free weights. Another reason is that free weights test your muscles more fully.

• Proper stretching technique. Unless told otherwise, slowly extend yourself until you feel the appropriate muscle is being stretched, then hold the position for 20 to 30 seconds. Most guys bounce and yank while stretching, or release the stretch after a few seconds. Bad habits.

• How much you need. The minimum amount of exercise time needed per week to gain significant health benefits is three 30-minute sessions, each session on a separate day, many doctors agree. Better yet is to do three days of a well-rounded routine that takes 90 minutes or so. Best of all is to rotate weight-lifting days with aerobic-exercise days.

• The workout sequence. There's much argument over this one out there in academia, but we've come to the conclusion that the best sequence has six parts.

1. Warm-up
2. Stretch
3. Resistance training
4. Aerobic exercise
5. Cooldown
6. Stretch

If you're doing your weight-lifting and aerobic workouts on separate days, we still advise a warm-up, stretch, cooldown and stretch sequence as part of each day's workout.

• The appropriate diet. Again, there is lots of debate on this. But our stance is that an active man should derive 60 percent of his calories from carbohydrate, 25 to 30 percent of calories from fat and 10 to 15 percent of calories from protein.

In addition, an active man should drink six to eight eight-ounce glasses of water per day.

Feeling smarter already? All part of the therapy to exorcise the gym-teacher demons from your soul. Peak conditioning is terrific to achieve and even better to sustain. Here is your definitive guide.

Neil Wertheimer
Senior Managing Editor,
Men's Health Books

Part One
The Peak Lifestyle

Defining Peak

Think of yourself as a man out of time. You may have a self-image as a turn-of-the-millennium kind of guy who drives to work, takes an elevator to his office, gets e-mail, sends faxes, eats microwaved dinners and watches satellite TV from his vibrating lounge chair. But your body knows you as a different person, someone completely out of place in the modern world.

To your genes, cells, tissues and organs, you're a man who walks or runs everywhere, climbs a tree or mountain when he needs some height, conveys messages in person, wrests his food from the land and only reclines to eat, rest or have sex. That's been the physical model for man ever since the time of those slope-headed guys with clubs you see on evolution charts. It has remained the model for man right up until times recent enough to be remembered by some of our living elders.

Our lives don't match our design parameters. And any time function doesn't follow form, you get problems. In this case, even though we work like pack mules to keep on top of our careers and family responsibilities, we've become (at least in the United States) a species of slackers physically. According to the National Center for Health Statistics, overweight prevalency rates went up a significant 8 percent between 1980 and 1991. In addition, according to Wayne Westcott, Ph.D., strength-training consultant to the national YMCA and senior fitness director for the South Shore YMCA in Quincy, Massachusetts, the latest research on the effects of aging on the body shows that the average rate for loss of muscle mass in the U.S. population is accelerating—it's now up to a loss of seven pounds per decade.

The Power Within

But population figures have nothing to do with you as an individual. The point is that you're a man with immense physical potential that's waiting to be set free. That's what this book means when it talks about peak conditioning: Each of us has a blueprint for strength, endurance, speed and agility that's far superior to what our physical states are like right now, says John Duncan, Ph.D., a leading exercise researcher and president of Wellmart, a wellness consulting company also in Denton.

Your mission is to develop your potential to a point that is reasonable for you—to set goals and make it happen. This book's job is to empower you to do it, by guiding you every step of the way, whether you've never exercised in your life or have been dedicated to workouts for years. "It's like that Army slogan: 'Be all that you can be,'" says Dr. Duncan. "Even highly trained men can improve." And if you're not trained, your potential is all the greater.

Consider this little-known but astonishing fact: If you're untrained, your muscles are more powerful right this minute than they appear to be. The reason? Your central nervous system—in the interests of preventing injury and keeping muscles working smoothly in ways they're most accustomed to—actually holds less-used but strong muscles back from unfamiliar movements or work. According to Dr. Westcott, you already have the capability within your muscles to be *40 to 60 percent stronger* than you seem. This latent power is unleashed within four weeks of starting a strength-training program, he says, as a phenomenon called the motor learning effect kicks in—and you've still barely touched your potential for growth of new muscle.

Your Fitness Spec Sheet

There's no end, it seems, to the good that physical conditioning does you. Studies find that exercise reduces the risk of major health problems like heart disease and cancer, lengthens your life, boosts energy, reduces stress and lifts bad moods. On a finer level, it causes lots of small but important changes in the body, ranging from increased insulin sensitivity (which helps to prevent diabetes) to higher levels of antibodies in the blood (which can help fend off disease).

All of which is great, but none of which you really need to think about when laying out your exercise plans. Conditioning is measured in just a few basic ways. All the other benefits of exercise fall into place automatically if you aim to be fit in these

Exercise Light: How Much Is Enough?

Ever since aerobics first became a buzzword back in the 1970s, the mantra about exercise was that nothing short of gasping for breath for at least a half-hour (preferably an hour), at least three days a week (preferably four or five), was going to do you any good. Not surprisingly, less than a quarter of the population found it within themselves to follow these guidelines.

Researchers are still singing that old tune if your aim is to reach peak condition, but they've added a harmonizing line: If you can't be a dedicated exerciser, simply becoming more active will confer most of the health benefits of vigorous workouts. For example, in a six-month study of walkers that John Duncan, Ph.D., a leading exercise researcher and president of Wellmart, a wellness consulting company also in Denton, calls "the first salvo across the bow" of conventional wisdom, slow walkers lowered their risk of cardiovascular disease just as much as fast walkers did, even though the faster, harder-working subjects became more fit. Other studies, including a similar experiment done with runners, have made similar findings.

As a result, the Centers for Disease Control and Prevention in Atlanta and the American College of Sports Medicine published a new, improved set of exercise recommendations in 1995. Two of their key points:

• The concept of "moderate-intensity physical activity" has been broadened to the point that stuff you wouldn't even consider exercise is said to make a substantial difference. Among the activities that the all-star team of researchers say qualify as health-promoting are playing table tennis, carrying a bag of golf clubs, fly-fishing while standing, mowing the lawn and painting the house.

• While it's still a good idea to exercise at least 30 minutes a day, it doesn't have to be all at once. Exercise accumulates, and every minute you spend climbing staircases, raking leaves, walking to and from your car and playing with your kids adds to the daily tally of active time.

Skeptics wonder if exercise advocates haven't simply lowered their standards to accommodate the slothfully inclined, but actually, they've come up with an additional standard for those who might never reach the higher bar. The crucial point is this: Exercise is dose-related—the more you do, the more you benefit in terms of fitness. That's a standard that hasn't changed, says Dr. Duncan.

---

fundamental areas, according to Alan Mikesky, Ph.D., director of the Human Performance Lab and associate professor at Indiana University-Purdue University Indianapolis.

Strength. Let's start here. Most men do. Strength is an inherently masculine trait, not only because we have more of it than women but because we measure ourselves against other men based on our physical power and build. (Remember those Charles Atlas ads in comic books where muscle-building "made a man out of Mac"?) Being strong means being able to make muscles work against some form of resistance, whether it's a barbell at the gym or a ladder in your backyard.

Strength tends to be measured in short-spurt activities like bench-pressing as much weight as you can in eight consecutive lifts. Do enough lifts and, over time, the muscles being used grow stronger and bigger. It's what exercise physiologists refer to as the overload principle: If you work muscles harder than they're accustomed to, they adapt by becoming stronger and more powerful. You keep muscles overloaded from workout to workout by increasing the weight lifted, the number of lifts or the speed of the muscle action.

Endurance. The terms *endurance, aerobic fit-ness, cardiovascular fitness* and *cardiorespiratory fitness* generally all refer to the same thing: the body's ability to generate energy for working muscles during sustained exercise. More than anything else, this depends on efficient delivery of oxygen, which comes down to the heart and lungs. The lungs take in oxygen and the heart pumps it via blood to muscles. There's a kind of alchemy here in which oxygen is used by the cells to help unleash the energy found in the foods we eat. The more efficient your body is at delivering oxygen and generating energy, the healthier and fitter you are.

Sustained-effort aerobic activities like running, swimming, biking or cross-country skiing not only tone muscle but also improve the capacities of the heart, lungs and blood vessels to deliver oxygen. In addition, they improve the ability of individual cells to use oxygen to generate energy.

Body composition. As a rule, fitness improves when the body has more muscle and less fat. The way to improve the muscle/fat composition is with strength or endurance training. Sustained aerobic exercise burns fat, while strength training increases muscle mass, which raises the body's daily calorie requirements.

Body composition is also a measure of health,

The Fast Fitness Test

It's a given: If you want to become better at something, you have to establish a starting point. Even if you think you're pretty fit, it's important to take stock of yourself.

The following tests provide quick, simple readings on the essential elements of conditioning, with the results gauged according to the criterion we all use in the real world: how well other men our age perform. Once you start exercising, however, keep in mind that the real benchmark is your own improvement.

Repeat these tests every now and then to measure progress (or lack thereof) and adjust your objectives accordingly, recommends Alan Mikesky, Ph.D., director of the Human Performance Lab and associate professor at Indiana University-Purdue University Indianapolis.

Chair Lifts

What it measures: Upper-body strength

Equipment needed: Sturdy bench or armless chair with four vertical legs

What to do: Sit on the edge of the bench or chair with your legs straight out so that your heels are on the floor and your toes are pointing up. Grasping the sides of the seat with your hands, carefully inch off and away from the chair so that you're supported by your heels and your hands. Lower yourself until your buttocks touch the floor. Hold for one second, then push back up. Repeat as many times as you can.

Average results:
Twenties: 10 lifts
Thirties: 9 lifts
Forties: 8 lifts
Fifties: 7 lifts
Sixties: 6 lifts

Slow Squat

What it measures: Lower-body strength

Equipment needed: None

What to do: Stand with your feet shoulder-width apart. Keeping your feet flat on the floor, very slowly bend your knees to lower your body toward the floor, taking 30 seconds to reach a point at which your hips are just below parallel with your knees. Take another 30 seconds to raise yourself back to starting position. If you feel you can't go the full minute, cheat on time, but try to complete the entire move.

Average results (in time to fatigue):
Twenties: 60 seconds
Thirties: 52 to 55 seconds
Forties: 44 to 50 seconds
Fifties: 38 to 45 seconds
Sixties: Less than 40 seconds

1.5 Mile Run

What it measures: Aerobic fitness

Equipment needed: A track

What to do: This test from The Cooper Institute for Aerobics Research in Dallas is intended for healthy, active people. Not there yet? Then work up

---

since sizable stores of fat in the body—especially in the abdomen, where it tends to collect in men—are associated with a number of serious problems that exercise helps alleviate, such as high cholesterol and heart disease, diabetes and some forms of cancer, according to Dr. Mikesky.

Flexibility. Flexibility is an unsung but crucial element of conditioning. Just ask any of the 31 million Americans with lower-back pain, a problem very often caused by tight, inflexible back muscles. Stiff muscles not only can cause cramps but also can constrain movement.

If you can't put muscles through their full range of motion, any type of conditioning you attempt is going to be shortchanged, because muscles only get more powerful within the range in which they're used. What's more, loss of flexibility tends to set in earlier than most other age-related changes, so that even a man in his thirties will start feeling twinges of

creakiness if he doesn't keep his muscles moving and stretching.

Tapping Your Potential

Two of the four exercise parameters are also basic forms of exercise: strength and endurance, each of which requires different kinds of activity, thanks to what's called the specificity principle. It says that the body responds in highly specific ways to whatever exercise you do, with very little overlap from one form of exercise to another. If you want to run a marathon, for example, power lifting won't necessarily help you. If you want to bench-press 150 pounds, biking won't get you there. If you want to improve your all-around fitness, you'll need to do a little of a lot of different things, but your improvements in any of them won't be as great as they would be if you concentrated on one at a time.

"It's difficult to have optimal levels of everything

to this by launching a walking program for several weeks first. The concept is easy: See how fast you can run 1.5 miles. If you have access to a 440-yard track, 1.5 miles is six laps running in the inside lane.

Don't push yourself to complete exhaustion while doing this. If you've been sick or get symptoms like chest pains when you start running, obviously consult with a doctor. Final notes: Don't eat for two hours before running, and be sure to warm up and stretch first.

Results (in minutes:seconds):
> Twenties: Superior—faster than 8:13
> > Good—8:14 to 12:51
> > Poor—slower than 12:51
> Thirties: Superior—faster than 8:44
> > Good—8:45 to 13:36
> > Poor—slower than 13:36
> Forties: Superior—faster than 9:30
> > Good—9:31 to 14:29
> > Poor—slower than 14:29
> Fifties: Superior—faster than 10:40
> > Good—10:41 to 15:26
> > Poor—slower than 15:26
> Sixties: Superior—faster than 11:20
> > Good—11:21 to 16:43
> > Poor—slower than 16:43

Triceps Pinch

What it measures: Body fat
Equipment needed: Ruler
What to do: Get a partner to hold the ruler. Extend your arm straight in front of you, palm up. Grab the skin on the back of your upper arm (the side facing down) between your thumb and your fingers, gently pulling it away from your arm, trying not to pinch too tightly. Have your partner measure the thickness of the skin held between your fingers and thumb (not the distance it's being pulled out).

Average results:
> Ages 20 to 40: ½ inch—good
> > ¾ inch—average
> Ages 41 to 60: ⅝ inch—good
> > ⅞ inch—average

Toe Touch

What it measures: Flexibility
Equipment needed: None
What to do: Sit on the floor with one leg straight in front of you and the other bent with the foot tucked against the thigh of your straight leg, so that your legs make a figure 4. Using the arm on the same side as the straight leg, reach as far as you can toward your toes.

Average results:
> Ages 20 to 40: Wrist to toe—good
> > Fingertips to toe—average
> > Fingertips to ankle—fair
> > Fingertips to sock line—poor
> Ages 41 to 60: Fingertips to toe—good
> > Fingertips to ankle—average
> > Fingertips to sock line—fair
> > Fingertips above sock line—poor

at once because different types of conditioning require different types of training," says Dr. Mikesky. "You have to decide what you want from training to design a program that will achieve satisfying results." Unless your objective is simply to increase your level of activity to reap some health benefits—and that's certainly a worthwhile goal—you're not going to achieve peak conditioning by simply deciding, "I'm going to exercise more." Vague ambitions lead to all-too-tangible disappointments. You need to make more focused choices.

Setting Goals

We know. You don't want to hear about goals. Exercise is about doing—it's running and throwing and lifting and going fast and breathing hard and strutting like a demigod. Goals are about thinking—they just kind of float around, if abstract thoughts can be said to do anything at all. Well, let us interrupt your yawn to divert your attention to the real issue here, which is *results*. To get them, you'll need both exercise and goals.

Everyone begins an exercise program with something in mind, even if it's vague. Maybe it's looking better, maybe it's feeling better, maybe it's living longer than your father did. There are as many motives as there are people. Setting goals is just a way of making what's in your head translate to your body while keeping your head interested for as long as it takes.

If you don't make decisions up front, you're more likely to give up when you don't perform as well as you'd like, because you don't have a tangible, realistic plan in place to get there, says Kate Hays, Ph.D., a sport psychologist and founder of The Performing Edge, a performance enhancement training company for athletes, performing artists and business people in Concord, New Hampshire. Not exactly a prescription for success. Goals give you the motivation to keep going when you start feeling bored, lazy or impatient with your progress.

"The main reasons people don't stick with exercise is that they either don't set goals or they can't meet the goals they do set," says Bess H. Marcus, Ph.D., associate professor of psychiatry and human behavior at Miriam Hospital and Brown University School of Medicine in Providence, Rhode Island. We're not talking five-year marketing proposals here—we're talking a few basic decisions on the actions you're going to take.

Scoping Out Your Life

Goals start with a reality check. If having impossible goals is almost as bad as having none at all, you need to take stock of your limitations and opportunities. You can make exercise work around reality, but not vice versa. According to Dr. Marcus, some of the more crucial considerations are:

Which twitch? Some men excel at sprints, others excel at marathons. Both sports involve running, but success depends on what your muscles are made of. There are two types of muscle fiber: fast-twitch and slow-twitch. Fast-twitch fibers contract rapidly and burn energy in short periods; they're used for anaerobic activities that require quick bursts of force like sprinting and power lifting. Slow-twitch fibers contract less rapidly and burn energy more gradually; they're used for aerobic activities like cycling and long-distance running. Your muscles contain a mix of both fibers, and both can be developed with training, but one type dominates. Bottom line: You'll get better results doing exercise that plays to your physiological strengths.

A crude way to tell which fiber type dominates your muscles is to look in the mirror, says Wayne Westcott, Ph.D., strength-training consultant to the national YMCA and senior fitness director for the South Shore YMCA in Quincy, Massachusetts. Generally, men who are *ectomorphs*—long and thin, with little fat—have more slow-twitch fibers and will do better with aerobic exercise. Men who are stocky, beefy *endomorphs* have more fast-twitch fibers and will do better with weight training. Still, there's another category of body type, the *mesomorph*, that's in between. To get a more precise handle on your twitch mix, take the test described in "How to Find Your Muscle Mix."

Your funhog quotient. One of the more noxious myths about exercise is that it has to be something you hate. Totally wrong. People who study exercise adherence, like Dr. Marcus, say you're only likely to succeed over the long term with activities you like. That doesn't mean exercise will ever feel like sipping mint juleps under a palm tree. You will work, you will sweat, but you will still enjoy it. How you'll do it depends on what you already consider fun. It's not just a matter of choosing in-line skating over rock climbing. "Fun could be socializing with others or enjoying an op-

How to Find Your Muscle Mix

Are your muscles made of mostly fast-twitch fibers, good for quick hits of power (think Arnold Schwarzenegger) or slow-twitch fibers, good for sustained, concert-length stamina (think Mick Jagger)? Your personal mix holds the secret to your natural success at different forms of exercise. To find it, take the following test, recommended by Wayne Westcott, Ph.D., strength-training consultant to the national YMCA and senior fitness director for the South Shore YMCA in Quincy, Massachusetts.

Using a bench-press machine or a bench with a barbell rack, start from a lying position and lift the heaviest weight you can manage in one controlled press above your chest. (Get a partner to spot you if you're using a barbell.) Rest five minutes. While you're resting, reduce the weight so that it's 75 percent of the amount you did on the first lift. For example, if you could press 100 pounds one time, you'd now cut the weight to 75 pounds. Now lie back down on the bench and do as many controlled lifts with this lighter weight as you can. Results, as determined by the number of lifts with the lighter weight:

Fewer than 8 repetitions: You're mostly slow-twitch and are likely to be an ectomorph, fast-moving and a natural at endurance sports. Having a thin frame, however, may make muscle-building a challenge.

8 to 12 repetitions: Your slow- and fast-twitch fibers are close to being evenly balanced, so you likely can build muscle fast *and* keep aerobically fit without too much effort, the characteristics of a classic mesomorph. You're the envy of all—but watch that gut.

More than 12 repetitions: You're mostly fast-twitch and are likely an endomorph with lots of strength but also a higher percentage of fat. You'll be good with weights, but you may need fat-burning aerobic exercise more. Enjoy the water? Your buoyancy and strength make swimming a good bet.

---

portunity to spend a rare moment by yourself doing what you want," she says. Either way, "if you enjoy it right then, you'll feel a lift afterward, and that's what will keep you going," she adds.

Time constraints. Some types of exercise require more time than others—or demand rigid schedule commitments. If your goal is to lose weight, for example, Dr. Marcus says you'll need to do fat-burning aerobic workouts for at least 20 minutes almost every day of the week. If you want to build strength and muscle at a gym, your workouts (including travel to and from) may take more time, but you'll have to do them only two or three days a week, she says. Pertinent questions to ask: If you elevated exercise to the status of a business meeting, where could you create openings in your schedule? Do you travel a lot? If so, try to choose an exercise that's easily done while on the road (like running) or that you can make arrangements for ahead of time (by, say, booking yourself into a hotel with an on-site gym).

Glory days. In some respects, a man with a long history of fitness finds it tougher to start a new program than someone who has never exercised in his life. "Men in particular may have really strong memories of who they used to be, and that can be a snag," says Dr. Hays. We often assume we can pick up our physical prowess wherever we left it last, especially if we were, say, captain of the football team or state cross-country champ in high school. Why is that a problem? We expect—and try—to do too much too soon, which can lead to injury or discouragement.

One strategy Dr. Hays suggests: If you're going to start an activity you excelled at in the past, make sure your current expectations and goals relate to your present lifestyle—fitness, time and energy.

Making Goals Work

At some point in your program, you'll ask yourself why you're doing this. Goals are for answering that question with reasons strong enough to keep you going. "Being healthy or fit or losing weight are really good reasons to exercise, but as primary incentives they're not enough," says James Gavin, Ph.D., professor in the Department of Applied Social Science at Concordia University in Montreal and author of *The Exercise Habit.* Here's how to make soft goals more firm.

Be specific. Unless goals are concrete, it's tough to tell when you've met them, says Dr. Marcus. Without that sense, there's no feeling of accomplishment or progress—reinforcements that are crucial for continued motivation. Instead of saying you'll take up running, say you'll run two miles twice this week.

Talk action. The best goals are about what you will do, not what you will accomplish by doing it. "Outcome goals can jump the gun or be unrealistic," says Dr. Hays. For instance, deciding you'll lower your resting heart rate to 60 beats per minute is specific, but it's not action-oriented. Focus more on process than outcome by deciding, for example, that you'll take three half-hour walks every week.

Think short-term. It's perfectly fine to have a

Matching Movement to Motive

You start with broad objectives. You narrow them into manageable nuggets. In between, there's another step: deciding what sports or activities you want to do. It has to be something you like, but it also has to be something that works. Here are ideas for achieving some goals, according to James Gavin, Ph.D., professor in the Department of Applied Social Science at Concordia University in Montreal and author of *The Exercise Habit*.

Look Better

You should do: Activities that emphasize overall body definition such as strength or circuit training.

You should minimize: Activities that target only limited areas of the body such as cycling and stair-climbing.

Lose or Maintain Weight

You should do: Moderate- to high-intensity calorie-burning activities of long duration such as running, speed walking, stair-climbing, cycling, swimming or rowing.

You should minimize: Activities that involve short, strenuous spurts of energy or low intensity such as body building, volleyball and easy splash-about swimming.

Stay Healthy in Years to Come

You should do: Moderate, low-risk, continuous and regular activities such as walking, cycling, rowing and swimming.

You should minimize: Non-continuous, competitive or risky activities such as body building, racquet sports and contact sports.

Improve Flexibility

You should do: Activities that use the whole body and put different areas through a range of motion such as swimming, cross-country skiing and yoga.

You should minimize: Activities that work limited body areas such as bowling and cycling.

Relieve Stress

You should do: Activities that distract, release or discipline the mind such as running, cycling, in-line skating and tai chi.

You should minimize: Anything that puts performance pressures on you such as highly competitive team or racquet sports and power lifting.

---

dream or ambition like "I want to ride 100 miles on my bike in a day." But to realize long-term goals, you'll need to concentrate day-to-day on accomplishing smaller objectives, which offer immediate gratification all their own, says Dr. Hays, as well as a sense of progress toward the big enchilada.

Seek control. What you're after in the on-going process of improving your skills and making progress is a sense of mastery, which eventually becomes a source of enjoyment and a motivating force. You won't get it by dwelling on things you can't control. Don't aim to bench-press as much as any other guy; keep your comparisons centered on how you're better than *you* once were, suggests Dr. Hays. Don't run a race to win; run it striving toward achieving your personal best. Don't bemoan your lacking the skills of someone more experienced in your sport; focus on how you enjoy the skills you have.

Measure your progress. How can you improve if there's no benchmark to tag it to? If you're weight lifting, keep track of when you add plates and how many. If you're running or biking, figure miles traveled and the time it takes. Write it down. Whenever you find yourself wondering what the use of exercising is, take a look at the record and see just where it's gotten you, recommends Dr. Hays.

Change when needed. You could set your goals all the right ways but still get bored. When that happens, start doing things differently. No need to start from square one with a totally new exercise. Just follow the FIT formula, says Dr. Hays, which entails making one of the following changes, but not two or more at once.

- Frequency: Change how often you do a particular activity or the number of repetitions at a given weight level.
- Intensity: Alter your speed or change the amount of weight.
- Time: Do a given exercise for a longer or shorter period or change the number of sets.

Set multiple objectives. You want to keep focused, but it doesn't hurt to have more than one goal going at once, as long as they don't conflict. You could aim to bike three times a week, and also to do a 100-mile ride in four months. "If you bomb on one goal, you might still accomplish another," Dr. Hays says.

Cut yourself some slack. Remember, exercise accumulates. "There used to be this all-or-nothing thinking where if you couldn't get in your run, you figured, 'Why bother with anything?'" says Dr. Marcus. "Now you can get in a ten-minute walk at lunch and the day is not a loss. Our studies find that you need goals, but you also need to give yourself some flexibility in meeting them."

Eating Right

Getting into peak condition is essentially a major renovation/remodeling project: You're constructing new muscle both to improve structural integrity and make things look better while simultaneously dumping fat like so much plaster debris. Projects like this require—in addition to time—abundant supplies of two essential commodities: raw material and energy. To get both, you need good nutrition.

"The nutrition component of any training program is just as important as the physical component," says Becky Zimmerman, R.D., a nutrition educator in private practice and a freelance dietitian at the National Institute for Fitness and Sport in Indianapolis. "But athletes at all levels of training often fail to follow through with it."

When you eat the right balance of nutrients, your body fuels muscles more efficiently, builds bulk faster and repairs injuries more easily. The bottom line is that you'll be stronger, faster and longer-lasting if you eat right. This isn't difficult, but it does call for a bit of know-how. What's important? "There are two basic things to look at: composition and timing," says Ellen Coleman, R.D., nutrition consultant with The Sport Clinic in Riverside, California.

What to Eat

First, composition, the cornerstone of any eating plan. There are six basic classes of nutrients, each of which matter for different reasons.

Carbohydrate. It's the powerhouse nutrient—"the preferred food for exercising muscle," says Zimmerman. Carbohydrate is crucial largely because of the way it's stored in the body—as glycogen, a substance that muscles use as fuel. Unlike other nutrients, carbohydrate in the form of glycogen is stashed directly in muscles, where it's immediately burned during exercise. Backup energy reserves of glycogen are stockpiled in the liver and float in the blood as glucose, but the on-site muscle supplies are most vital. Without them you run out of energy, which makes your performance fizzle. For example, one study in which men were asked to exercise to exhaustion found that those who ate a high-carbohydrate diet could keep going almost three times longer than men who ate mostly fat.

Keeping muscles stocked with energy requires constant replenishing of carbohydrate. It takes about 24 hours for muscles to refill their glycogen stores, provided you take in enough carbohydrate to top off the tank. If you don't—and you continue a regular schedule of vigorous exercise—your glycogen supply at the start of every workout will be progressively lower. Next thing you know, you're chronically fatigued.

Carbohydrates should comprise at least 60 percent of your diet. The best are complex carbohydrates, which burn slowly and evenly. These tend not to be highly processed, and as a result also have a lot of vitamins and minerals. Good high-carbohydrate foods include whole-grain breads and cereals, pasta, apples, bananas, oranges, pears, potatoes, corn, peas and beans.

Protein. Protein's role in fitness is often misunderstood, but it is misunderstanding based on a truth: that protein is crucial for building and repairing muscle. Protein is like lumber: It's a basic structural component, and nothing gets bigger or stronger without it. Working on the assumption that more is better, weight lifters and athletes in training often boost their intake of protein or amino acids (which make up protein), but this isn't necessary and may even hinder performance.

Some studies do suggest that men engaged in strength training or endurance training need more protein than nonexercising men. In fact, an active man's need for protein may be slightly higher than the Daily Value (DV). That doesn't justify an increase in protein intake, however, because if you're eating a typical American diet, you're already getting two to three times more protein than the government standards call for. For example, a 150-pound man needs 55 grams of protein a day—the amount in just one eight-ounce serving of lean steak. An eight-ounce glass of milk gives you 8 grams more; a serving of bread provides another 3 grams. It's easy to see why getting more than enough protein is a no-brainer.

Eating these typically elevated amounts isn't necessarily harmful, but if you start chugging raw eggs or eating, say, protein supplements purported to boost muscle gain, you run a number of risks.

- By getting more protein, you're likely to eat fewer calories of carbohydrate and more of fat. If an active body doesn't get enough carbohydrate, it starts tapping protein for energy, by breaking down muscle—exactly the opposite of what you want. Concentrating on carbohydrates helps *preserve* protein.
- Excess protein produces waste products that need to be excreted, which puts greater demands on the kidneys and draws energy from your workouts.
- Protein or amino acids from supplements aren't as easily digested as protein from food and may cause irritation, cramps and diarrhea.

Protein should comprise 10 to 15 percent of your diet, says Zimmerman. To determine the number of grams of protein you need each day, multiply your pounds of body weight by 0.37. For example, a 175-pound man needs slightly under 65 grams of protein daily. In addition to milk and meat, good sources of protein include fish (7 grams of protein per ounce), yogurt (8 grams per cup), eggs (6 grams per egg) and peas (4 grams per half-cup).

Fat. Fat gets a bad rap. Yes, we tend to get too much of it, and yes, it wreaks havoc in excess. But if your diet is balanced at 60 percent carbohydrate and 10 to 15 percent protein, the remaining 25 to 30 percent you get from fat isn't likely to be a problem. In fact, you need it.

Any man with a few extra inches of padding knows that fat does an excellent job of storing calories, which would be important if we spent all day chasing bison. Theoretically, the average guy has enough carbohydrate energy in his body to walk about 20 miles, but has enough fat energy to walk from Boston to San Francisco three times. When you exercise, you burn some of that fat for fuel, which helps spare your carbohydrate stores, which will enhance your endurance. Fat is also important as insulation in the cold and for carrying fat-soluble vitamins in the body. Fat wants to be our friend.

The problem is that we want to be fat's friend so much that fat is compelled to hurt us to make us back off. Does any self-respecting man want to play this role in a relationship? Go easy on high-fat fare. Remember that fat comes in two general ways: from animal products and from oils. So drink skim milk; opt for baked and broiled over fried; cut back on meat portions; trim skin and visible fat off chicken, turkey and beef; substitute fruit spreads for butter; and eat low-fat cheeses, recommends Zimmerman.

Water. Even though it has no calories, it's the most critical of nutrients. Water carries all-important oxygen and nutritional fuel to working muscles, clears out waste and dissipates body heat, to name just a few of its vital functions. It's also lost at a rapid rate when exercising. During prolonged activity (particularly aerobic), water is lost as sweat at an hourly rate 285 times greater than sweat losses at rest, while the rate lost through breathing is 7 times greater during prolonged activity. When running at a training pace, it's easy to lose up to two quarts of water an hour. That kind of dehydration has a definite impact on performance: Losing just 2 percent of your body weight in water can cut your capacity for prolonged effort by 10 percent.

There's nothing complicated about drinking water, so long as you get enough. That means not only drinking while you're working out, but all day long. A typical guy should drink six to eight eight-ounce glasses of water a day. If you're bigger or more active than the common Joe, drink more. And don't wait for thirst to hit before imbibing, says Zimmerman. By the time you're thirsty, you're already slightly dehydrated.

Vitamins. The word is derived from "vitality," but vitamins have no usable energy of their own. Rather, they make possible a wide array of complicated processes involving energy creation from other nutrients, along with cell function, muscle and bone growth, blood formation, brain/muscle interaction—the kind of stuff your biology teachers used to fill entire blackboards with. We've all known vitamins are important ever since our moms fed us chewables. But what do we need now?

Research suggests that an exercising body uses certain vitamins differently than a sedentary one, but it isn't clear whether this translates to an increased need, or whether taking extra doses of vitamins will improve physical performance. A number of studies over the years, for example, have suggested that taking vitamin C in amounts ranging from 50 to 200 milligrams a day boosts endurance and increases work capacity. But, as one research review points out, most studies involving vitamins and performance have not been designed or controlled well, making any conclusions . . . well, inconclusive.

One thing researchers agree on, however, is that it's important to get vitamins in food, not pills, because food contains other substances that either make vitamins work better or provide beneficial effects all their own. "Variety is very important," says Roseann Lyle, Ph.D., associate professor of health promotion at Purdue University in West Lafayette, Indiana. "You'll get everything you need if you eat a lot of fruits and vegetables and foods that are high in starch." The U.S. Department of Agriculture's ubiquitous food pyramid

Performance Boosters

Let's say your diet is perfect. Can't you do something more to enhance your performance? Certainly, plenty of potion-, pill- and powder-makers claim you can. Most of these claims are bogus, says Melvin Williams, Ph.D., a leading expert on ergogenic aids, as they're called, and professor in the Department of Exercise Science, Physical Education and Recreation at Old Dominion University in Norfolk, Virginia, and former director of the Human Performance Laboratory there. "But there may be exceptions," Dr. Williams says. Here are the substances that he says may offer a competitive athlete some small benefit (as for the just-trying-to-stay-in-shape regular guy, these likely won't be of any use).

Sodium bicarbonate. That's baking soda to you and me. It's been shown to buffer the formation of waste products in muscle that contribute to fatigue. The theoretical result is greater capacity for short bursts of power, usually lasting one to two minutes. In one study, runners who took baking soda before an 880-meter race averaged almost 3 seconds faster times than runners who didn't take baking soda. Dr. Williams says a 155-pound man would need about four level teaspoons for an ergogenic effect, which should be taken one hour before a competition. The downside is that it can cause stomach cramps and diarrhea.

Caffeine. Hey, it boosts performance at work, why not during a workout? "It has definite benefit for endurance," Dr. Williams says. In one well-known study, cyclists who took 330 milligrams of caffeine (the amount in about three cups of coffee) boosted their endurance 20 percent over cyclists who drank decaf. The downside is that it gives you the jitters and may dehydrate you. To utilize this substance most effectively, Dr. Williams suggests that you avoid all caffeine for three days before a competition. Then an hour before the competition, you can take 300 to 350 milligrams of caffeine in tablet form, or roughly two or three seven-ounce cups of coffee.

Chromium. It's purported to boost muscle growth. Two studies by one researcher found that men in strength training who took 200 micrograms daily of chromium picolinate (the form most often sold in retail stores) gained lean body mass and lost fat at levels significantly better than similar men who didn't take chromium. Other studies find no effect. "It probably merits more research," Dr. Williams says, especially since chromium is lost in sweat and not easily absorbed from food. At this point, there have been no adverse effects reported from its use. If you'd like to try it, Dr. Williams says you should take no more than 200 micrograms a day, which is the estimated safe and adequate daily intake amount recommended by the Food and Drug Administration.

Creatine. It forms a high-energy compound stored in muscle, theoretically boosting strength and power. Research is promising, but equivocal, says Dr. Williams: At a 1995 conference, for example, of eight papers presented on creatine, half found a performance benefit and half didn't. No adverse effects other than weight gain have been reported from its use. Dr. Williams says that most athletes who do use it take 20 to 25 milligrams per day for five to seven days prior to a competitive event.

All these substances are available in health food stores and should only be taken for the purpose of enhancing your performance in periodic competitive events, not your everyday workout session, says Dr. Williams. Be sure to check with your doctor first before using any of these substances. Dr. Williams also suggests that you experiment with a substance in practice sessions before you use it for a competitive event.

recommends three to five servings of vegetables and two to four servings of fruit every day.

Minerals. Last and least are minerals. We say least not because minerals aren't important—they're crucial for providing structure for bones, for maintaining vital functions like heartbeat and muscle contraction and for regulating things like cell activity. But the body needs minerals only in tiny amounts. In fact, many minerals, including sodium, magnesium and iron, can have harmful effects in excess.

The most important thing to know about minerals is that a good diet, balanced as we've outlined here, will give you all you need. There is one mineral, however, that is of special concern for active men, and that's zinc. This single mineral is important for an astonishing number of different metabolic functions including digestion, wound healing and taste. Exercise makes the body lose zinc in sweat and also boosts the amount excreted in urine. One of several studies on zinc loss in athletes and military trainees found that 23 percent of male runners had below-normal concentrations of zinc in their blood. So try to eat foods high in zinc, such as moderate amounts of lean beef and pork, skinless poultry and seafood such as oysters, crabmeat and tuna, recommends Zimmerman. Whole grains, beans and legumes are also good sources. Avoid supplements: Too much zinc can hinder the body's absorption of copper, and it can also

Ten No-Fail Foods

Dietitians are fond of saying that there are no bad foods—if everything is eaten in the right amounts. Still, diet decisions are always made at the moment, with the question: Should I eat this or not? You can't go wrong with these food choices, says Becky Zimmerman, R.D., a nutrition educator in private practice and a freelance dietitian at the National Institute for Fitness and Sport in Indianapolis.

Cereal. It tastes good and is easy to prepare, while being low in fat and high in carbohydrate and fiber. Unsweetened is best (some sweetened brands get up to 43 percent of their calories from nutrient-poor sugar), but even the kid stuff that turns your milk pink is fortified with vitamins and minerals.

Bananas. Think of a banana as a carbohydrate stick. It's also high in fiber and potassium, one of the minerals you need. Best of all, its prepackaging allows mess-free toting.

Low-fat yogurt. A good source of protein and calcium. If you add extra fruit to fruit-on-the-bottom brands, you can get an extra helping of vitamins, minerals and fiber.

Oranges. Vitamin C. Enough said.

Potatoes. A classic powerhouse of carbohydrates. Eat the skin and you have a helping of vitamin C as well. Be careful with the condiments, though: Heaping on butter or sour cream drowns an otherwise good thing in fat. Some alternative toppings: salsa, low-fat melted cheese, cottage cheese or salad dressing, cooked vegetables or baked beans.

Bagels. High in carbohydrates and, if you buy whole-grain, they are high in minerals and fiber as well.

Pasta. More carbohydrates. Just forgo oily sauces in favor of tomato and vegetable sauces, which provide vitamins and minerals that the pasta lacks.

Broccoli. When food gurus talk about dark green vegetables, think broccoli. It has vitamin C, calcium and minerals like magnesium.

Tuna. An exceptional source of protein: One six-ounce can of it contains about 40 grams. If you combine it with low-fat mayonnaise and celery, it makes a great sandwich spread.

Lean beef. There's nothing wrong with beef as long as you limit it to small portions. A roast beef sandwich is full of protein, zinc and iron. Just don't make the beef the central ingredient: Balance it with thick, whole-grain bread, tomato, lettuce and mustard.

lower levels of "good" HDL cholesterol. If you do take supplements, don't take more than the DV amount of 15 milligrams a day.

When to Eat It

If you get the basics of composition down, timing is a secondary concern, but a real one if you're interested in peak performance. There are several basic principles.

Fast before a workout. You don't have to starve yourself, but it's wise to avoid eating 45 minutes to an hour before exercising. "Even carbohydrates take at least an hour to digest," Coleman says. Fats take even longer: two to four hours. When your body diverts energy to digestion, it's robbing muscles of power and making your workout less effective.

Drink fluids constantly. If you're hungry before a workout, have a small snack such as fruit or juice instead of eating a meal. Immediately before exercising, drink at least one cup of water, then keep sipping one-half to one-quarter cup every 15 to 20 minutes during exercise. Top off your workout with another full cup. Remember, throughout the day you should get a total of at least eight eight-ounce glasses.

Refuel immediately. Studies find that muscles replace glycogen stores most efficiently within two hours after exercising. If you wait longer, the body's resources concentrate more on muscle repair, and glycogen storage slows or even stops—by the second two hours after exercise, for instance, glycogen replacement dwindles by 50 percent. Zimmerman recommends eating a half-gram of carbohydrate for every pound of body weight 15 to 30 minutes after a workout. A large banana, large bagel or 12-ounce glass of fruit juice each provide 30 to 40 grams. Eat the same amount again after two hours have passed.

Eat breakfast. It's vital for replenishing blood glucose and glycogen stores depleted while you sleep. Men should eat 300 to 400 calories at breakfast—an amount easily covered by toast and jam, cereal with skim milk and fruit, according to Zimmerman.

Get enough. Graze on high-carbohydrate fare throughout the day to make sure you're eating enough, says Zimmerman. You heard right: If you're eating a high-carbohydrate diet, you may actually be in danger of not getting enough calories. Carbohydrates have only half the calories of fat gram for gram, so you need to eat twice as much of them to achieve the same calorie intake. And as you become more fit, your body will need more energy: Muscle burns more calories than flab even when idling.

But don't get too lost in the details. "You can't emphasize the basics enough," says Dr. Lyle. "Eating a variety of healthy foods that are high in carbohydrate and low in fat will keep you prepared for whatever you want to do."

Getting Rest

Nothing seems more contrary to the idea of reaching peak performance than resting. After all, isn't resting what you're doing when you're slouched on the sofa tossing back a Bud and watching war flicks on TNT? Isn't it what exercise pundits are always hounding us to get off our butts and stop doing?

Well, yes. In fact, so much attention goes to butt-from-sofa extraction that you almost never hear about how crucial rest is to the success of any exercise program. We're going to assume you're beyond the need for prodding—that you're dedicated enough to being active that it's now more important for you to hear what, outside the world of elite athletics, is rarely recognized as crucial.

Training for peak performance seems a simple deal: You work out, you improve. It stands to reason that if you work out harder and more often, you'll get better faster. But that's not always the case. Studies of swimmers, for example, find that training 3 or 4 hours a day confers no greater benefit than training for just 1 or 1½ hours a day. In fact, the higher training levels significantly reduce muscle strength and sprint performance.

You don't have to train at elite levels for adequate rest to be an issue. For any regular exerciser, "if you want to steadily improve, you need to balance muscle overuse, which is training, with underuse, which is rest," says Houston training consultant Ronald Sandler, D.P.M., co-author of *Consistent Winning: A Remarkable New Training System That Lets You Peak on Demand.*

Recovery Movement

The need for rest harkens back to the overload principle that drives your gains: If you regularly work the body harder than it's accustomed to, it adapts by building ever greater strength or endurance. Fine. But what's really going on here?

Actually, exercise doesn't build muscles up, it tears them down. When muscles are worked intensely, they become marred by tiny tears and other forms of microscopic damage. Muscles sore? That's microtrauma you're feeling. Muscle-building kicks in after the exercise is over. "When damage occurs, there are processes for repairing it—repairs that make the muscle better than it was before," says Dennis Wilson, Ed.D., head of the Department of Health and Human Performance at Auburn University in Alabama. "There needs to be some kind

of rest or reduction in exercise for tissue to renew itself." It's what athletes call recovery.

Recovery happens not only between exercise bouts, but while you're exercising. If you're lifting weights to build strength, for example, it's important to rest between sets to let your muscles recuperate as fully as possible. "If you don't, you'll reduce the amount you can lift with each set, which means your strength gains will come much harder," says Mike Stone, Ph.D., president of the National Strength and Conditioning Association.

How much rest and recovery you need depends on your goals, how fit you already are and your training potential. It's a truism among exercise experts that each person will adapt differently to the same workout, depending on individual makeup. "There are many ways to structure recovery," says Dr. Wilson. Still, there are some easy-to-follow general principles.

Allow more recovery for heavy exercise. If you take a brisk walk every day, the 24 hours between outings will probably be more than adequate for recovery. If you do a three-mile run, however, it's wise not to run the next day—unless you're already accustomed to running ten miles at a stretch. "Intensity is the key," says Dr. Wilson. It's sensible to take a day of rest between high-intensity workouts: For example, you would exercise on Monday, rest Tuesday, then exercise again on Wednesday. One way of measuring intensity is with metabolic equivalents, or METs (see "The Intense-O-Meter" on page 14). Each person's need for recovery may vary, but as a rule, the higher an activity's MET value, the more likely it will demand a day off after you do it.

For strength, rest more. When lifting weights, the amount of time you rest between sets helps determine the effects of your workout. If you're trying to build

The Intense-O-Meter

One way to measure exercise intensity is perceived exertion: how much work you think an activity is. But, like any opinion, yours may be different from the next guy's. A more precise measure is how much oxygen a given activity requires, expressed in metabolic equivalents, or METs. As a rule, higher-MET activities demand more recovery time than lower-MET ones. Here are different activities and their MET values. Get to know your METs. It pays.

Lying down or sitting	1
Getting dressed	2
Making the bed	3
Playing golf	4
Ballroom dancing	4.5
Level walking at 4 mph	6.5
Chopping wood	6.5
Downhill skiing	8
Playing basketball	9
Playing handball	10
Level running at 8.5 mph	12
Swimming a crawl at 2.5 feet per second	15
Swimming a crawl at 3 feet per second	20
Running a 4-minute mile	30

Pushing or Punishing?

Everyone has off days. How can you tell if you're overtraining or just going through the run-of-the-mill blahs? Dennis Wilson, Ed.D., head of the Department of Health and Human Performance at Auburn University in Alabama, suggests these methods.

Check your habits. Have you recently made a significant change in your program? Are you constantly trying to keep up with someone who's better at your sport than you are? Do you always exercise at the same pace, never lightening your pace or intensity? If you've answered yes to any of these, you've fallen into classic overtraining patterns and are probably pushing yourself too hard.

Monitor your mood. The single best indicator of overtraining is an otherwise inexplicable plunge into the emotional toilet. Mood often deteriorates before physical performance does.

Take your pulse. Overtraining typically makes your resting heart rate go up over time. To keep track of it, take your pulse in the morning before you get out of bed, counting the number of heartbeats in one minute. A persistent rise of the same amount over a period of weeks may indicate a problem.

strength, a relatively long wait of three to five minutes between sets will allow you to pump heavier weights and make gains more quickly, according to Dr. Wilson.

For endurance, rest less. If you're building muscular endurance with your weight routine, you'll be using lighter weights and more repetitions, which allow you to take shorter between-set rests of one minute or less. According to Dr. Wilson, not resting at all between stations may actually provide an effect that closely mimics aerobic activities.

Progress gradually. Whether you're lifting weights or doing aerobic activities, it's important not to overtax yourself. As a rule, don't make more than a 10 percent increase per week in sets, repetitions, weight or, for aerobic exercise, pace or distance, recommends Dr. Wilson.

Don't fret about losses. Dedicated exercisers often fear that any tapering off will undo hard-won progress. But you lose nothing with short rests—or even relatively long ones.

Studies have found that runners and swimmers who cut back their training by 60 percent showed no loss of endurance even after two to three weeks. Another study showed that strength losses weren't noticeable even a month after a three-week training program stopped.

The Overtraining Syndrome

Maybe you're the kind of guy who *likes* working yourself hard every day. What harm is there in continually pushing your limits?

It depends on how fond you are of feeling chronically tired, having trouble sleeping, being sick all the time with colds, flus and infections or feeling depressed. These are some of the signs of overtraining, a clinical condition in which you've pounded yourself so hard for so long that you've gone beyond your body's ability to quickly recuperate, says Dr. Wilson. Overtraining can also produce potentially more serious symptoms as well, such as high blood pressure and increased heart rate.

It's no coincidence that these same symptoms are tied to emotional stress. By overtraining, you physically stress yourself beyond your ability to cope and you burn out, just as you do after weeks or months of unrelieved out-of-control pressure at work. This relationship—in case you're thinking only elite athletes get overtrained—may make overtraining more common in nonelite, dedicated recreational athletes, according to doctors who treat the condition. That's because, unlike top competitors, with their sponsors and patrons, average Joes have to mix their training with the additional stresses of workaday life.

Treating overtraining is difficult. For one thing, its

How Exercise Affects Sleep

You've had a tough workout, you've set a personal distance record, you've hauled furniture all day: Better turn in early, right? Well ... maybe. A review of different studies concluded that a single bout of exercise might, at most, make you sleep an extra ten minutes—barely a blip on the slumber charts.

Overall, being sleepy and being weary aren't the same thing, says Patrick J. O'Connor, Ph.D., who has studied the interaction of sleep and exercise as an associate professor in the Department of Exercise Science at the University of Georgia in Athens. Your body could be sore and aching, and you could feel physically exhausted, but that's a muscle matter, not a sleep issue. Muscles can rest even when you're awake. "If you're getting good sleep, exercise won't affect your normal needs or patterns much," Dr. O'Connor says.

But what constitutes "good" sleep? It varies from person to person, but most of us feel refreshed after seven or eight hours—assuming we get those seven or eight hours when it makes sense to our bodies. Sleep is governed by a number of daily rhythms, such as internal temperature, the release of hormones and the perception of daylight. Everybody's rhythms are a little different, says Dr. O'Connor. While it's broadly true that we sleep at night and are awake during the day, if you go to bed at 10 P.M. when you're accustomed to turning in at midnight, your sleep may suffer. But don't worry that you could be sleeping at a more optimal time than you do. "What we're accustomed to and what our bodies want are usually close to the same," Dr. O'Connor says.

Although exercise doesn't much affect our need for sleep, it does appear to improve sleep quality and energy levels. One study, for example, found that physically fit people went to bed later, fell asleep faster and spent less total time asleep, yet awoke feeling less tired than more sedentary people. Another study found that sedentary people say they feel tired during the day almost twice as often as active people do.

Bottom line, there's no need to head for the sofa after a workout. Of course, if you want to, there's no harm. Just be sure to keep daytime naps short. "If you sleep for two hours in the middle of the day," Dr. O'Connor says, "you might have trouble sleeping at night."

symptoms overlap with so many other conditions (Lyme disease is one), that it's often hard—but not impossible—to spot (see "Pushing or Punishing?"). Once it's identified, the main remedy is rest or reduced activity, says Dr. Wilson. In many cases, if the overtraining was minimal or caught early, a few days' recovery may be all that's needed, he says. If you're suffering from bona fide overtraining syndrome, however, recovery can take up to 12 weeks.

Preventing overtraining is easier—and wiser. If you're hard-driving, here are some precautionary steps to take.

Mix it up. You can work out every day as long as you're not constantly stressing the same muscles in the same way. Do upper-body exercises one day and lower-body exercises the next. Or get what's called active rest by alternating heavy workouts (like a ten-mile run) on a Monday with light workouts (like a two-mile walk) on a Tuesday, says Dr. Wilson. If you're a serious athlete in training, though, you may very well utilize the same muscles on successive days—with good results. It really depends on your fitness level, he says.

Eat more carbohydrate. Remember, if muscle-powering glycogen stores aren't constantly replenished, your energy will dwindle further with every workout. Think you're already getting enough? Get more anyway, keeping your plate colorful with lots of fruits and vegetables, especially if you're doing endurance training, recommends Dr. Wilson.

Get enough sleep. It's equal parts recovery and stress-resistance. Studies find that people who say they average less than six hours of sleep a night are three times more likely to say they're under great stress almost every day than those who sleep seven or eight hours a night. Both stress and sleep loss can lower your immunity, an important contributor both to fatigue and respiratory illnesses like colds and flus. In one study, 23 men who were cheated out of four hours' sleep in a lab suffered 30 percent drops in natural killer-cell activity, a key measure of immune-system strength.

In the end, men who exercise excessively make both cautionary and inspiring examples: They have problems we almost wish we had. For most men, the main issue isn't spending too much time exercising. It's eking enough time out of our busy schedules to get what little exercise we can.

Making Time

People say they can make time," a guy in the foyer of a restaurant was saying into the receiver of a pay phone. His voice had the desperate urgency of a man whose margin of excusability was quickly narrowing to nothing. "I have children, a job," he said. "I've tried to make time. *It doesn't work!*"

Raise your hand if you have not at least occasionally felt the same way. Anybody? We thought so. Now tell yourself you're going to exercise three times a week for an hour, minimum. Great idea, but when will you do it? "Lack of time is the number one barrier to exercise," says Bess H. Marcus, Ph.D., associate professor of psychiatry and human behavior at Miriam Hospital and Brown University School of Medicine in Providence, Rhode Island.

In one sense, the guy on the phone was right: You can't make time. There's only so much of it in a day. But you can make choices about how you spend it. In fact, you already do, says Pam Kristan, founder of The Practical Matters, an organizational skills consulting firm in Boston. "If you're not making decisions about your time consciously, decisions are being made for you," she says.

You have to control your time or it will control you—and the really important things in your life won't get the attention they deserve. "If exercise is important to you, eliminate the idea that you don't have time for it," says Denise Dudley, Ph.D., executive vice-president of SkillPath, a management training firm in Mission, Kansas. "Instead, say 'I *do* have the time—and I will find it.'" Here's how, say the experts.

Uncover Hidden Time

"The best way to fill time is to waste it," a French author once said. You don't have to kill time as ably as the French to appreciate that much of our existence is squandered on inefficiencies. Little pockets of hidden time are available to us throughout each day. All you have to do is tap them. Some ways to do it:

Take charge of the trivial. We waste 50 to 70 percent of our workday on unimportant stuff like drop-in visitors and phone calls. Get control by:

- Standing when someone enters your office to discourage unscheduled chats
- Getting straight to business with a question like "What can I do for you?" rather than inviting conversation with a more open-ended "How are you?"
- Making calls just before lunch or closing time, when there's maximum incentive to keep talk short
- Eliminating phone tag by setting up appointments for call-backs

Energize the twilight zone. You know it and surveys confirm it: the hour between 4:00 and 5:00 P.M. is one of the least productive times of the day. Take advantage by reserving late afternoon for low-key necessities like planning the next day or cleaning out your hard drive.

Get real. Studies find that most people optimistically underestimate how much time their tasks will actually take. When planning, don't generalize from those rare occasions when all goes perfectly. Coldly plan for surprise setbacks and snafus. Then, for good measure, add 25 percent more time.

Identify black holes. Most workplaces have offices where material goes in and never comes out. The people inside may be overwhelmed, disorganized or both. Whatever the case, by sitting on stuff that eventually makes its way to you with a "yesterday" deadline, they're holding you up and wasting your time. If the problem is an organizational one, it's not your co-worker's fault—maybe you're too good at picking up the slack. Diplomatically make sure the boss knows about logjams; he's the one best able to unclog them, but he may not know they exist.

Play a mind game. Create a sense of found time by imagining your boss decreeing that all workers spend an extra hour each week at a meeting. Then cancel the meeting.

Adjourn permanently. Regular staff meetings for "touching base" can kill hours at a stretch. But if there's no specific reason to meet, there's no justification for a meeting. Lobby your boss to eliminate all standing meetings in favor of short, issue-oriented conferences. When meetings are scheduled, establish not only a starting time, but an ending time.

Don't do lunch. "Lunches are one of the biggest time wasters in corporate culture," Dr. Dudley says. "You cannot get out of one in less than 1½ hours." If the lunch is for pleasure or political gain, indulge. Often, though, lunches are simply a rote gesture that both parties erroneously assume is required. If clients have a simple business agenda, tell them you'd be happy to discuss it in a 20-minute meeting.

Keep your wallet closed. After TV viewing and eating, the most frequent leisure activity in America is shopping, according to a University of Maryland survey. "Shopping doesn't just entail the actual buying," Kristan says. "It includes making decisions, returning items that don't work out, assembling things, fixing them later if they break. If you spend less, you'll find a lot of time opening up."

Simplify your workout. Finally, is the problem that you lack time for a workout—or for *your* workout? "The more complicated it is, the more impediments you'll have to doing it," says Dr. Dudley. Do you have to drive a long way to a gym? Consider using weights at home. Are you doing three sets at each of your weight stations? Consider shortening your workout time by eliminating one set or doing fewer stations—you will need less time for each workout but may end up exercising more often.

Know Your Priorities

When it comes to actually doing what you want, nothing is more important than setting priorities. With a numbing array of activities, obligations and entertainments clamoring for our attention, having a sense of priorities helps us recognize what we truly value and then sift the treasure from the fool's gold. Knowing you want to exercise isn't enough. "Priorities aren't about deciding what to do, but about saying no to the rest," Kristan says. Here's what our experts recommend to get your priorities straight.

Check what you do. The things you actually spend your time on are, in fact, your priorities. But they may not be the priorities you would consciously choose. You won't carve more meaningful time for yourself until you recognize that watching reruns of the old *Dick Van Dyke Show* on Nick at Nite seems to top your de facto list of important stuff.

Go on a mission. If you have a sense of long-term purpose, your most important tasks or activities will, by definition, be those that move you closest to your goals. To better focus on the overriding objectives that should govern your actions, write them down in a mission statement such as "I will be more fit." List different missions in order of importance. Before committing time to anything, ask: "How will

Foolproof Prioritizing

You have five projects screaming to be done at once. Which should you do first to make best use of your time? Here's how to decide, according to Denise Dudley, Ph.D., executive vice-president of SkillPath, a management training firm in Mission, Kansas.

1. Make a list of all your tasks, listing items in order of their long-term importance. No ties allowed; you have to make judgments.

2. Give each item an additional urgency value, according to the following scale:

- Needs to be done immediately = 1
- Needs to be done soon = 2
- It can wait = 3

3. Multiply the importance ranking by the urgency value. The resulting scores will tell you in what order you should do your projects.

this further my most important goals?"

Look to the future. When making decisions about how to spend your time, picture yourself six months from now. Ask yourself which choice will later make you feel the best, or which will create the most problems if you don't choose it.

Distinguish urgent from vital. Important matters fall into these two categories. Urgent stuff clamors loudly for our attention: an impromptu meeting with a company honcho, a project that's late, a knock at the door. We usually attend to urgent matters first, even though they're often not important in the long run. Better to focus on what's vital—tasks such as planning, staffing and organizing that have greater importance over the long haul and ultimately deliver greater satisfaction. (For a simple prioritizing formula, see "Foolproof Prioritizing.")

Get Organized

Organization isn't about neatness. It's about saving time. Consider that men spend an average of six weeks a year just looking for stuff. There has to be a better way. And there is, according to our organizational experts.

Begin life with the four Ds. Dump, delegate, do or delay. These are your options for incoming material. Avoid choosing "delay"; it leads to an overload of matters on hold, which you'll waste time reconsidering later.

End the paper chase. Only 20 to 40 percent of the paper thrown at you each day is worth your concern. Sure you can file stuff, but there's a cost there too: By one estimate, each file cabinet takes about

Life's a Batch

When is the perfect time to exercise? It depends a lot on what the rest of your schedule looks like. The trick to making your workout time as efficient as possible is to do what management experts call batching—combining activities that are the same or have similar elements. If you've ever postponed errands so you can do them all in one trip, you understand batching. A cousin of batching is substitution, in which you work out instead of squandering tick-tocks on some time-sucking waste of energy. Here are some specific batching suggestions from Denise Dudley, Ph.D., executive vice-president of SkillPath, a management training firm in Mission, Kansas.

Tie workouts to shower time. Why waste time taking more than one shower in a day? If you normally shower in the morning, exercise early, then combine your pre-workday and post-workout lathers. If you normally shower at night, work out then. If you normally shower in the morning and at night, eliminate one of them and work out any time you please.

Do the commute. Is there any part of your day that's a bigger waste of time? How much of your car/train/bus/subway trip could be self-propelled? Just because it's not a workout per se doesn't mean it's not exercise.

Dodge traffic jams. Find a gym close to your office. Go there right after work while everyone else spends their drive time parked in their cars on the freeway, desperately trying to dial someone on the cellular who can lend significance to this abysmal span on the clock. An hour later, emerge from the gym and count all the green lights you whiz through on the way home.

Become a midday miracle. We've already said what a terrific time-waster lunches can be. It takes no more than 10 to 15 minutes to get through a brown-bag lunch. Even allowing another 20 minutes for changes and a shower, that still gives you a minimum of 25 to 30 minutes for actual exercise.

Be a social activist. When you get together with buddies, don't watch football—*play* it, or get a game of basketball going or play a round of tennis. When you're doing the quality-time thing with the family, make a point of actually doing something—taking a hike, going for a bike ride, playing soccer.

Do what's necessary. Who says you can't have it all? If your weights are in the basement and your TV is in the living room, do you need to have your conflicting desires constantly doing the angel-and-devil dance on your shoulder? No you do not. Get a crummy little TV—black and white if that's what it takes—and put it in the basement. You'll never have to miss another *Seinfeld* rerun.

$2,000 a year to maintain—and a lot of that cost is your time. Try to keep only material you'll someday act upon by:

• Making files action-oriented. Establish a roster of slots numbered 1 to 31, one for each day of the month. If you can't act on a memo immediately, put it in the folder for the day when you can. Every morning, pull out that day's folder, and you'll find a small number of purposeful papers at the ready.

• Putting all papers you don't know what to do with in a box or slush file. Go back to this collection occasionally and throw out anything you haven't needed for six months.

• Keeping your pile of unread material to six inches high or less.

Don't overplan. In time-management circles, they're called planner nerds: people who can't go to the john without checking their daybooks first. Remember that schedules and to-do lists have their uses but are counterproductive when you're constantly erasing and re-penciling as the unexpected inevitably occurs.

Getting Started

Teddy Roosevelt, that manliest of presidents, used to preach what he called the doctrine of the strenuous life—a doctrine defined not so much by what it was as by what Roosevelt said it was the opposite of: a life of "ignoble ease."

None of us likes being called ignoble, even if we have to look the word up. But the wise man knows that jumping suddenly from the sofa to a strenuous life can lead to injury, not to mention ignominy, another two-dollar word you want to avoid.

From the last several chapters, you know what's involved with living a peak lifestyle. In the next section, you'll learn how to achieve it. But between the knowing and the doing, we need to say a few words about getting started. Triathlon legend and three-time Ironman champion Scott Tinley sums it up: "Do nothing you're not prepared for," he says.

We'll be brief, but it's worth knowing the following tips.

Get an inspection. You wouldn't take your car on a road trip without checking under the hood for loose belts or leaking fluids. Likewise, if you're taking your body on a high-intensity trip to peak performance, it's worth making sure that there's nothing wrong with the machinery that could cause an unpleasant breakdown. If you're young and healthy, there may be no reason to see a doctor (although a routine preventive visit with your physician every three to five years is a good idea), says Morris Mellion, M.D., clinical associate professor of family practice and orthopedic surgery at the University of Nebraska Medical Center and medical director of the Sports Medicine Center in Omaha, Nebraska. You should, however, seek a medical stamp of approval if:

• You're over 40. You may be in fine shape, but there's no escaping the fact that your odometer has turned over; you can expect a few problems to start showing up. If nothing else, visiting your doctor periodically for a preventive evaluation gives him a baseline against which to measure the payoff of exercise in subsequent exams.

• You're at risk for heart disease. Exercise improves the heart, but if it's vulnerable to heart attack, overstressing the cardiovascular system is potentially disastrous. Heart patients need to proceed under a doctor's guidance. Major risk factors are if any parents or siblings developed heart disease before age 50, a total cholesterol level of 200 or more, and having diabetes or a blood pressure of 140 over 85 or more. Other signs to have checked out include shortness of breath with mild exertion, dizziness, palpitations or a known heart murmur.

Start low, go slow. "Guys like to hammer themselves when they do something," says Alan Mikesky, Ph.D., director of the Human Performance Lab and associate professor at Indiana University-Purdue University Indianapolis. It feels great immediately afterward. But then you get sore. "Most people can't stand hammering themselves every workout," Dr. Mikesky says. "After a few times, you lose your enthusiasm—or you get injured." If you're just beginning or have laid off a regular program for more than six months, start by doing less than you think you can. Slowly raise the demands you make on yourself, increasing the intensity, duration or frequency of your exercise no more than 10 to 15 percent per week.

Seek expert guidance. Even if you're armed with the best of knowledge and intentions, it's a good idea to have your program designed by someone else. A gym staffer or personal trainer can tell you if your goals are unrealistic, guide you on proper form and tailor your program to your needs. Don't worry that you're signing on to a long-term dependency. "Even if you buy just one session with a personal trainer, it will be 25 to 50 bucks well-spent," says Dr. Mikesky.

Make an investment. *Any* money you spend on your fitness program will increase the value of what you're doing, providing a strong (but not fail-safe) motivation to keep active. Beyond trainers and gym memberships, it's hard to resist the allure of cool, expensive equipment. (See Setting Up a Home Gym on page 312.)

There's a dilemma here, however: If you're new to something, how do you know you'll like it? If you're taking up biking, should you immediately blow as much as you can afford on a new steed? It's a tough call that's ultimately yours to make, but here are some thoughts to guide you.

• Rent first. It's probably not a good idea to spend gobs of dough on big-ticket items without a few trial runs. Start with day-long excursions with a bike (or kayak or snowboard or skis) from a local outfitter. If you enjoy your experience, you'll keep coming back for more, and the financial advantage of owning your own gear will quickly become apparent.

• Get good gear. When you do buy, invest in quality that's appropriate for what you intend to do, advises Kate Hays, Ph.D., a sport psychologist and founder of The Performing Edge, a performance enhancement training company for athletes, performing artists and business people in Concord, New Hampshire. "You won't get full value out of equipment without a certain investment," she says. If you take up running but start with inferior shoes ("just until I know I like it"), you'll feel lead-footed and possibly pained. That won't be encouraging. "A moderately priced pair of shoes can make all the difference," Dr. Hays explains. "You need good-enough stuff, but it doesn't have to be top of the line." If you're buying a bike, don't spend $2,000 on an elaborate rig, but don't spend $200 on a discount department store special either.

• Consider buying used. Stores that sell pre-owned gear are becoming more common. Or check the classifieds for people who bought more hardware than they were ready for—and are now ready to sell.

Include your friends. You're not in this exercise thing alone. It helps to have someone around with whom you can share your progress, enthusiasm and disappointments. Part of this involves what sport psychologists call values clarification. "If you tell someone, 'This is what I'm planning,' you're more likely to actually do it," Dr. Hays says. And who should this someone be? "A friend—it might be your wife or girlfriend—who will be interested in your plans or reasons for exercise. Sometimes guys get so competitive with each other that exercise becomes a contest instead of a process," she says.

Choose workout partners carefully. Having a male workout partner can help foster motivation, but, again, make sure competitiveness doesn't end up making the whole experience unpleasant or tougher than you really want. Remember, exercising should be fun.

Fortify against intimidation. Starting a new sport, joining a gym for the first time, trying a new activity—all can be intimidating initially. You may only be paying attention to the people who seem to be able to do what you're doing so much better than you. There's a certain dork factor, which is determined by how you feel and think about yourself. To feel more comfortable, work on listening to the negative things you tell yourself and substitute some internal cheerleading, says Dr. Hays. Instead of saying, "I'll never be able to do that," say, "In a week, I'll be doing better than I am now." Anticipate the times and places where you feel the most self-conscious and think of positive words to tell yourself ahead of time.

Build armchair enthusiasm. One way to feel more at ease with a new sport is to learn more about it. Read magazines or books. Talk to people at shops that sell gear. You can build a sense of knowing the ins and outs of an activity without committing your ego to actually doing it in public until you're ready.

Mark your calendar. You're psyched, you're pumped, you're ready to go. At least *now* you are. But two to four months from now, it will be a different story. Count on it. In fact, *plan* for it. Studies find that half the time, regular exercise programs fizzle after six months, with most of those people dropping out after four to six weeks.

This isn't necessarily bad: Incredible gains can be made in six weeks, and it's possible to hit many of your goals in that amount of time. Figure you'll eventually get bored and apathetic, but take it not as a sign to bail out, but as a sign to set new goals and do something more interesting—and demanding. Persistent progress requires persistent effort. "Nothing's for free," Tinley says. "If there's no sacrifice, there's no reward."

Part Two
Achieving Peak Conditioning

Weight Lifting

At first glance, nothing could seem more simple than lifting weights. Up. Down. Up. Down. It's rudimentary nearly to the point of boneheadedness in its apparent lack of complexity. But if the world were so readily reducible to crude appearances, sexuality would be pretty simple too. In. Out. But we know there's more to it than that.

The variables include position, speed of movement, how often you do it, how intense it is, how long you draw things out . . . excuse us, we're talking about *weights* here. Weight lifting—more properly defined as resistance training, in which muscles are called on to work against a resisting force—isn't difficult, but there are some subtleties to be aware of if you're going to be successful with it.

The benefits of being successful are plain to see and quick to make themselves known. "When you've been lifting, you can actually feel that your muscles are more pumped up by the time you walk out of the gym," says Bruce Craig, Ph.D., director of graduate studies in exercise science at Ball State University in Muncie, Indiana. It's a temporary effect caused when working muscles become engorged with blood (the sensation lasts about a half-hour), but in a matter of weeks, this pumped-up feeling becomes more permanent and more visible.

"People who continue going into the weight room just keep looking better," says Tom Baechle, Ed.D., chair of the exercise science department at Creighton University in Omaha, Nebraska. "In the first three weeks you'll see some toning. In eight weeks you'll see size gains." There's just one caveat: "Muscle cells are pretty stupid," Dr. Baechle says. "They have a short memory and need to be shocked on a regular basis," not only to keep them improving, but to remind them of what they've become.

The Muscle Menu

To shock muscles, they need to be subjected to stresses they're not accustomed to. What kind of stress you put on them depends on what you're trying to achieve. There are three basic goals to strive for with resistance training, and each has a unique program, says Dr. Baechle.

Strength. Physiologists define strength as a measure of how much weight you can lift one time. If you aim for strength, you generally won't be able to sustain muscular movements for extended lengths of time, and your muscles won't be as big as they could be had you followed a program designed to maximize size.

Program principle: lifting very heavy weights a low number of times.

Size. Muscles get bigger when you lift, thanks to hypertrophy, a process in which existing muscle fibers increase in size. (The process is fueled in part by testosterone, which is generally accepted as the primary reason men's muscles are bigger than women's.) If you build mass, you'll also build strength, but the two don't correlate exactly. In fact, bodybuilders—despite their size—may not be as strong as power lifters who train sheerly for strength.

Program principle: lifting moderately heavy weights a moderate number of times.

Tone. When people talk of "toning," three concepts often get interchanged: muscle tone, muscular endurance and cardiovascular endurance. Here's how to make sense of it all.

Toned muscles are muscles that are firm, lean and well-trained. The usual path to muscle tone is training for *muscular endurance,* defined as a muscle's ability to sustain movement for a relatively long period of time. See the well-defined, lean leg muscles of a long-distance runner? All that running has made his muscles toned.

To achieve *cardiovascular endurance,* you need muscular endurance, but the two aren't necessarily the same. Cardiovascular endurance refers to the heart and lungs' ability to efficiently move oxygen-rich blood to the muscles, and oxygen-deficient blood from exercised muscles back to the heart and lungs. (Running three miles requires a good level of cardiovascular endurance.) In contrast, muscular endurance is about keeping *any* muscle working for extended periods of time without undue fatigue, whether the work challenges the heart or not (doing 20 push-ups).

Toned muscle is not bulky. It's what a

Free Weights or Machines?

It's largely a matter of personal choice, based on these considerations.

• Machines do a superior job of guiding muscles through a range of motion with proper form—a particular asset on exercises that take the muscle through an arc, such as leg and arm curls, or flies that work the chest. Because they're more controlled and generally keep the weights at a distance from the lifter, you're less likely to get hurt using machines, and you don't need a spotter. Because machine exercises typically demand less skill, they're ideal for beginners.

• Free weights require more control and therefore call more muscles into action to help guide the barbell or dumbell. For that reason, free weights develop areas that might not be touched on a machine. They're also superior for developing tendon and ligament strength, all of which makes free weights the tool of choice for serious lifters. "Free" means these weights are unrestricted in their movement, which can cause injury—but won't if you perform them with good form in a slow, controlled manner.

A Safer One-Rep Max

Determining proper resistance by straining to lift as much as you can in one repetition is decried as unsafe, but it can be done. You just need to exercise care. One way to do it is to start with a series of easier lifts. Wayne Westcott, Ph.D., strength-training consultant to the national YMCA and senior fitness director for the South Shore YMCA in Quincy, Massachusetts, recommends the following procedure, which both prepares muscles for maximum exertion and tires them out slightly to buffer against overexertion under heavy loads.

• First do ten warm-up lifts using a light weightload that's about 30 percent of your body weight (for a 150-pound man, that would be 45 pounds). Rest two minutes.

• Do five lifts with a load of 50 percent of your body weight. Rest two minutes.

• Do one lift with a load of 70 percent of your body weight. Rest two minutes.

• Continue doing single lifts with two-minute rests in between, adding 20 percent of your body weight with each lift, until you find the maximum load you can lift once.

wrestler needs to stay fast and quick—but not what a football lineman strives for when building brick-wall beefiness or strength for "combat" in the line.

Program principle: lifting light weights a high number of times.

Getting the Most from Your Workout

Whatever you're trying to achieve, there are a number of essential elements to any weight-lifting program, and manipulating these elements helps train muscles to do what you want them to. Here are the imperatives.

Load up. To challenge your muscles adequately, you have to lift enough weight. One benchmark for establishing the right resistance is based on the one-rep max, the heaviest weight you can lift in a single repetition. The ideal resistance for a beginning strength development program (in terms of safety and effectiveness) is 75 percent of your one-rep max, says Stephen Alway, Ph.D., director of the neuromuscular lab in the anatomy department at the University of South Florida College of Medicine in Tampa. For example, if you could bench-press 100 pounds once, the best weight for this exercise would be 75 pounds. Few exercise scientists actually recommend putting everything you have into one lift, especially if you're just starting a new program with untrained muscles.

"It's a good way to injure yourself," says Dr. Alway.

An alternative to the one-rep max is to aim for a weight that makes targeted muscles fatigue within 40 to 70 seconds, says Dr. Baechle. Assuming each repetition takes approximately four to six seconds, that gives you about 8 to 12 lifts. This isn't just guesswork: Studies find that most people working at 75 percent of their maximum resistance will fatigue within this range of repetitions, with the average being about 10 lifts.

Count off. How much weight you use is directly related to how many times you plan to lift it. The idea is simple: You can't lift heavy weights as many times as light ones. If a safe and effective resistance is something you can lift in 8 to 12 repetitions, it's fair to wonder: Which is best, 8 or 12? The answer depends on your goals and your progress—and it may not be limited to this range.

According to Dr. Baechle, who had a 16-year career as a competitive power lifter before receiving his doctorate, the 8- to 12-rep range is actually most ideal for building size. Studies confirm that if you're building strength, you'll need heavier loads and fewer lifts—in the range of 3 to 8 repetitions. For muscular endurance, you'll need to lighten weights enough to do 12 to 20 repetitions, says Dr. Baechle.

As for where in these ranges you should be, the rule of thumb is to start with lighter loads and try to

How to Begin

You're starting a weight program after months or years of not training. You decide to launch a commonly followed program doing three sets of ten reps at ten exercise stations. Consider what this means: "That's doing 300 reps more than you did the day before," says Tom Baechle, Ed.D., chair of the exercise science department at Creighton University in Omaha, Nebraska. "What you'll feel the next day is excruciating pain, which will make it obvious that there is a better approach to training."

There may be latent power in your muscles just waiting to be unleashed, but give your body a break. "Muscles are usually stronger than the tendons that support them," says Stephen Alway, Ph.D., director of the neuromuscular lab in the anatomy department at the University of South Florida College of Medicine in Tampa. "You need to rebuild tendons, blood vessels and muscles gradually." Here's what to do for an opening gambit.

Stick to one set. "It's silly to start with three," says Alan Mikesky, Ph.D., director of the Human Performance Lab and associate professor at Indiana University-Purdue University Indianapolis. "One set is enough of an overload during the first three weeks."

Start light. Use a weightload that you could lift for 15 repetitions, but stop at 12, says Dr. Alway. "In your second workout, add five pounds at most and aim to do 12 reps, as long as it's not so gut-wrenching it feels like your life will be over if you do 13."

Listen to your pain. If you're sore after the first workout, wait until you're not sore before you work out again, advises Dr. Alway.

Cut loose after three weeks. By this time, you should have established a resistance load that's challenging, but not so heavy it will make you sore. Add sets and follow the program you envision. "If you held back at the beginning and didn't tear yourself up too badly, you should be at full power," says Dr. Alway.

perform more repetitions in each workout, says Dr. Baechle. Let's say you're lifting enough weight to make 8 repetitions difficult. As you get stronger, you'll be able to do more. When doing 12 reps at that weight becomes easy, add more resistance. To avoid injury and soreness, many physiologists advise adding no more than 5 percent of the weight you're already lifting. If that's not possible (for example, moving from 15-pound dumbbells to 20-pounders represents a 33 percent increase), limit repetitions to as many as you can do with perfect form, gradually adding reps as strength improves.

Finish fatigued. To tap your muscles' full potential for development, doing one set of lifts isn't enough. At least that's what most trainers will tell you. "You won't find any successful competitive lifter who does just one set," Dr. Baechle says. However, there's some debate among physiologists about how much extra work—and time—is really necessary. Some studies, for example, suggest that exercising your muscles to fatigue in just one set of 8 to 12 repetitions builds strength and size just as much as three sets do.

The bottom line is this: How many sets you perform depends on just how serious you are and how much time you have. "Most of us can achieve our potential for muscular fitness with only a single set per exercise," says Wayne Westcott, Ph.D., strength-training consultant to the national YMCA, senior fitness director for the South Shore YMCA in Quincy, Massachusetts, and one of the researchers who has done studies to prove this. But limiting yourself to one set may cheat muscles of maximal gains possible beyond what's required for basic fitness.

Research shows that to make maximal gains, you need multiple sets, theoretically because additional effort challenges extra muscle fibers that would otherwise get off easy. The most common recommendation of serious weight trainers is to do three to five sets of the most important exercises and one to three sets of the others, says Dr. Baechle. If you're bodybuilding (striving for mass and muscle definition), extra exercises are needed to stimulate additional size. For example, two sets of biceps curls might first be done on a machine and the other sets with dumbbells to stress as many different muscle fibers as possible.

If you're short on time but still want to give your muscles an added kick, one compromise is to exhaust muscles in one set, then reduce the weight by ten pounds and immediately do a few more repetitions. In a two-month study of exercisers who limited lifts to one set, Dr. Westcott found that men and women who added this small measure of extra work during their second month of training developed 40 percent more strength than subjects who continued training with just one set.

Whatever you do, aim to make your last set the hardest: Your final lift is the benchmark for your progress. Let's say you're doing three sets of 10 repetitions. If you feel you can do 12 on the first set, stop at 10; otherwise, you might use up energy you'll need to complete the next sets. "You should never fall short by more than two repetitions," says Alan Mikesky,

Ph.D., director of the Human Performance Lab and associate professor at Indiana University-Purdue University Indianapolis. On the last set, however, push to do as many as you can.

Rest up. As covered in Getting Rest on page 13, it's important to allow muscles to recover not only between workouts (allow at least one day), but between sets. Again, what you do depends on what you're trying to achieve. The longer you rest between sets, the more your muscles recover and the harder you'll be able to push them on the next set. That's why long rests of two to five minutes are ideal for building strength, says Dr. Baechle. To build size, which involves the use of moderate weight and repetitions, you also want moderate rest between sets—30 to 90 seconds. If you're after endurance, the idea is to keep muscles working with little rest, and you should aim to break only 20 to 30 seconds between sets.

Think big. Major areas of the body—chest, back, legs, arms—aren't individual muscles, but muscle groups. An effective workout will exercise big groups of muscles first, leaving smaller muscles like the biceps and triceps for last. There are a couple of reasons for this.

First, it's efficient, since a single exercise such as a leg press works many different muscles at once, including the quadriceps, hamstrings, buttocks and calves. Other big-muscle exercises are the bench press and overhead press. Be sure not to perform a smaller muscle exercise, such as one for the triceps, before a larger muscle exercise like the bench press or overhead press. "If you start with the biceps and triceps, those muscles will be fatigued when you need to use them during the bench press," says Dr. Craig. "That means you won't get as much out of the more important exercise."

Go slow. Hefting heavy objects is never something you should rush, since rapid movements put tremendous pressure on both muscles and tendons, making you vulnerable to injury. But slow and steady movements are important for other reasons as well: Slow, controlled lifting stresses muscles more thoroughly and ensures that momentum isn't taking work away from you. "You want a controlled up-and-down movement," says Dr. Mikesky.

It's especially important to be smooth and slow when you're lowering the weight. You might assume that muscle development comes mostly from lifting up, since that's the part that seems hardest. Research shows, however, that the lowering—also known as the negative or eccentric phase—may actually be more crucial. You'll find lifters, in fact, who do nothing but negative movements, lowering a heavier-than-usual barbell to the chest during a bench press, for example, then having a spotter lift it back up.

Some physiologists say eccentric exercises build

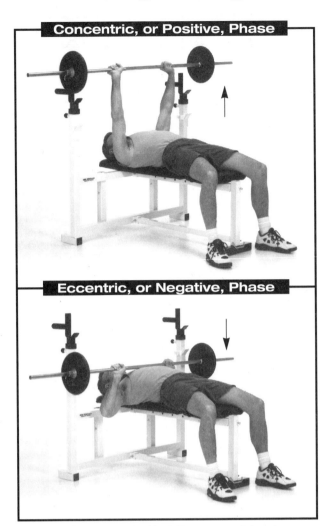

Research suggests that the eccentric phase of a lift may provide greater muscle gain. Experts suggest taking twice as long in this part of the lift as in the concentric part.

Program Principles at a Glance

Strength
- *Resistance:* Heavy
- *Repetitions:* 3 to 8
- *Sets:* 3 to 5
- *Rest:* 2 to 5 minutes

Size
- *Resistance:* Moderate
- *Repetitions:* 8 to 12
- *Sets:* 3 to 5
- *Rest:* 30 to 90 seconds

Tone
- *Resistance:* Light
- *Repetitions:* 12 to 20
- *Sets:* 2 to 3
- *Rest:* 20 to 30 seconds

Supercharging Your Program

Once you've established your basic program, try giving your workouts an extra kick: Physiologists agree that adding variety in order to challenge muscles in new ways provides superior results. Here are two ways to do it, according to Tom Baechle, Ed.D., chair of the exercise science department at Creighton University in Omaha, Nebraska.

For strength: pyramid training. The idea is to make each set progressively heavier, with fewer repetitions performed on each set. For example, after a warm-up set at your usual weightload, you might increase the load to 75 to 80 percent of your one-rep max on the second set, 85 percent on the third set and 90 percent on the fourth set. If your one-rep max is 150 pounds, here's how the sets would progress.

First set: 110 pounds, warm-up
Second set: 120 pounds, six to eight reps
Third set: 130 pounds, four to seven reps
Fourth set: 135 pounds, one to three reps

For size: compound sets. Sometimes referred to as supersets, compound sets build more bulk and better definition by hitting the same muscles from different angles with different exercises. Often, one exercise takes the muscle through an arc, while the other moves in more of a straight line. For best results, you proceed from one exercise to the next without resting. Examples of compound sets are bench presses followed by dumbbell flies for the chest, or barbell curls followed by dumbbell curls for the biceps.

---

muscle as much as 20 percent faster than concentric, or positive-only lifts. "Coming down is not as normal a movement as pushing up: It stresses the tissues differently and more damage is occurring," says Dr. Craig. His research has shown that greater amounts of muscle-building growth hormone are released during eccentric exercise than concentric.

Emphasizing the down phase makes the most of the eccentric movement built into every lift you do. Some exercise physiologists recommend a six-second lift consisting of two seconds up and four seconds down, says Dr. Baechle. (The only exception might be if you're, say, a football player training for power, an explosive form of strength that's keyed not only to how much force you can produce but how fast you can exert it.)

Make changes. By the time you get bored with a routine, your muscles are way ahead of you. What used to shock them now makes them yawn. Or maybe they're just tuckered out. Giving muscles an occasional wake-up call or change of pace is known as periodization. You do it by tinkering with any of the elements we've just outlined, says Dr. Baechle. Do more sets. Use different exercises. Add or subtract repetitions. Rest less or more. Lift faster or slower. Change the order of the exercises in your workout. Exercise your upper body one workout and your lower body the next.

Just keep in mind that there's a proportional relationship between many of the key components. If you do fewer reps, you should add weight. If you add sets, you might need to lighten the load or rest more between sets. Overall, "the number one principle," Dr. Mikesky reminds us, "is to overload the muscle beyond what it normally encounters."

The Effects of Time Off

To continue making gains in strength, size or endurance, it's important to be persistent with your workouts. Whipping your muscles into better and better shape requires at least three workouts a week. But as with aerobic exercise, doing less won't blow your whole program. In fact, you can put yourself into a holding pattern indefinitely with minimal effort and not lose any of your gains. "For maintenance, you can get by with as little as one workout per week, doing one set per exercise," states Dr. Mikesky. "With any less than that, strength will deteriorate over time."

Granted, this happens slowly: If you completely slack off for a few weeks, you might still be able to handle your usual workout, but you'll pay a penalty in soreness. The important thing, Dr. Mikesky says, is to continue to be able to lift the same load from one workout to the next. "You cannot sacrifice that intensity," he says. If you do, you've allowed a loss—and more than usual soreness is one sign of it.

If you've gone two weeks without a workout, don't despair: You can get back into top form in just one or two weeks, if you go back to a three-times-a-week schedule. To avoid soreness or injury from your first few workouts back, initially reduce your weightload by 10 to 20 percent, suggests Dr. Baechle. Do one set fewer than usual and cut your repetitions by two or three.

Above all, don't get frustrated when the dramatic gains you made at the beginning of a program begin to taper off. "It's like with golf," says Dr. Baechle. "A neophyte might cut 20 points off his game in a year, but if a pro shaves just one point in a year, he's had a great year."

Aerobic Exercise

Aerobic exercise is the stuff of life: It's about blood and air, the two things we can't go without for more than a few moments. If you don't want to be so philosophical, think of it this way: Aerobic exercise is the stuff of *living*, because it's also about having energy and stamina—not only to keep up an activity for long periods without fatiguing but also to keep active and healthy far into your twilight years.

Fitness fanatics sometimes toss around superlatives like "fountain of youth" when describing aerobic exercise. Such terms actually aren't far off the mark when you consider just one significant benefit of aerobic exercise: its ability to prevent heart disease, the top killer of men in the United States. A regular program of aerobic exercise lowers blood pressure, knocks your ratio of good-versus-bad cholesterol into a healthier balance, makes the heart pump blood more forcefully, reduces body fat and can prevent diabetes. Bottom line, men between the ages of 35 and 74 who keep aerobically active have a 64 percent lower risk of suffering a first heart attack than more sedentary men, according to one large study.

Unlike weight training, which targets specific muscles or areas of the body one at a time during short, intense exercises, aerobic exercise works large muscle groups for sustained periods. (As a rule, any exercise that causes your heart to beat fast and can be sustained for more than 20 minutes is a good aerobic exercise.) "But in a sense, you're still targeting one muscle—the heart," says Laura Gladwin, who chairs the board of certification and training for the Aerobic Fitness Association of America.

To understand why, you'll need a basic anatomy lesson. Muscles need two ingredients to do their work—oxygen and glucose (a simple form of sugar that is the end result of the digestive process). The longer the exertion, the more muscle cells need of both. While muscles maintain small stores of fuel, they are unable to store oxygen. So it is up to your heart and lungs to deliver a steady flow of oxygen via the bloodstream. And when you exert your muscles for a long time, muscles also need extra fuel. That, too, is delivered via the bloodstream.

So where do lung and heart fitness fit in? Easy: The stronger the heart is, the more efficiently it can pump oxygen-rich blood to oxygen-hungry muscles. The more powerful your lungs are, the better they can get oxygen into the bloodstream. So the more aerobic training you do, the more you'll fine-tune your heart and lungs, the two main engines of your body's speed, strength and power, says Alan Mikesky, Ph.D., director of the Human Performance Lab and associate professor at Indiana University-Purdue University Indianapolis.

The trick is to keep going without working muscles so hard that their need for oxygen exceeds the ability of the lungs and heart to efficiently provide it—a task that gets easier as your conditioning improves.

What It Takes

Your ability to improve your aerobic fitness is limited by your genes and your current level of conditioning. Still, anybody can improve aerobically if they follow well-established guidelines regarding three fundamental factors.

How hard: the intensity factor. It's critical both to work yourself hard enough to make a difference and to pace yourself. The whole idea with aerobic exercise, after all, is *sustained* activity. "If your oxygen demands are greater than what you can handle," says Gladwin, "you'll have to slow down or stop to catch your breath."

Fortunately, each of us has an onboard intensity meter. Heart rate, oxygen consumption and exercise intensity all go up in direct proportion to each other when your body becomes active. Gauging your heart rate gives you a first-hand measure of how hard you're working.

The optimal intensity level for aerobic conditioning is 70 to 85 percent of your maximal heart rate—the rate at which your heart just can't pump any harder. Maximal heart rate tends to be fairly consistent from one person to another, although it varies with age, declining about 1 beat per year after adolescence. You can calculate your maximal heart rate by subtracting your age from 220. If you're a 40-year-old man, that would give you a maximal heart rate of 180

Progressing by the Numbers

If you're new to aerobic exercise (or you've completely laid off for a few months or more), it's wise not to start full-tilt at your target heart rate in the interests of avoiding overexertion or injury, says B. Don Franks, Ph.D., professor of kinesiology at Louisiana State University in Baton Rouge. Instead, take it one step at a time.

1. Start by walking (or running or biking) at a pace that's easy for you, no sweating or heavy breathing necessary. Go for about 15 to 20 minutes at least three times a week, picking up the pace as it feels comfortable. For the moment, forget about your heart rate.

2. When you can comfortably walk about three miles, figure your target heart rate, the rate at which your heart should pump during exercise. If you want to skip the math, just set a pace at which you're breathing hard but can still hold a normal conversation. Hold this pace for 20 minutes or so three days a week. Note how much distance you generally cover at this speed.

3. When you're comfortable with your pace, set a higher distance goal and increase your mileage by 10 to 15 percent a week, keeping pace consistent. When you meet your mileage goal, work on increasing speed, keeping mileage the same.

Getting Your Body Ready

Just contemplating a spin on a bike or a dash to the corner market makes your heart beat a bit faster and causes alertness hormones and brain chemicals to start churning. But your body can't do all the preparation it needs on its own. You have to help it out. Prescription:

Before, stoke the fire. Warm muscles are limber muscles, and keeping loose reduces the risk of injury and soreness. Before starting any strenuous activity, do a five-minute warm-up of walking or rhythmic limbering movements like jogging in place and shaking your arms. "It's like a rehearsal," says Laura Gladwin, who chairs the board of certification and training for the Aerobic Fitness Association of America. "It readies the body for more vigorous movement." Hold off on stretching, which won't benefit cold muscles.

After, turn down the burner. After you've finished exercising, do a light cooldown activity such as walking. "You need to bring blood that has pooled in your extremities back to the heart," says Gladwin. "If you bring your body to a complete halt after vigorous activity, you could become lightheaded or even faint," she says. Now that your muscles are warmed and pliable, do some gentle stretching to improve flexibility.

---

beats per minute. To determine a target heart rate that's at least 70 percent of that, you'd multiply 180 by .70, which gives you 126 beats per minute.

Remember, this is how hard your heart should pump while you exercise. To get a handle on what it feels like to work out at your target heart rate, you'll need to take your pulse during your workout. "Don't do it for a full minute, because your heart rate slows as you rest and it won't be accurate," says Ben Hurley, Ph.D., director of the Exercise Science Labs at the University of Maryland, College of Health and Human Performance in College Park. He suggests taking your pulse for ten seconds, then multiplying that measure by six for the minute-long value.

How long: the dirt on duration. As a rule, to qualify as a sustained activity, an aerobic workout should last at least 20 to 30 minutes. There's nothing wrong with exercising for longer periods, but once you get beyond 30 to 40 minutes, you tend to decrease your intensity, which may lower the return on your time investment if your goal is to increase your cardiovascular fitness, says Dr. Hurley. "If your condition improves to the point where you can go for a longer period, it makes more sense to raise the intensity level than to draw out the exercise."

That's the long of it. With the short of it, the story is slightly different. If you exercise for less than 20 minutes, you don't get much aerobic benefit—unless you exercise again for a short period later in the day. Remember, the American College of Sports Medicine now suggests that if you can't fit a 20-minute workout into your schedule, you instead exercise for, say, 5 minutes, four times a day. What's important is that exercising in short bursts is said to confer health benefits akin to those of more lengthy aerobic workouts. But that's different from becoming aerobically conditioned. To achieve optimal gains in your level of cardiovascular fitness, you'll still need to exercise for a solid 20 to 30 minutes at a stretch.

How often: What's the frequency? How many times a week must you work out in order to see improvement? This is one place where your current condition comes into play. Some studies find that if you're so sedentary that *any* increase in activity would be a major improvement, significant changes in cardiovascular condition can be made with as little as one workout per week. But don't be lulled by such extreme scenarios. For most men, the majority of research finds that getting an optimal training response—continually notching closer to peak aero-

A Man's Armchair Guide to Aerobic Exercises

No exercise is perfect. But some are more perfect than others—for you. To help you figure yours, here's a rundown of some random pluses and minuses.

Biking

Hits: Wind-in-your-hair speed. Exercise doubles as transportation. Good bikes are cool. Equipment available for indoor workouts.

Misses: Reason to wear Spandex. Yahoo motorists make road riding scary if not dangerous.

Running

Hits: Can do anywhere, anytime. Need minimal equipment. The most spiritual of exercises, if you believe the hype.

Misses: Impact injuries common. Shoes must be replaced regularly.

Walking

Hits: Can do anywhere, anytime. Need even less equipment than running. Injuries nil. The only exercise virtually guaranteed to lengthen your life.

Misses: Low on speed and action. For conditioning, you may need to pick up the pace.

Cross-Country Skiing

Hits: Highest calorie-burner. Works both upper and lower body. Equipment available for both outdoors and indoors.

Misses: Indoor equipment hogs floor space. Outdoors, snow and skiable land required.

Stair-Climbing

Hits: Low-impact. Can do year-round.
Misses: Dull.

Step Aerobics

Hits: Low-impact. Equipment simple.
Misses: Annoying videos or classes generally required.

Dance Aerobics

Hits: Few guys—high babe ratio.
Misses: Few guys—you look like a dweeb.

Swimming

Hits: Low-impact. Exceptional fat-burner. Doesn't make you hot and sweaty.
Misses: Pool required.

---

bic condition—requires at least three workouts per week, says Dr. Hurley.

Here, too, it's not necessary—or even desirable—to work out more than that. A number of studies find that training four or five times per week provides little or no benefit beyond exercising three times. "However, working out every day is okay, as long as you don't overtrain," says Dr. Hurley.

Measuring Up

It doesn't take long for aerobic exercise to make a difference—a fact that you'll feel in terms of general well-being, but which you also can easily quantify. When it comes to measuring aerobic progress, again, "let your heart rate be your guide," says Dr. Hurley.

In this case, it's not your heart rate while exercising that's important, but your heart rate *at rest*. A sedentary man's resting heart rate is high because an unconditioned heart has to work harder at all times than a conditioned one, just to keep a body alive while it's horizontal watching ESPN. With training, your resting heart rate goes down. A middle-aged, out-of-shape man averages between 80 and 100 beats per minute, while highly conditioned endurance athletes fall more in the range of 30 to 40 beats per minute. A resting heart rate of 60 is normal for a moderately active person. Let's say you're at the low end of the sedentary scale, with a resting heart rate of 80. If you start a program of endurance training, that rate

will drop by about one beat per minute each week. After ten weeks, your rate will drop to about 70—already halfway to levels typical of active people.

To find your resting heart rate, don't take your pulse right before exercising: Your body knows what you're about to do and raises your heart rate in anticipation. In fact, says Dr. Hurley, the only time you're reliably at total rest is just after you wake up. Lie quietly before taking your pulse for a full minute.

Maintaining Your Gains

Some men make aerobic exercise one of life's givens: It's something they love and will always carve time for. For many of us, however, maintaining a continuous program is a challenge. That's not necessarily bad. Don't fall into the trap of thinking that anything less than a maximal effort is worthless. In fact, if you make mere maintenance your goal, you can get by with considerably less effort without losing anything you've gained.

The key to maintenance isn't keeping up your schedule, but keeping up your intensity. Studies find that if you exercise hard, you can reduce both the frequency and duration of your workouts. For example, you could go from training six days a week to two, or from 40 minutes a day to 13, and show no decline in performance. If you back off your intensity, however, fitness levels decline significantly, even if you work out just as long and just as often.

Cross-Training

Cross-training is the most natural thing in the world: You've been doing it all your life and probably still are. If you ran your dog on Monday, biked around the neighborhood with your kid on Wednesday and moved furniture all afternoon on Saturday, in essence, you've been cross-training—mixing totally different forms of exercise.

Unless you've participated in serious athletics, the idea that cross-training is a radical or novel concept—or even deserves to be conferred a category all its own—might seem odd. For understanding, recall the specificity principle, which declares that if you want your muscles to do a particular thing well, you must train them in just that way. Runners get better by running, lifters get better by lifting and never the twain shall meet. It's a tiresome view of training that nevertheless inspires relentless dedication from athletes for the simple reason that it works.

Recently, however, this single track to excellence has been branching into alternate routes, inspired in part by bored athletes who found that working a little variety into their programs seemed to help rather than hinder them. One is Gordon Bakoulis, a member of the U.S. 1991 World Marathon Championship Team and author of *Cross-Training: The Complete Training Guide for All Sports*—an elite runner who also bikes, swims and lifts weights.

"Doing activities other than running spares me pounding, breaks up the monotony and gives me a chance to work different muscles, which helps prevent injury," Bakoulis says. "People ask how it actually helps make me a better runner, but it's not like swimming or biking has some direct benefit. It's more that it provides a sense of balance and just overall makes me *feel* better."

Physiologists who have studied cross-training say Bakoulis is on the right track. "Cross-training will never be better than specific training for a given sport, but it has many benefits for people who are interested in superior overall fitness," says Hirofumi Tanaka, Ph.D., research associate in the Department of Kinesiology at the University of Colorado at Boulder. For peak conditioning as we've defined it, it's just what the doctor ordered.

The Best of Both Worlds

The underlying concern about cross-training is that by trying to do many things at once, you end up doing none of them well—that is, when performed together, one form of exercise robs another of its effectiveness.

In reality, evidence for this is mixed, which is good news: Even in instances where activities interfere with each other, the effect isn't as significant as many coaches and trainers long believed. Although the consequences of cross-training have not been thoroughly investigated, a number of studies have been done on how various activities relate to others. Following are some of the conclusions to date.

It's never wrong to be strong. Research on strength training consistently shows that it won't interfere with aerobic development. "Aerobic capacity is limited primarily by the heart's ability to pump blood to muscles," says John P. McCarthy, Ph.D., a former bodybuilder and NASA research physiologist who's now a post-doctoral fellow at the School of Physical Therapy at Texas Women's University in Houston. "Strength training affects muscles locally but has minimal effect in terms of oxygen uptake." And the effects that strength training *does* have on the heart may improve cardiovascular function. One study, for example, finds that weight training on its own can lower resting heart rate and blood pressure.

The caveat is that strength training won't necessarily improve performance in aerobic sports. For example, weights are often used to develop the upper-body strength required for competitive swimming, but research fails to find consistent evidence that strength in the gym translates to strength in the water. One study, for example, found that when weight training was added to swim training, the weight lifters' stroke strength improved no more than that of men who just stuck with swimming. Other studies, however, find that weight training *will* help cycling performance. It all

How to Mix and Match

Cross-training means different things to different people. An elite athlete looking to infuse new activities into his training may want to choose sports that work the same muscle groups used in his primary avocation. But those of us who are just looking for a little variety in our pursuit of overall fitness are better off choosing activities that are *not* similar. Beyond the idea that you should do both aerobic and resistance training, here are some rules of thumb for combining sports, as recommended by Gordon Bakoulis, a member of the U.S. 1991 World Marathon Championship Team and author of *Cross-Training: The Complete Training Guide for All Sports.*

Combine upper- and lower-body activities. If all you do is run and bike, your lower body gets all the attention while your upper body languishes. Adding an upper-body sport makes for more balanced fitness. Some possible matches: walking, running, biking or team sports combined with swimming, rowing, kayaking or tennis.

Emphasize skill and movement. Some sports are rote. They're movement-oriented, you've known how to do them for a long time and no special skills are involved—walking, riding a bike and swimming, for example. Some sports demand higher levels of skill: Even if you have raw talent, you'll always be trying to improve. Adding such sports—tennis, skiing, racquetball, golf, basketball, softball—to your routine engages your body and brain in ways that are different than more repetitive sports where you let your mind wander.

Match stressful with less-stressful. If you add one joint-pounding sport to another, you may end up having to give up both because of an injury. Better to choose new sports that are easier on your joints than the activities you already pursue. If you run or play tennis or basketball, add more forgiving sports like biking, rowing or walking.

---

depends, Dr. Tanaka says, on how closely your movements in the weight room mimic the movements of your sport.

Aerobic exercise undercuts strength—maybe. Unfortunately, aerobic exercise doesn't appear to be as benevolent toward strength programs as strength programs are to aerobic exercise. A number of studies found that strength gains are compromised when aerobic exercise is added to weight training. It's not that you won't get stronger; you just won't get as strong as you would by doing strength training alone. "The impairment isn't great, but it is statistically significant," reports Dr. Tanaka.

These findings may be skewed, however, according to Dr. McCarthy. He points out that studies often require cross-training subjects to do two programs at full tilt simultaneously: The cross-trainers are exercising more than the people to whom they're being compared and, it's safe to assume, are more tired. "Exercising up to six days a week, as some of these studies require," he says, "is just not realistic." When Dr. McCarthy conducted a study of sedentary men in which exercisers—whether they were only lifting weights, only doing aerobic exercise or combining the two—all stuck to a three-day-a-week program, he found no difference in strength gains between the weight trainers and the cross-trainers.

All aerobic exercises are not equal. You might assume that one form of aerobic exercise will improve cardiovascular endurance as well as another, but some activities appear more complementary than others. How well a combination of activities works depends in part on how fit you are before starting: Studies find that less-trained men or average exercisers interested in fitness show greater improvements from cross-training than do men who are already highly trained.

Beyond that, to get the most out of multiple activities, it makes sense to combine forms of exercise that use the same muscle groups. For example, running and cycling seem to complement each other well: Runners who take cycling tests and cyclists who take running tests all show substantial increases in oxygen uptake after training. (Caveat: Cycling helps runners more than running helps cyclists.) Dissimilar activities like running and swimming, however, "may have little practical benefit" if you're highly trained, concludes one research review.

Cross-training burns more fat. Aerobic exercise gets all the glory for fat-burning and weight loss, but strength training has tangible benefits of its own. Not only does strength training raise the body's fat-burning metabolism during the workout but adding muscle—which requires more fuel to maintain than fat does—keeps the metabolism firing at a higher rate even when you're resting. Together, strength and aerobic training are dramatically superior at burning fat than either one alone.

In one study of men and women who ate the same diet, for example, those who split their half-hour workouts into equal parts strength training and aerobic conditioning lost twice as much body weight as those who did only aerobic exercise.

Flexibility

Few of us look at an example of physical perfection like Michelangelo's *David*, and say, "I'll bet *he* could reach past his toes." Our appreciation of conditioning generally doesn't stretch that far.

That's understandable, but unfortunate, because flexibility is not only the easiest element of fitness to develop but it's also extremely important—especially for men. "In my experience, men's muscles tend to be much tighter than women's," says William D. Bandy, P.T., Ph.D., associate professor of physical therapy at the University of Central Arkansas in Conway. For active men in particular, that can cause problems.

- Stiff muscles that are subjected to sudden elongation during exercise or sports can more easily become torn or strained.
- Tightness in muscles can cause pain elsewhere in the body. Tight calves, for example, can cause knee pain, shin splints and foot pain. Tense muscles at various points in the lower back can cause pain to radiate throughout the entire torso.
- Lack of flexibility can cause muscular imbalances. A tight hamstring, for example, can make the thighs work harder at keeping the body properly aligned, which may cause knee pain.

Beyond that, feeling stiff makes you slow down, move more carefully, act more tentatively—it's the first way a young man starts to feel like an old one. "Some tightness results from a loss of elasticity with age, but for most people, it's simply because they're inactive," says Michael Kaplan, M.D., Ph.D., director of the Rehabilitation Team in Catonsville, Maryland. "We're not talking about an unavoidable situation," Dr. Kaplan says. "People who work at it can stay flexible well into old age."

Requirements for Resilience

Working at it takes more than exercise alone: You need to stretch. "You can be very strong and very fit and still not be flexible," Dr. Kaplan says. As with other types of training, improvement in flexibility depends on subjecting muscles to more than they're accustomed to—by making muscles work through a range of motion in a controlled and systematic way. You don't need to add a second workout to what you already do, but merely take ten minutes or so for stretching. To do it properly, follow these guidelines.

Soften up. When muscles are cold, they're stiffer. Light exercise before stretching warms muscles and makes them more pliable, improving the stretch and reducing the risk of muscle strain (which makes warming up a good idea whether you stretch or not). "You shouldn't exercise so much in a warm-up that you fatigue yourself before your workout," says Bryant Stamford, Ph.D., director of the Health Promotion and Wellness Center at the University of Louisville School of Medicine in Kentucky. He recommends a walk or slow jog for ten minutes or so. "You should just be verging on a light sweat," he says. If the weather is hot and you're already sweating, you can shorten your warm-up exercise to about five minutes (although going the full ten minutes won't hurt).

Stretch, but don't strain. You want to extend the muscle far enough to make a difference, but not so far that you cause muscle fibers to tear. Stretch until you feel a slight tug, but don't push beyond that point.

Put muscles on hold. Hold each stretch for 30 seconds. In studies, Dr. Bandy has found that how long you hold a stretch has a direct bearing on improved flexibility. Holding for 15 seconds is no better for elasticity than not stretching at all. Holding for 30 seconds has significant benefit, with measurable weekly improvements. Holding for 60 seconds, however, provides no greater benefit than 30 seconds.

Banish bouncing. Stretches should be slow and steady, not fast and jerky. Some athletes such as gymnasts do use bounce stretches, but only because their bodies already are extremely elastic. Bounce stretches pose a particular potential for injury because when you lengthen a muscle, electrical impulses involuntarily signal the muscle to snap back in a contraction. "The body actively resists overstretching," Dr. Bandy says. Stretching too far too fast puts excessive strain on muscles; it's the difference between bending a tree branch slowly and giving it a hard snap. Slow, steady stretches over time make muscles adapt to ever-greater lengthening.

Shoulders

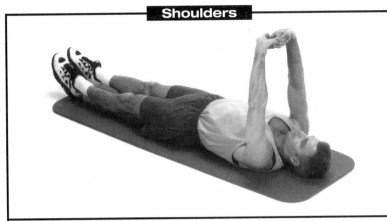

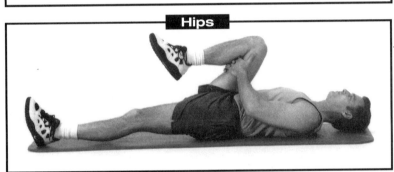

Hips

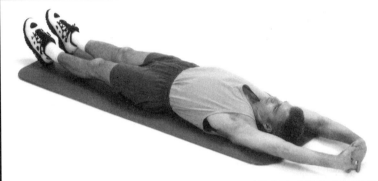

Lower Back

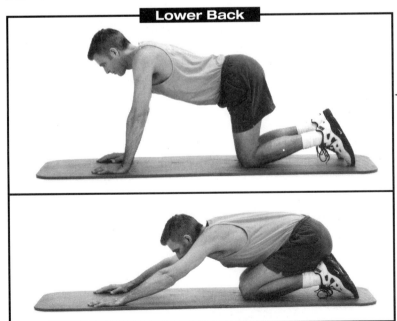

Seven to Remember

There are plenty of useful stretches you can do, as any yoga course will teach. But a basic overall stretching program need only hit several major muscle groups, particularly in the lower body, where the vast majority of flexibility-related problems occur. Here are some good basic moves that hit all the important areas.

◄ Shoulders

Lie on your back on the floor and point your toes. Extend your arms straight above your face, interlocking your fingers, with your palms pointing toward the ceiling. Keeping your arms straight, slowly lower your hands until they rest on the floor behind the crown of your head. Hold.

◄ Hips

Lie on your back with your legs straight. Interlacing your hands behind your right upper thigh, pull your right knee toward your chest and hold. Return to the starting position and repeat with your left leg.

◄ Lower Back

Get on your hands and knees, with your hands directly under your shoulders. While keeping your hands in place, sit back onto your heels, feeling a stretch along your back. Your arms will be outstretched.

Philosophies of Flex

Here in the Western world, we don't get too excited about flexibility, which is one of the reasons we need it so much. In the East, however, flexibility is practically a religion—or, at the very least, a crucial element in various disciplines involving both mind and movement. But you don't need to subscribe to a lot of spiritual and philosophical tenets to get benefits from the techniques involved in two of the best-known and most accessible of these disciplines.

Yoga. Its image is that of incense-burning mystics in flowing robes, but yoga doesn't need to be exotic. Practicing it entails moving your body through a range of poses that not only increase flexibility but also build strength, balance, speed and endurance. Traditional yoga emphasizes breathing, with poses held for sustained periods, which allows plenty of time to contemplate the universe. One form of yoga, however, ashtanga (also known as power yoga), keeps you moving fluidly through poses without pausing, providing an intense workout.

Tai chi. The grace and control of tai chi was initially inspired by the movements of animals. It's a kind of slow-motion calisthenics in which you're supposed to be relaxed, yet fully aware of your body as it moves through a variety of positions. Tai chi is categorized as a martial art, although there's nothing explosive or aggressive about it. Rather, the discipline extols quiet, inner strength. As with yoga, balance and breathing are important, and its benefits include increased flexibility, muscle tone—and maybe even wisdom.

It's tough to learn either yoga or tai chi by looking at pictures or reading descriptions. The best form of instruction is to get lessons from somebody whose moves you can follow and whose coaching can ensure good technique. Look in the Yellow Pages under yoga, martial arts or karate, or check with the local YMCA.

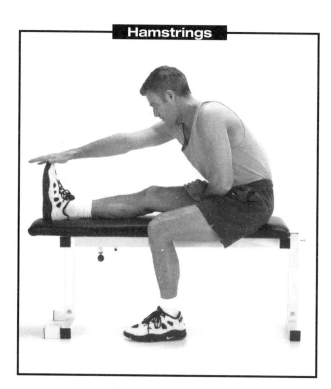

Hamstrings ▲

Sit on the edge of a bed or bench with your right leg extended on the bench and your left foot on the floor. Rest your right hand on your right knee, then slowly slide your fingers to your toes, reaching as far as is comfortable. Hold. Repeat with your right leg on the floor and your left leg on the bench. (This position takes stress off the lower back, unlike similar exercises in which you sit on the floor.)

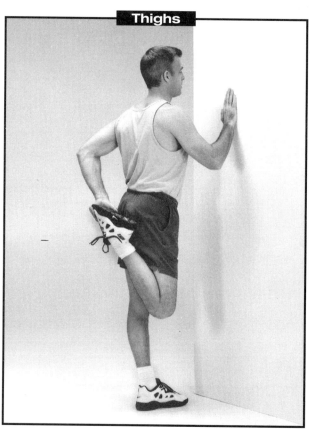

Thighs ▲

Stand touching a chair or wall for support. Bending your right knee, grab your right foot with your left hand and pull your foot up so that your heel presses against your buttocks. Hold and repeat with your left leg.

Calves

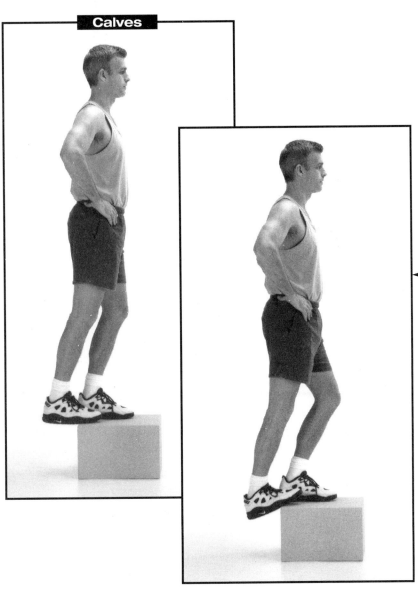

◄ Calves

Stand on a step with the heel of your right foot protruding over the edge of the step. Drop your right heel below the level of the step until you feel a tug. Hold, then repeat with your left heel.

Groin

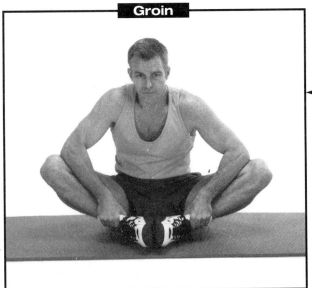

◄ Groin

To do a butterfly stretch, sit on the floor with your legs bent frog-style, the soles of your feet pressed together. Gently press your knees toward the floor with your hands or elbows. Hold.

Mental Conditioning

If ever there was a poster boy for mental toughness, it's Dan Jansen. When he slid up to the starting line for the 1,000-meter speed skating event at the 1994 Olympic Games in Lillehammer, the world cringed. We knew his story. He'd blown opportunities to win medals at both the 1988 and 1992 Olympics. He'd slipped again in the 500-meter at Lillehammer. He was an aging warrior, and this was his last chance to strike at the gold. Everyone knew he was physically capable of winning the event. But the baggage of personal tragedy and defeat stepped up to the line with him. The question was, would he carry the baggage into the event, where it would encumber and trip him up, or would he leave it behind and slash his way down the track unburdened?

Jansen's answer to the global village of doubters watching his performance that day was to shatter a world record and win a gold medal. His victory lap holding his eight-month-old daughter, now a revered bit of Olympic iconography, brought "tears of joy" to the face of the man who trained Jansen to accomplish mentally what his body was already prepared to do, sports psychologist James Loehr, Ed.D.

According to Dr. Loehr, the mental and emotional discipline that made Jansen a champion can help any man trying to make the most of his physical potential. In fact, he says, fortitude of the mind is an essential part of peak conditioning. "Mental toughness is the ability to bring to life whatever talent and skills you have—on demand," says Dr. Loehr, president of LGE Sports Science in Orlando, Florida. "That may come down to an ability to fight sleepiness, or to stay relaxed and calm or to not surrender your spirit when the odds are against you."

Even in noncompetitive exercise, when you're in the right frame of mind, you'll keep focused, push harder—and be better able to cut yourself slack when that's what your body demands. Bottom line, your physical efforts will count more if your mind is helping out. "Nothing happens in the brain that doesn't affect the rest of the body," says Jonathan Robison, Ph.D., an exercise physiologist, nutritionist and executive co-director of the Michigan Center for Preventive Medicine in Lansing.

Dr. Loehr likens body and mind to hardware and software: You can have fast, powerful hardware, but it's worth little if you lack equally powerful software to make it go.

Giving Yourself a Mental Edge

Sweating, groaning, gritting your teeth: There was a time when a man's goal in life was—outside of sex—to avoid the kind of physical labor that produced these sorts of responses. Even today, beneath the surface, many of us are conflicted about working out. "For a lot of men, it's just one more thing we have to do," says Dr. Robison.

What we tell ourselves and how we feel about exercise—even as we do it—can have a bearing on how successful we are at it. According to Richard Gordin, Ed.D., professor of health, education and recreation at Utah State University in Logan, here are some tricks of the trained for achieving a frame of mind in which you *want* to excel at exercise.

Hail what's hard. The better you are at pushing yourself beyond your normal limits, the closer you'll come to peak conditioning—a truth that's easy to accept while reading it chair bound, but another matter when your muscles feel like they're turning to jelly and you're pushing to eke out one last lift. What's to keep a sensible man from giving his muscles the relief they're screaming for? An attitude that celebrates the struggle. Dan Jansen once feared and loathed the 1,000-meter because it was difficult for him. "It's not the thing you *can* do that makes the difference, but the thing you can't," says Dr. Robison. "When you're working the hardest, think, 'This is the part that really counts.'"

Daydream for endurance. Some of the most effective performance-boosting mental techniques involve focus—but not necessarily concentration. When it comes to endurance training, a *lack* of focus actually has remarkable power, says Michael Sachs, Ph.D., associate professor of physical education at Temple University in Philadelphia. Psychologists call it dissociation, a kind of controlled daydreaming that takes your mind off what you're doing, makes your workout more pleasant and prevents you from getting bored—all of which make it easier to continue a sustained effort.

In one study, exercisers who were asked to spend 15 minutes cycling were divided into two groups. One group was to concentrate on their exertion levels while pedaling; the other group was to try to remember the names of every teacher they'd had since kindergarten. The actual exertion levels of both groups were the same, but those whose minds were busy scouring their scholastic past rated their exertion levels significantly lower than the self-focused group. Other dissociation techniques might include writing letters in your head, doing math puzzles or counting telephone poles.

Concentrate for weights. The opposite of dissociation is association, which is more useful for weight lifting, an activity that requires presence of mind for both safety and effectiveness. "By concentrating on the specific muscle being exercised, you're more likely to put more energy into your effort and execute your movements with better form," Dr. Sachs says.

Play a mental movie. Use of imagery, or visualization, has become a staple among athletes, and for good reason: Numerous studies find that mentally rehearsing movements before doing them can boost physical performance. It works on a couple of levels. First, research suggests that picturing an action has a direct impact on the nerves that make muscles move. Some scientists have measured a 30 percent contraction in the biceps of test subjects who merely envisioned flexing the muscles. It's easy to see how this can have tangible benefits. In a grip-strength test, for example, subjects who imagined themselves squeezing a pressure-measuring meter could actually apply more force to it than subjects who mentally prepared by whipping up hostile feelings or counting backward out loud.

Beyond that, however, visualization seems to have an effect on motivation and interest. In one study, a group of men and women who had never golfed before were taught to putt and told they'd later be tested on their ability. Participants were divided into two groups: One got putting imagery training and the other didn't. The imagery group spent significantly more time practicing, adhered better to a training program outside of the lab and set higher goals than the other group. Not surprisingly, the imagery group also performed better. Here are some tricks for making mental projections, according to Dr. Gordin.

- Remember a previous event when things went well and focus on it. Recall all the feelings and sensations you can remember, including details like the smell of the air, the feel of your clothes, the sweat on your back.
- Play the mental movie as *you* would experience it, from inside your head, not as some outside observer. Imagine events unfolding in real time, not in slow motion.
- Don't put your vision on pause to revisit certain moments, but play it through, then repeat the whole thing from start to finish.

Know what you want. When you enter the gym or start a run, avoid open-ended objectives such as "Today, I'll do my best." One study involving a sit-up endurance test found that exercisers who were challenged to do a precise, high number of crunches significantly outperformed those who were simply told to do the best they could. Yet preliminary screening had shown all the subjects to have roughly equal potential. "By limiting yourself to what you *think* your best is, you can shortchange your true abilities," says Dr. Sachs.

Further, your true abilities may surprise you, even when your goals are well-defined. One coach tells of waiting at the gym for another guy to finish with the 40-pound dumbbells. The coach started his workout, which felt tough, but he pushed through and finished. Only after he was through did he discover that he was mistakenly lifting 45-pounders—something he says he wouldn't have been able to do if he had known.

Speak well of yourself. With specific goals come specific disappointments, backslides and failures. But it's important to accept these moments for what they are: temporary setbacks and not indictments of your overall condition. "When expectations are not met, there's a tendency to start using poor self-talk, which is important to recognize," says Dr. Gordin. Thoughts such as "What's wrong with me?" or "I can't do this" or "This isn't working" can bog down your performance and poison your attitude toward your next workout. "Don't dwell on what you can't do, because it will get in the way of what you can," says Dr. Gordin. "Instead, say, 'I'm having a hard time, but I'll do better on the next station or the next day.' Say to yourself, 'This is not like me.'"

Control socializing. There's a lot to be said for working out with partners. They can motivate you to show up for your workout, encourage you to push harder, give you new ideas and just make the time pass more pleasantly. But people around you can also be a distraction. "Gyms are the bars of the 1990s," says Dr. Robison. "I've seen people spend their whole time talking, which isn't going to benefit anyone."

Getting Into the Flow

Maybe you've had one of these moments. You're running a race or riding your bike and everything seems to click. You're in control, you feel good, time seems to stand still. It's called flow, and it has become something of a catchphrase in the working world.

In the realm of physical activity, researchers have tried to identify what causes flow and how it might be induced to improve performance. Here are some of the essential elements, according to Richard Gordin, Ed.D., professor of health, education and recreation at Utah State University in Logan.

- Wanting to perform. The motivation could be anything—demonstrating excellence or power, securing your place in the culture of a certain sport, achieving mastery of a skill. Whatever it is, you have to want to be there.
- Feeling good beforehand. You need to look forward to what you're doing, or at least feel

comfortable playing the part. Feeling well-prepared and highly fit is one way. Indulging in the clothing, paraphernalia and gear associated with your sport may be another.

- Having a plan. We have already told you plenty about the importance of specific goals. Here it is again.
- Enjoying the environment. Location, location, location. You have to enjoy or be comfortable in your surroundings. If you feel out of place in a gym full of bodybuilders, or you ride your bike where you fear being struck by a car, or you jog where you might get mugged, flow gets dammed.
- Focusing. Flow is a kind of engrossment that comes from enjoyment. Thoughts beyond what you're doing at the moment must be pushed from your mind.

When lifting, focus on what you're doing. Keep conversation limited to what's pertinent to your workout. If someone strikes up a conversation, tell him you'll be happy to talk later—after you're finished with the business at hand.

Sticking with an Exercise Program

When Baltimore Orioles shortstop Cal Ripkin broke Lou Gehrig's phenomenal record for straight games played, he was characteristically modest. All he did, he explained, was show up all the time.

Strictly speaking, that's all it takes for you to get into peak condition as well. Keep showing up at the gym, keep running or biking or rowing or jumping rope or whatever it is you do. Sounds easy. But Cal knows, and you know, that just showing up takes a discipline and mental fortitude all its own. It's perhaps the most important part of mental conditioning because without the work there is no reward.

We've covered some of the essential ways to bolster your commitment in previous chapters, such as Setting Goals on page 6 and Getting Started on page 19. A brief review from our experts:

- Have fun. Who wants to do something he hates? Only a guy who's getting paid for it, which you're not. "Exercise should feel like an avocation, not a vocation," Dr. Sachs says.
- Mix it up. Take different routes, use different weight stations, learn new sports. Barring a Zen-like affection for repetition, variety is crucial to continued interest.

- Seek approval. The odds are stacked against you if your family or friends aren't supporting your efforts. If their support is too passive, enlist some help by, say, having a friend regularly inquire about your progress: In a six-week study of walkers, those who got calls about their program every week stuck with their programs at a rate 17 times greater than those who received no calls.
- Get advice. Remember the importance of realistic goals? A trainer or coach will keep grandiose ambitions in check and help ensure you don't sandbag yourself with an injury.

Beyond these guidelines, there are a number of other mental tricks for keeping up your motivation, inspiration and perspiration.

Lay your money down. A study at Michigan State University in East Lansing found that people who bet $40 that they could stick with their program had a 97 percent success rate, while less than 20 percent of exercisers who didn't make a bet were able to stick with their routines.

Remember the big picture. Short-term goals are most effective at keeping you active from day to day, but long-term objectives are important, too. "When you meet your short-term goals, there needs to be something else moving you forward," Dr. Robison says. Examples:

- When I retire, I want to be fit enough to hike in the mountains.
- I'm not going to have a heart attack at age 50 like my dad.

- Exercise makes me confident and gives me energy. I'm not going to let anything take that away from me.

Get technical. The more you know about exercise and the equipment that goes along with it, the more confident you'll be, says Dr. Gordin. Visit stores and look at cool gear, even if you're not buying. Read magazines. Talk to people. Do anything that makes you feel less like a rank amateur and more like an old pro.

Don't obsess. When you're tyrannized by your exercise goals, you don't find meeting them any fun. If you feel compelled to beat or match your previous time every day you run, fine. But if you want to stop to pet a dog or talk to a neighbor, that's fine, too. "Most people hear a coach in their heads," says James Gavin, Ph.D., professor in the Department of Applied Social Science at Concordia University in Montreal and author of *The Exercise Habit*. Feel free to shut the coach up every now and then.

Fight disillusionment. About three weeks into an exercise program, men often find themselves saying, "Who am I kidding?" It's the toxic by-product of a noxious stew of thoughts that arise from loss of initial excitement, creeping feelings of inadequacy around fitter men and the discouragement of not having an Adonis-like body after nine workouts. "Men often feel like outsiders who haven't earned their stripes," Dr. Gavin says. You need faith that things will get easier as you get fitter. Studies find that how you feel in the gym is influenced by how much work you've done there. One group of researchers found that highly active people feel exercise is easier than sedentary people do, even when both work at 60 to 90 percent of their maximum capacity. With ease comes confidence and satisfaction.

Isn't that what it's about: confidence and satisfaction? Those are the marks of a champion, even among the nonelite. As Dr. Loehr says, "Everyone should think of themselves as an athlete."

Peak Technique

Walk into any gym, and you'll find guys who don't know what they're doing. This, at least, is the impression of Barney Groves, Ph.D., who would know. He is associate professor of physical education at Virginia Commonwealth University in Richmond, has taught weight training for more than 30 years and is still active in competition. "I like coaching or teaching people who are walking into the weight room for the first time," he says. "Regular lifters usually have bad habits I have to break them of first."

He's talking about matters of form and technique, the art of executing exercises properly. Practicing proper technique is important with weight lifting as well as with every form of exercise, for two reasons. First, it reduces your risk of injury by placing stress only on muscles, bones and tendons that can take the punishment. Second, it cuts down on inefficient movement that can undermine your strength gains, reduce your endurance or slow your speed.

Rules for Resistance

One of the most important elements of resistance training is its ability to target specific muscles—which isn't going to do you much good if those muscles are targeted poorly. Throughout this book and in The Core Routine on page 121, we offer pointers and correct common errors of form on the most basic weight-lifting exercises. No matter what you're lifting, though, there are three principles you should follow, says Dr. Groves.

Don't lock up the joint. Locking elbows or knees during pushing movements such as shoulder presses and leg presses takes some of the weight off muscles and puts it on bones. That gives muscles a rest, which reduces the stress necessary for maximum results. Beyond that, the bone-against-bone contact may irritate or damage the joint, especially if it locks abruptly. Always keep movement slow and controlled. If your joints tend to hyperextend (bend beyond a straight line), be especially careful not to lock out.

Control your breathing. Ever notice how some guys tighten their lips, hold their breath and make veins pop out of their faces while they lift? Don't do it. Lack of oxygen during exertion can make you black out. As a rule, breathe out when lifting a weight and breathe in when returning to your starting position. If you feel that the internal pressure of holding your breath helps you through your lift, hold briefly through the hardest part of the repetition, then exhale.

Get a grip. Correct grip technique is important in resistance training. Your thumb should wrap around the bar; it should never be on the same side of the bar as your fingers. (See "Proper Grip Technique.")

Aerobic Retraining

We know what you're thinking: Of course I have to be careful about proper technique when lifting bars of solid iron over my head. But I've been running, riding a bike and climbing stairs for, oh, a few centuries now. Is there really anything more I need to learn about these?

Think of it this way: You learned how to read, write and do arithmetic a long time ago. Then along came books on tape, word processors, calculators. Technology created a new wrinkle on old skills, and you had to adapt to make the most of it.

So it is with the exercise equipment we often use to mimic common aerobic activities—treadmills, stationary bicycles, stair-climbers, rowing machines. Technology has given us a way to exercise without getting wet, stepping in dog poop or getting thrown by a pothole.

Again, this book is filled with tips on proper technique, so if you turn to the Bicycling or Running chapters, for example, you'll learn the winning form for each of those pursuits. But to make the most of the indoor machine equivalents, you have to learn how to use them first. And just as you spent a few frustrating hours learning to use your new computer so you could balance your checkbook or print your résumé, so you have to learn the subtle nuances of working out on exercise machines. The following, then, is a review of what experts observe to be common errors in exercise-machine use.

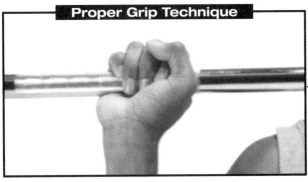

Proper Grip Technique

Correct: Thumb wraps around bar

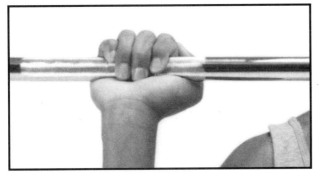

Incorrect: Thumb on same side of bar as fingers

◄ **Proper Grip Technique**

Get a grip. Grab a bar by wrapping your thumb on one side and your fingers on the other, the way you might hold a beer can. This will provide stability and control, unlike "the death grip," as Dr. Groves calls it, in which thumb and fingers are both placed on one side of the bar. "It's very dangerous because if the bar slips, it will fall," he says. Also make sure your hands are evenly spaced on the bar, so that weights are balanced and muscle-stress is evenly distributed.

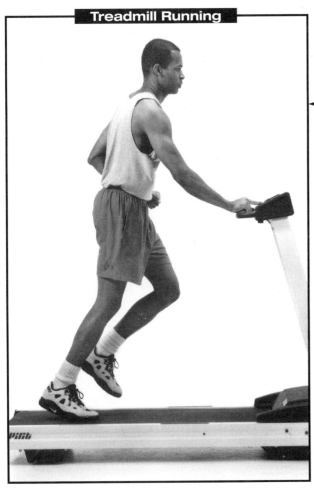

Treadmill Running

◄ **Treadmill Running**

Look straight ahead. Unlike solid ground, which is all around you when you run, a treadmill is relatively narrow. "I tell people not to look to the left or right when they're on a treadmill," says Budd Coates, marathon runner, trainer, exercise physiologist and special consultant to Runner's World magazine. "You'll start to drift in whatever direction you're looking. Outside, that's fine. Indoors, you could run right off the treadmill and take a spill."

Know your place. While you run, your speed and tempo are bound to alter slightly. "That's a problem on treadmills. Slow down a little, and you could fall off the back. Go a little too fast, and you could catch your foot on the front of the treadmill belt," says Coates. Make a mental note to check your positioning every so often. "Just reach out occasionally to touch the front panel of the treadmill," says Coates. "If you can barely touch it, you're drifting too far back. If your hand is brushing against the panel while you run, then you're too close."

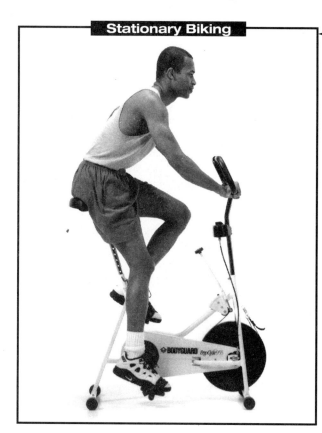

Stationary Biking

◄ **Stationary Biking**

Set the seat. It's a common mistake to hop on an exercise bike and just start pedaling at whatever height the seat is already set. But it's worth taking the three seconds required to custom-adjust your seat, says Michael Schreiber, D.O., staff physician at HealthFitness America at The Sports Club/L.A. in Los Angeles. Proper seat height gives you a more efficient stroke. Further, consistently keeping the saddle too low can put pressure on the knee, which can cause irritation, swelling and pain. When your seat is properly positioned, your knee should be only slightly bent at the bottom of your stroke.

Get straight. Maybe it's boredom, maybe it's tiredness, maybe it's a desire to get a better view of the aerobics class, but something usually compels us to lean over on the bike, rounding our back and shoulders and resting our arms on the bar or display board. It may seem like a more relaxed position, but it's not: "I see a lot of problems from the stress this position places on the lower back and neck, especially in people who are also raising their heads to watch TV," says Dr. Schreiber. Ride in an upright position with your head in line with your spine, or, if your bike offers the option of double or adjustable handlebars, lean straight from the hips when grasping the lower position.

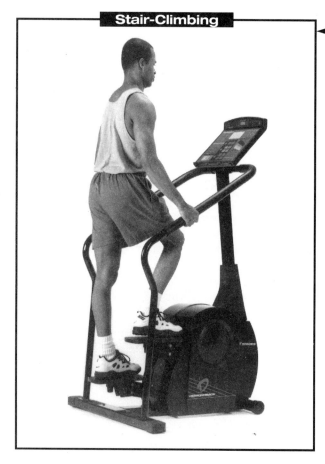

Stair-Climbing

◄ **Stair-Climbing**

Go deep. A lot of people take shallow, mincing steps on stair-climbers, thinking the speed of their movements makes them work harder, but think about it: Is this the way you'd climb a real set of stairs? In a study comparing two different rates of climb, researchers at Illinois State University in Normal found that taking deep, slower steps burns 5 percent more energy than taking shallow, fast ones. Longer steps work larger muscle groups, make the heart beat faster and spur delivery of more blood and oxygen. The ideal step depth? About the same as you'll find on your front porch: eight to ten inches.

Stay off your toes. There's room for your whole foot on the pedal, so take advantage of it: One survey of 212 stair-climber users in seven fitness clubs found that 39 percent experienced tingling in their feet. It's a common problem that comes from stepping with the toes, which puts pressure on the nerves in the ball of the feet. Be sure to keep your feet flat on the pedals and wear shoes with shock-absorbent soles; try loosening the laces to increase blood circulation.

Don't lean. Bending over creates the same kinds of problems on stair-climbers as it does on stationary cycles, says Dr. Schreiber: pain or stiffness in the lower back and neck. Even if you're imagining yourself climbing the bell tower at Notre Dame, you're not Quasimodo: Keep an upright stance on the stairs.

Rowing

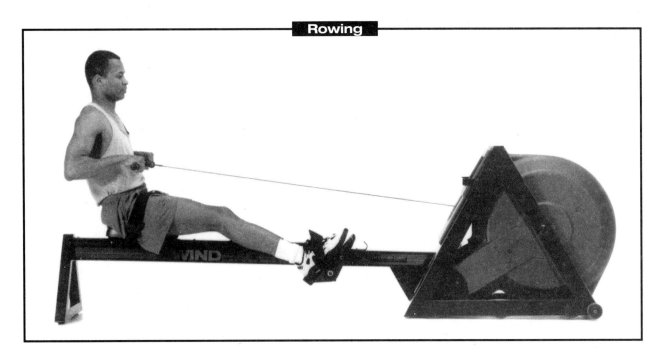

Rowing ▲

Back off. A lot of men throw too much of their back into rowing—and therefore too little of their arms and legs, which are the parts a rower is designed to work. If you drive rearward with your back first, you also leave yourself vulnerable to muscle strain. One clue that you're doing it wrong: You've pulled the cable back, but your arms are still extended in front of you. Proper form entails a fairly precise sequence of movements, says Dr. Schreiber. With your upper body pitched slightly forward, push back with your legs first. Then lean slightly back and pull the handle toward your gut with your arms. As you return to the starting position, extend your arms, bend your legs and lean slightly forward again.

Part Three
Achieving a Peak Body

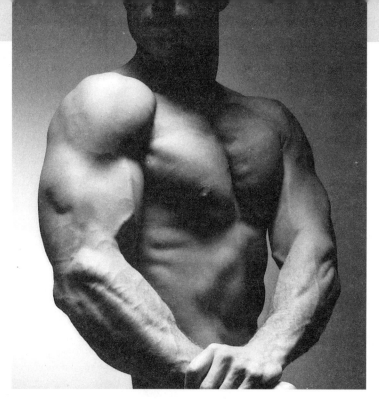

Arms

We need strong arms for any number of physical and psychological reasons. In terms of health, being well-armed can save you from the kind of back pain that so often plagues men later in life, simply by virtue of the fact that, the more lifting your arms do, the less your back will have to deal with. Arms also serve as the strongmen that back up your hands, powering your grip while putting thrust behind a well-aimed throw or blow.

Plus, big arms are a great accessory of manhood, helpful when you want to see how you measure up to another guy. There aren't a lot of appendages you can expose in public to make that comparison, but you can always roll up your sleeves.

Arms and the Man

"Next to the chest, the arms are about the single biggest area of the body where guys want big muscles," says Jeffrey Stout, Ph.D., assistant professor of exercise physiology at Creighton University in Omaha, Nebraska.

And no wonder. Few muscles are nicer to flex, for example, than the biceps, those great cannonball muscles on top of your arms, just above the elbow. Biceps allow you to bend your arm, not only so you can actually make a muscle for your girlfriend, but also so you can cock your arm for a throw or pull your weight in a tug-of-war match.

While the biceps are the high-profile muscles on the arms, they'd be pretty useless without the triceps, which run beneath the biceps and make up about 60 percent of the muscles in your arms. If you were to flex to show off your bulging biceps, and you didn't have triceps, you'd be stuck in that position. "The triceps are what allow you to extend your elbow joints; they're just the opposite of the biceps," says Edmund Connors, a certified strength and conditioning specialist in Hingham, Massachusetts. The triceps enable you to extend a hand in greeting, throw that winning touchdown pass or keep danger at arm's length.

Meanwhile, those of us who grew up watching Popeye can appreciate the value of powerful forearms. Since these muscles provide essential grip strength, keeping them well-toned is what makes us strong to the finish in any sport involving our arms, which is most of them (see Hands and Forearms on page 58).

Winning the Arms Race

The problem is that the arm muscles are deceptively hard to develop. You might work your arms out every other day at the start and, noticing that they quickly look better and feel stronger, think, "Hey, my arms are getting bigger." But Dr. Stout says what you're looking at isn't muscle growth, but a quick adaptation by your arms that gives them a toned appearance. "Toning is certainly better than nothing. But once you get up to a basic level of tone, most guys plateau. It can take a long time to stimulate the muscles to where you start to notice a significant increase in muscle size," he says.

Unless, of course, you take some shortcuts, the kind that bodybuilders and professional athletes use to build powerful arm muscles safely and efficiently. Here are some tips to help you, next time you heed the call to arms.

Make your arms last. As a general rule of thumb, save your serious arm workouts for the end of your weight-lifting routine. "You use your arms for a lot of exercises, especially back, chest and shoulder exercises," says Dr. Stout. "If you work your arms first, they'll be worn out when it's time to work these other muscle groups.

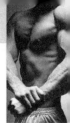

You'll end up cheating yourself."

Avoid a biceps bias. As nice as they might look, bulging biceps alone do not a strong arm make. "Try not to focus too much on the biceps," says Connors. "You need to work them, but not to the point where you have no time to work the triceps, which is what a lot of guys tend to do." If you don't work out these muscles in equal measure, you'll actually end up weakening your arm. "If the biceps are much stronger than the triceps, you'll create a muscle imbalance that could cause a tear or other injury when you're in the middle of heavy activity involving those muscles," warns Dr. Stout. For every biceps exercise you do, try to do at least one set of a triceps exercise.

Don't fret your forearms. Forearms are certainly an important part of your arm strength, the vital link in channeling upper arm power to both your hands and whatever sporting implement you're using. Forearms also have major muscular responsibilities in their own right—they're the secret to a great grip, and they also help you pilot and aim whatever you're throwing or swinging.

But their location on the arm also gives them a distinct workout advantage. "They get a workout from virtually every exercise involving your arms," says Dr. Stout. You also work them during chest exercises and shoulder exercises where you're gripping a bar. Even when you're on a circuit machine like a leg press, you're working your forearms because you're gripping the handles on either side of the machine.

"So I wouldn't sweat doing specific exercises for them," says Dr. Stout. "They get a great workout, and the more your upper-arm strength increases, the greater the load they'll be required to help hold, so they get stronger along with your upper arms." (For you diehards who want specific forearm exercises to improve your grip, see Hands and Forearms on page 58.)

Don't alternate—isolate. For more advanced lifters, there's a technique to assure that the arms are getting worked to their maximum, called isolation exercises. The idea is to work individual muscles until they are completely fatigued. Doing alternating exercises like dumbbell curls can work the arms individually, but there's a better way, and you'll need one hand free of weights to do it.

As Dr. Stout explains, the trick is to work the muscles in each arm until they can't do any more lifts on their own, then use your free arm to help the fatigued limb do just two or three extra lifts. These are called forced reps, and they're the secret to arming yourself with more bulk and muscle. By doing the forced reps, you're pushing the arm to total exhaustion, then pushing it one step further. "It's during those forced reps that the muscle really stretches, and that's what will stimulate it to grow," explains Dr. Stout.

Use some strong-arm tactics. It's a fact of life that one of your arms tends to be stronger than the other. That's another important reason for exercising one arm at a time with dumbbells. "If you work them together, the weaker arm tends to cheat by letting the stronger arm do more work," says Connors.

When you isolate, be sure to make your stronger arm work to its individual limit. "Make sure it does more reps than the weaker arm. If the weaker arm can do 15 reps, you know the stronger arm can do at least one more rep, so do it," says Dr. Stout.

Peak Points

When you're doing arm exercises, keep the following points firmly in mind. Use them as a mental checklist; recite them like a mantra in your head. If you can follow these simple rules, you'll go a long way toward eliminating your chance of injury and maximizing your muscle-building.

Don't rock the boat. You may be a swinger in all other aspects of your life, but avoid this kind of motion with any arm exercises you do. "If you swing or rock the weight while you're lifting, you're cheating, because momentum is doing the work, not your muscles," says Edmund Connors, a certified strength and conditioning specialist in Hingham, Massachusetts. In addition, the more you let momentum handle the load, the less control you have over the weight, and the more likely you'll be to drop the thing on your toe.

Give your arms the cold shoulder. With any lifts that work the biceps or triceps, your shoulder muscles are bound to feel the urge to step in and lend a hand. Resist the urge. "If you try to get other muscles involved, you're going to expose yourself to all sorts of problems, such as tendinitis or overuse injuries in the shoulders," says Jeffrey Stout, Ph.D., assistant professor of exercise physiology at Creighton University in Omaha, Nebraska. If the weight is just too much for your arm muscles to lift by themselves, swallow that pride and start with a smaller weight.

Back out of it. For the same reasons, don't send a back in to do an arm's job, warns Dr. Stout. One of the reasons you want stronger arms is to help keep your back from doing any heavy lifting; don't sabotage your efforts by using your back muscles to help in an arm exercise. That is a perfect set-up for back injury.

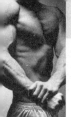

Biceps

Barbell Curls ►

"This is the basic lift everyone knows," says Connors, but it's absolutely essential for crafting cannonball biceps.

Stand, and grab the barbell so your palms are facing up; your hands should be about shoulder-width apart. In the starting position, your arms should be extended, so the barbell will be at about thigh-level.

Now, with your back straight and your elbows close to your sides, lift the barbell, curling it up toward your collarbone. Lower the barbell back to the starting position—that's one rep. Keep your wrists straight and do the curl slowly; if you move too fast, your body will start rocking, and momentum will be doing all the work. That's cheating.

Barbell Curls

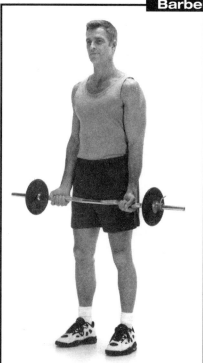
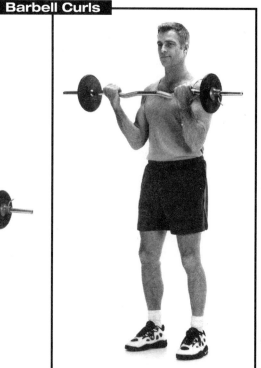

Preacher Curls

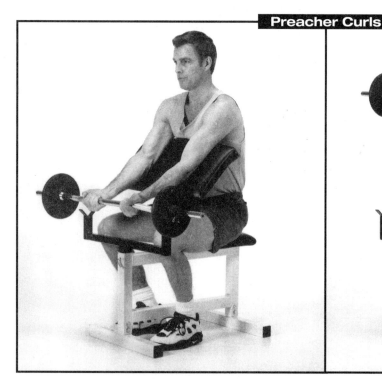
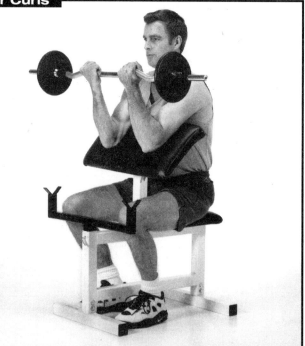

Preacher Curls ▲

As arm exercises go, the so-called preacher curl is a tough one since it isolates your arms for some serious lifting and makes it nearly impossible for you to cheat by letting your shoulder or back muscles help with the lifting.

To do it, you need to use a preacher bend platform—an accessory found on some weight benches. Put your arms over the platform (the platform should be up under your armpits). Hold the barbell with your palms facing upward, hands about shoulder-width apart.

Now raise the barbell toward your chin. Don't raise your elbows, and keep your wrists locked.

Dr. Stout recommends starting out with lighter weights than you'd normally use during a regular curl. "This is a tough exercise—you don't want to overdo it," he says.

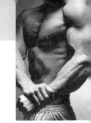

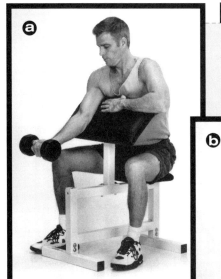

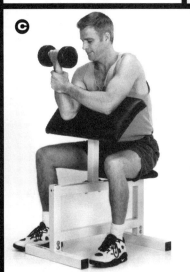

Ultimate Peak

When the usual curls and kickbacks just don't cut it for you anymore, it's time to call the preacher.

The chapter describes the preacher curl, which uses a barbell and a preacher bench to isolate the biceps muscles. Even tougher, however, is the one-arm preacher dumbbell curl, particularly when you use your free hand to work your exercising arm to exhaustion.

◄ One-Arm Preacher Dumbbell Curls

ⓐ Position yourself on a preacher bench and hold a dumbbell in your right hand, with your upper arm flat against the slanted pad. Grip the dumbbell so your palm is facing up.

ⓑ Now, with your wrist straight, slowly curl the dumbbell up toward your chin. As you do this, keep your elbow against the bench, eyes forward and feet firmly planted on the ground. Lower and repeat.

ⓒ Select a weight that will thoroughly fatigue your arm in 8 to 12 repetitions, suggests Jeffrey Stout, Ph.D., assistant professor of exercise physiology at Creighton University in Omaha, Nebraska. Then immediately force yourself to do 2 more reps. It is these extra reps that stimulate muscle growth. Take your left hand and use it to support your right wrist as you force yourself to do 2 more reps. "As long as your free hand acts as a spotter, you'll contract and stretch the muscles safely and slowly, without injuring them," says Dr. Stout.

Hammer Curls ►

Sit at the end of your bench, knees bent, feet shoulder-width apart. Hold the dumbbells so your palms are facing your body.

Curl the weight up toward your shoulder—as though it were a hammer you were lifting in order to drive a nail. Don't rotate your wrists. Keep your shoulders back and your back straight. You can alternate this exercise—first curling with your right hand, then your left.

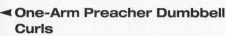

Hammer Curls

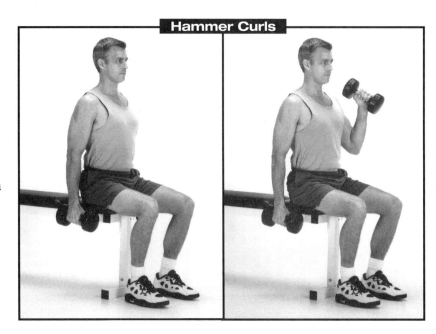

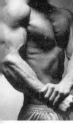

Concentration Curls ►

Sitting at the end of your bench with your feet shoulder-width apart, lean forward and put your right arm between your legs. Your elbow and upper arm should be resting against your thigh. Keep your free hand on your other knee. Extend your arm, holding a dumbbell with your palm facing up.

Slowly lift the dumbbell to your shoulder. Brace your elbow against your thigh and lean on your free hand if you need support.

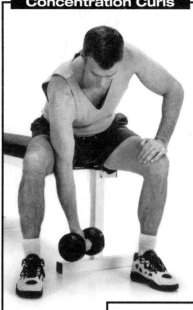

Concentration Curls

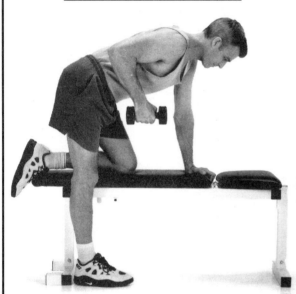

Dumbbell Kickbacks

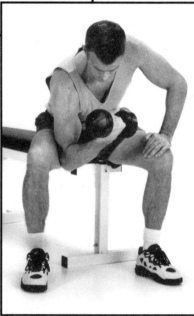

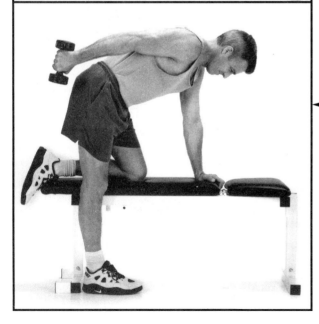

Triceps

◄ Dumbbell Kickbacks

To work your triceps, hold a dumbbell in your right hand, palm facing your body. Rest your left knee and hand on a weight bench, then raise the dumbbell up toward your chest. Your elbow should be pointing toward the ceiling; your back should be straight. This is only the starting position, pal. Now it's time for the real exercise.

Straighten your arm out behind you, extending the weight away from your body. Keep extending until you feel your triceps fully contract, then bend your arm and return the weight to your side.

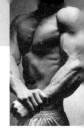

Seated Triceps Press

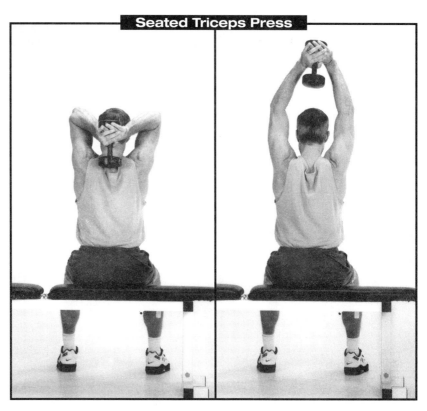

Seated Triceps Press ►

Sitting on a weight bench, position a dumbbell behind your head. Interlace your fingers to hold the dumbbell at one end, underneath the weight.

Now extend your arms and push the dumbbell straight up. Keep your back straight, and lift slowly—you don't want to drop the weight on your head. Then bend your arms to lower the weight. Keep your arms bent near your head, elbows pointing up.

Overhead Triceps Extensions

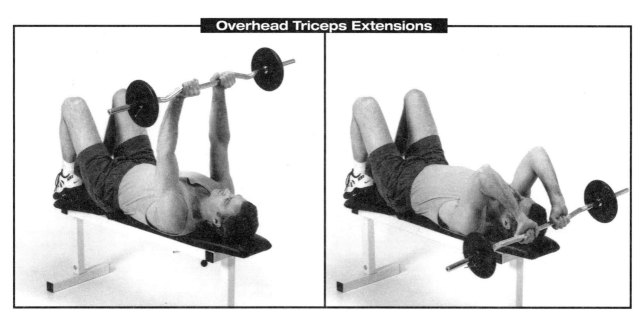

Overhead Triceps Extensions ▲

Get on your back on the weight bench. Make sure your back is in full contact with the bench. If your lower back arches when your feet are on the floor, pull your feet up to the end of the bench. Hold a barbell above your chest, arms extended. Your hands should be only four to six inches apart, palms facing away from you.

Now slowly lower the weight toward the top of your head, bending your arms at the elbows. Extend your arms back out to the starting position.

FACT The largest biceps in the world were flexed by Denis Sester of Bloomington, Minnesota. His right biceps measured 30¾ inches.

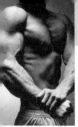

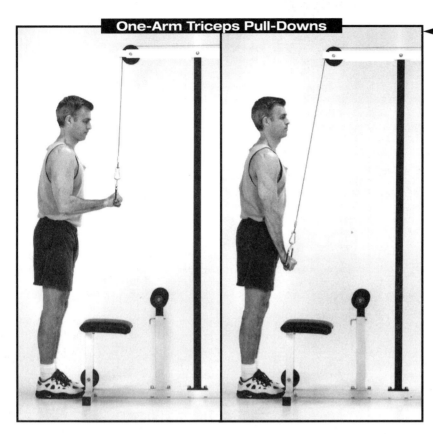

One-Arm Triceps Pull-Downs

◀ **One-Arm Triceps Pull-Downs**

If you're working out at a health club, try this on the triceps pull-down machine.

Stand facing the machine, gripping the middle of the handle with your right hand, palm facing away from you. Keep your arm bent, elbow close at your side.

Now pull down on the bar and straighten out your arm. Keep your elbow close to your body, wrist locked and straight. As with the other one-armed exercises, once you've exhausted your arm, you can make it do a couple of extra forced reps by using your left hand to help complete the reps. Then switch arms.

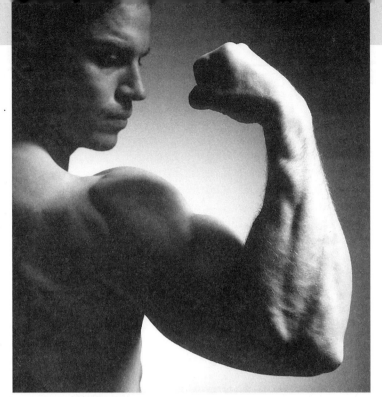

Arm Joints

If you've ever twisted your elbow, sprained your wrist or jammed your finger, you've learned the hard way just how important your arm joints are. The arms may be the tools of industry in our life, but the arm joints are the infrastructure without which nothing gets done.

To understand why joints get injured, it helps to know some anatomy basics. A *joint* is where two or more bones come together. *Ligaments* are strong, rubbery strands that connect one bone to another. *Tendons* are strands that usually connect muscles to bones. *Bursae* are tiny sacs of liquid that help keep ligaments and tendons from rubbing against each other or against bone and prevent excess wear.

Picturing that, it's pretty simple to understand joint injuries. Mostly, they're muscles, tendons or ligaments tearing or straining, leaving you with a muscle pull or an outright sprain. In minor cases, you'll have a hot, achy feeling and limited motion, but in a few weeks it will heal on its own. A larger injury—like a major rip—can mean a lifetime of limited motion. It is the stuff of ruined sports careers.

Obviously, you don't want this to happen to you. The answer? First and foremost, you need to take steps to strengthen and stretch your key tendons and ligaments. Here's the program.

Fixing Fingers, Elbows and Wrists

All of your arm joints—from your elbow to the last joint on your little finger—are tough to protect but easy to ruin. Keeping them safe involves a two-tier exercise approach. You do need to build the surrounding muscle, but at the same time you have to be working the joints through range-of-motion exercises—lightweight routines that get the joint used to the activity it will be performing. We're not talking about weight lifting here. Strengthening your joints is a different animal entirely from strengthening your arm muscles. With the few exceptions listed below, arm-joint exercises should be done with very light weights and high reps (12 to 20). Here are some key ways to make your joint ventures go smoothly, from the elbow down.

Keep arm strength balanced. "If you don't spend some time pre-training the elbow—making sure the muscles on all sides of it are strong, you can end up getting all sorts of problems, such as tennis elbow or golfer's elbow," says Dan Hamner, M.D., director of sports medicine and rehabilitation for the New York State Athletic Association and visiting professor of rehabilitation at New York Hospital in New York City. As Dr. Hamner explains, both of these elbow ailments are a result of overused and undertrained muscles and tendons. Microtears in the weak point of a tendon, where it attaches to muscle or bone, cause inflammation and pain.

If you're not doing so already, spend some time working on your triceps, biceps and forearms. Basic biceps curls and triceps extensions ought to be enough to keep the muscles around your elbow strong and protected. "Just be sure to pay attention to each muscle in equal measure," says Jeffrey Stout, Ph.D., assistant professor of exercise physiology at Creighton University in Omaha, Nebraska.

"Too many men focus on one exercise—biceps curls, for example—and don't spend any time working the triceps or the forearms," says Dr. Stout. That's just asking for an elbow injury, because you're creating a strength imbalance between the muscles, which can weaken the joint. Strive for balance in your workout and you won't elbow yourself out of the game. Keep these joint-friendly tips in mind, too.

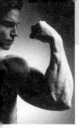

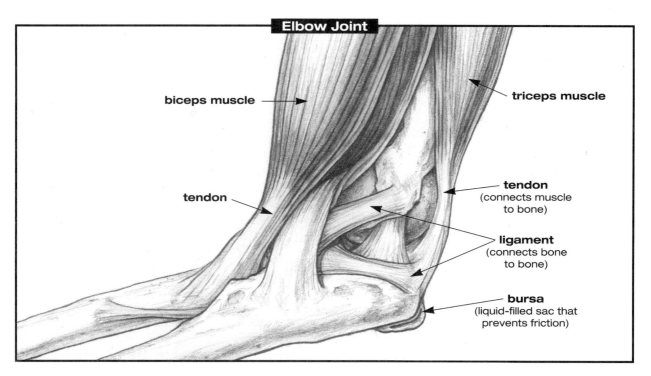

Elbow Joint

biceps muscle

triceps muscle

tendon

tendon
(connects muscle
to bone)

ligament
(connects bone
to bone)

bursa
(liquid-filled sac that
prevents friction)

Roll with the blow. Don't stick your arm out. Learn how to fall. "If you're cycling or skating, or playing any game where you're likely to get knocked down, you can train yourself out of the old instinct of sticking your arm straight out to break your fall," says Dr. Hamner. Good idea—breaking your fall that way has caused countless elbow and wrist injuries.

Instead, Dr. Hamner suggests doing somersaults and tumble drills. "Professional cyclists do this a lot: When you go down, instead of sticking your arm out, you tuck your chin into your chest and as you go down, roll over your shoulder. That distributes the impact and minimizes your chance of injury," says Dr. Hamner.

Don't lock yourself out. When you're lifting weights, it's only too tempting to lock your elbows at the apex of the lift, offering your muscles a brief rest. But it's a rest you're enjoying at the expense of your elbows. They're not designed like a deck chair—built to unfold, lock out and bear heavy weights.

"When you're doing an exercise, lift the weight just until your arms are almost fully extended, then hold it there, with your elbows unlocked, before you bring the weight back," says Dr. Hamner. Not only are you sparing your elbows weight they weren't meant to carry but you're also giving your muscles an even tougher workout—which was what you were trying to do when you picked up that weight in the first place.

Get a grip. The wrist is the key to our manual dexterity: It gives us snapping power when we swing a racquet or bat, and it helps us to fulfill the manly function of opening tightly sealed lids and faucets.

The secret to keeping your wrists strong, though, lies not in the wrist, but in the hands and forearms. "You can strengthen them—and protect your wrist—by doing basic grip exercises," says Todd Ellenbecker, P.T., clinical director of Physiotherapy Associates Scottsdale Sports Clinic in Arizona and a member of the U.S. Tennis Association's Sports Science Committee. Use spring-loaded devices, putty or even a tennis ball—try to do at least 10 to 20 squeezes with each hand every day.

Jam it? Tape it. Jammed fingers are among the most common of joint injuries, usually occurring when the bones of an individual finger smash into one another, causing swelling in the joints.

"If you jam a finger, the best thing you can do is to try to keep the joint stabilized by taping it with medical adhesive tape—just wrap it around the jammed finger or knuckle," says Dr. Hamner. Not only does this stabilize the joint but the tape can decrease swelling. Just be careful not to wrap your finger too tightly. If it swells excessively or becomes numb, loosen the tape.

Note: If your finger swells excessively, turns blue and can't be bent without sharp, excruciating pain, chances are that's not a jam—that's a break. Get to a doctor to check alignment, suggests Dr. Hamner.

Pull your finger. Another quick anti-jamming device is to grab the injured finger between your thumb and index finger, then pull gently on it for five seconds, says Dr. Hamner. Rest five seconds, then pull again. This stretches any tissue that was compressed during the injury and helps pull the joint into better alignment.

Elbows

Elbow Stretches

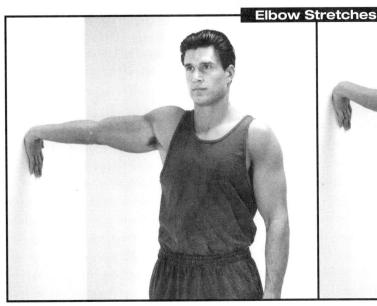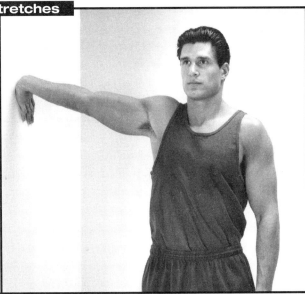

Elbow Stretches ⋀

Is your elbow getting sore after nine holes of golf or a quick tennis match? Try this stretch before, during and after.

Stand next to a wall. Extend your arm straight out to the side so your hand touches the wall. Place your palm flat against the wall, fingers pointing down.

Keep your palm pressed to the wall and slowly raise your arm up until you feel a stretch in the forearm. To work the muscles on the outside of the elbow, turn your hand around so the back of your hand is pressed gently against the wall. Now raise your arm up until you feel a stretch in the forearm.

Double-Jointed or Double Jeopardy?

They were the schoolyard freaks, and we loved them: the boy who could bend his thumb forward to touch his wrist, the guy who could bend his knees the other way and strut like a chicken, the kid who could cross his legs behind his head and walk on his hands.

"Cool!" we gushed, and we tried to imitate them. We grunted and strained and tried to contort our bodies, but it was no use. Either you were born double-jointed or you weren't.

Maybe you should be glad you weren't.

Actually, there is no such thing as being double-jointed. The clinical term is joint hypermobility. "That means the joints, and the connective tissue around them, are much looser than normal, giving you an unbelievable range of motion," says John Baum, M.D., professor emeritus at the University of Rochester School of Medicine and Dentistry in New York and a researcher into the phenomenon of joint hypermobility.

As Dr. Baum explains, although hypermobility can be a side effect of serious joint-related diseases, in most cases it's something you outgrow. "Some kids will start out with very loose joints, but they usually tighten up as they get older," he says. Chances are the kid who could cross his legs behind his head would dislocate a hip if he tried it today.

However, if you are one of the few men who carries hypermobility into adulthood, Dr. Baum warns that you need to be particular about your fitness and leisure pursuits. "Other men may envy you because you don't need to stretch as much or because you have incredible dexterity with a ball or racquet. And we've found that hypermobile people have distinct advantages in gymnastics and dancing. But if you have joint hypermobility and you play more rigorous sports, you actually need to work harder than the rest of us tight guys," says Dr. Baum.

Specifically, you have to do more weight training and range-of-motion exercises with light weights, focusing on the muscles that surround your loose joints. "If you don't and you get hit or injured in some way, your hypermobility becomes a liability. Without strong surrounding muscles to hold the joint in place, it could get severely damaged or ruined," he warns.

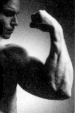

Wrists

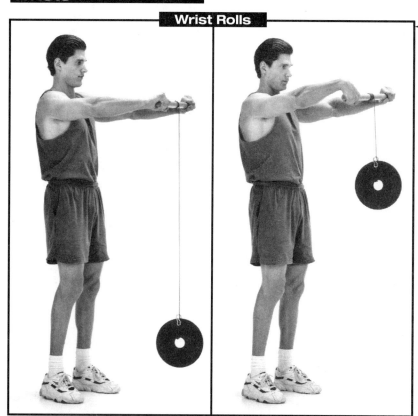

Wrist Rolls

◄ **Wrist Rolls**

A good wrist-protecting exercise is the wrist roll, Dr. Hamner says. You'll need a wrist roller, which you can find in most gyms—it's a short dowel or rod with a chain or cord attached in the middle. You attach a weight plate at the bottom of the chain. You could even make one yourself if you have a two-foot long dowel, a short length of chain and Olympic weight plates.

Stand upright, feet shoulder-width apart, holding the roller in both hands, palms down, with your arms extended in front of you. The weight should be dangling in front of you.

Now slowly roll the weight up with your wrists. Use long, exaggerated up-and-down movements with your wrists to get their full range of motion. Keep the rest of your body stationary—don't sway your body or drop your arms. When the weight has reached the top, slowly lower it using the same motion. Do 10 to 12 reps.

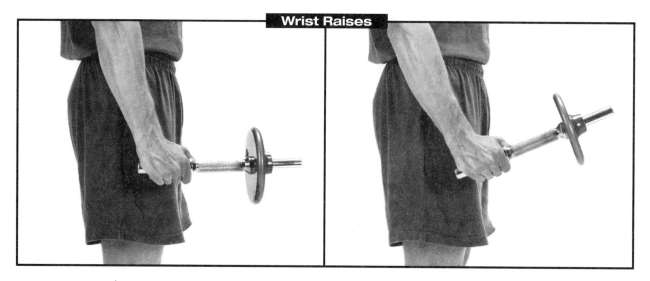

Wrist Raises

Wrist Raises ▲

Physical trainers call this lift radial deviation, since it's working the muscles and tendons around the radius bone of your forearm—all major supporters of your wrist. Ellenbecker says this exercise is a great toner and wrist trainer. He calls it a prehabilitation exercise—a routine that will keep the wrist from getting hurt when you *really* work it out.

Stand with your right arm at your side, grasping a hammer or a dumbbell with a weight on one end only—that weight should be in front of your hand. Hold the weight so your thumb is pointing straight ahead of you.

Slowly raise and lower the weight through a comfortable range of motion. Don't move your elbow or shoulder—all movement should occur at the wrist. Do 10 to 12 reps, then switch hands.

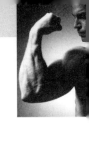

Reverse Wrist Raises

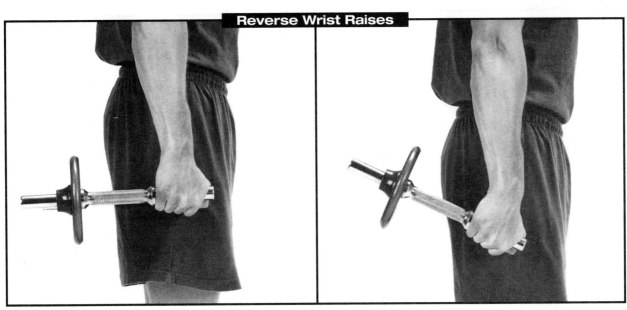

Reverse Wrist Raises ▲

Also known as ulnar deviation, this prehab exercise works the muscles and tendons around the ulna, the forearm bone right next to the radial bone. Therefore, it strengthens the other side of your wrist.

Stand with your right arm at your side, holding the same weight you used for the wrist raise—only now the weighted end should be behind your hand. Your thumb should still be pointing forward.

Now slowly raise and lower the weight, using only your wrist. Again, don't move your elbow or shoulder. Do 10 to 12 reps, then switch hands.

FACT It's okay to crack your knuckles—or any other joint for that matter. The cracking sound you hear is nothing more than fluid in your joints shifting and gas escaping. Don't worry: It won't cause arthritis.

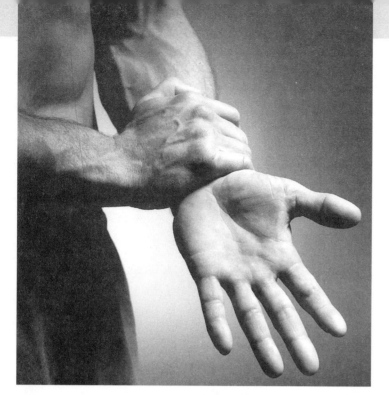

Hands and Forearms

On their own, hands don't have all that much strength. A man's hand is home to over two dozen bones and at least as many ligaments and joints, all balled up in a space not much bigger than a fist—that doesn't leave a lot of room for powerhouse muscle.

Not to worry. Although your hand muscles play a big role in grip strength, the true power behind a viselike grip comes from the wrists and forearms, according to Dan Hamner, M.D., director of sports medicine and rehabilitation for the New York State Athletic Association and visiting professor of rehabilitation at New York Hospital in New York City.

"You can certainly strengthen the hand muscles you use for gripping, but doing exercises that also work the forearms and the wrists are going to support and increase hand strength far better than if you tried to focus on your hands alone," says Dr. Hamner.

In fact, one of the fringe benefits of a regular weight-training regimen is that almost every exercise you do helps work your grip.

"All barbell and dumbbell lifts require you to keep a good grip on the weights—otherwise, you'll drop them on your foot," says Dr. Hamner. "And that in itself is a good grip-trainer. Plus, on many machines that work the legs, you often have handles to grab on to, so you can work your hand strength while you're working your legs. Each time you inhale, you can give a strong hand squeeze to the hand grips, and each time you exhale, focus on working your legs."

And it doesn't stop there. "Any sport where you're swinging a club or bat or racquet is going to be good for hand strength," according to Todd Ellenbecker, P.T., clinical director of Physiotherapy Associates Scottsdale Sports Clinic in Arizona and a member of the U.S. Tennis Association's Sports Science Committee. "And the more you play, the better your grip can get."

Still, there are worthwhile exercises you can do that focus on the hands. Some of these exercises—especially those involving the wrist—do more than bulk up your grip; they also protect your joints from harm. "Wrist rolls and similar wrist exercises, for example, are good ways to work your hand and forearm muscles while pretraining the joint to withstand injury," Ellenbecker says. Unless we specify otherwise, follow a toning regimen for hands—that is, do high reps (12 to 20) of low weights.

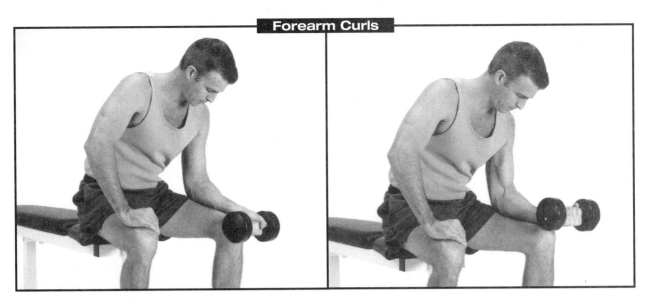

Forearm Curls

Forearm Curls ▲

Sit at the end of a bench with your legs slightly wider than hip-width apart. Your right hand should be on your right knee, and you should be holding a dumbbell in your left hand, with a palm-up grip. Your left wrist should be slightly over your left knee, so you can bend your wrist through its full range of motion. The top of your forearm should be resting against your thigh, and your upper body should be upright, but you may lean slightly into your left leg for comfort.

Curl the dumbbell up toward your body as far as you can. Don't let your arm rise up off your thigh. At the top of the curl, hold for a second, then lower to the starting position. Finish your reps, then switch hands.

You can also do this with both hands and a barbell.

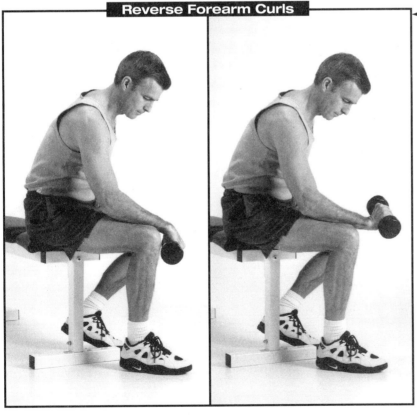

Reverse Forearm Curls

◄ Reverse Forearm Curls

Sit at the end of a bench with your legs slightly wider than hip-width apart. Put your left hand on your left knee. Hold a dumbbell in your right hand, palm down. Hold your wrist slightly over your knee, so you can bend your wrist through its full range of motion. Rest the bottom of your forearm against your thigh; hold your upper body fairly upright, but you can lean slightly into your right leg for comfort.

Curl the dumbbell up toward your body as far as you can. Don't let your arm rise up off your thigh. At the top of the curl, hold for a second, then lower to the starting position. Finish your reps, then switch hands.

Use a lighter weight for this lift than you would for a standard forearm curl. Also, you can modify this exercise using both hands and a barbell.

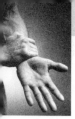

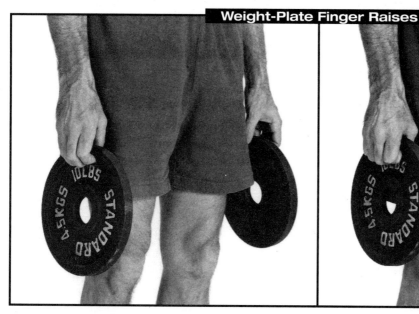
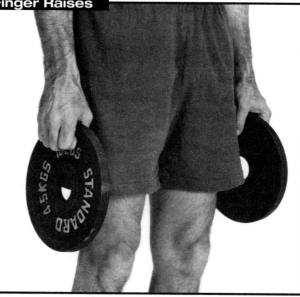

Weight-Plate Finger Raises

Weight-Plate Finger Raises ▲

This is an excellent grip-trainer and a killer workout for the forearm muscles that power your grip, according to Chip Harrison, strength and conditioning coach at Pennsylvania State University in State College.

Hold a 10-pound Olympic weight plate in each hand by grasping the raised edge of the plate with your fingers

with your thumb against the flat side of the plate. Stand straight, palms inward, arms by your sides. Straighten your fingers and lower the plate.

Now close the fingers, raising the plate as high as you can. As you get stronger, switch from 10-pound plates to 25 or even 45.

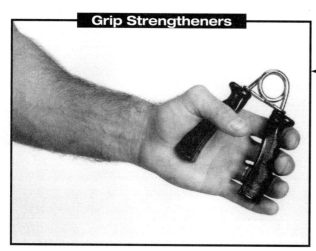

Grip Strengtheners

◄ Grip Strengtheners

For a classic hand workout, get yourself a spring-loaded gripper device that offers moderate resistance. Now squeeze it closed. Release and repeat. How's that for simple? Go for the most reps possible, then switch hands. The beauty of this exercise is that you can do it while watching television or talking on the phone—anywhere, anytime, for a fast, effective hand workout.

FACT People usually have about the same grip strength in both hands. But if they are active in one-sided sports, such as tennis or baseball, their dominant hand can have up to 22 pounds (ten kilograms) greater grip strength.

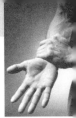

Man and Machine

The most common—and one of the most convenient—hand-strength trainer is the simple grip exercise, where you clench and unclench . . . something. The question is: What's the best tool to test your grip against? You don't necessarily have to use those old spring-loaded grippers. Here's a look at some of the new possibilities, from grippers to great goop.

• New grippers: Newer products like the Gripmaster allow you to work each finger individually, while forearm strengtheners like the Power Stik get the wrists and forearms into the workout.

• Balls: Squeezing a sphere can be just as effective as using a gripper, and may be cheaper, too.

While there are many excellent rubber exercise balls out there, you may find an old tennis ball works just as well for you, according to Todd Ellenbecker, P.T., clinical director of Physiotherapy Associates Scottsdale Sports Clinic in Arizona and a member of the U.S. Tennis Association's Sports Science Committee.

• Putty: Exercise putty allows you to customize a grip-strength tool that fits your hand precisely—and you can work all your fingers more easily. Our favorites include Power Putty (which comes in a fist-shaped container that looks cool on a desk) and Reflex, fluorescent-colored putty that makes for a colorful workout.

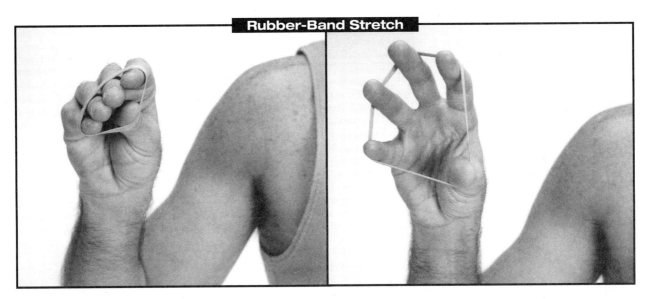

Rubber-Band Stretch

Rubber-Band Stretch ▲

In the midst of all your efforts to work your hands so they can clamp down harder and harder, don't forget to work the muscles that help you unclench your hands. They're called the antagonist muscles, and they run along the top of the hand, wrist and forearm. Probably the best way to work them is not with some exotic piece of exercise equipment, but with a simple rubber band.

Make your hand into a "C" shape and wrap the rub-

ber band around the ends of your fingers and thumb. When you relax your hand, the rubber band should pinch the hand closed (if it doesn't, find a stronger one or wrap the band around your fingers twice).

Now slowly force your hand open. You'll feel the muscles in the top of your hand doing their thing. Do about ten repetitions, then switch hands. When the rubber band breaks, get a stronger one.

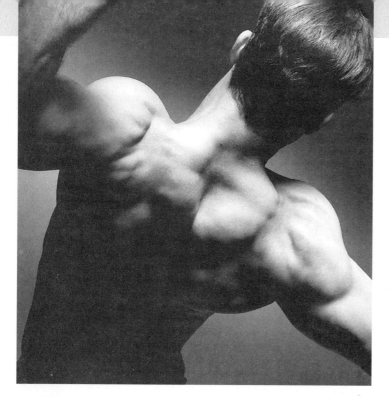

Shoulders and Neck

Shoulders aren't just a simple set of muscles; they're a complex bodily construction—an intricate collection of joints, bones, nerves and muscles that helps support and protect the upper back and neck. And while they're at it, they help to give your arms a wonderful range of motion.

The major players in your shoulder muscles are the trapezius and the deltoid. "When you raise or rotate your shoulders, you're using the trapezius," says Allen Kinley, assistant strength and conditioning coach at Texas A&M University in College Station. These muscles also keep your neck strong and well-supported. Your delts help your arms with lifting and pulling. At the same time, they cover your rotator cuff, a band of muscles and tendons that encapsulate the shoulder joints and are key to your mobility.

Getting the Bold Shoulder

As a complex juncture of joints and muscles, shoulders are a feat of biological engineering. Unfortunately, it is their complexity that makes them an easy mark for monkey wrenches of every stripe.

"You know how they say the more sophisticated a machine is, the more things there are that can go wrong with it? Well, that's partly true where shoulders and certain exercises are concerned," says Todd Ellenbecker, P.T., clinical director of Physiotherapy Associates Scottsdale Sports Clinic in Arizona. As Ellenbecker explains, many of the things we do can wrack the shoulders if we're not careful. Lifting objects overhead, pulling or pushing very heavy objects—these can injure shoulder muscles and joints if our shoulders aren't strong.

"That's where pre-training comes in," says Ellenbecker. "If you pre-train your shoulders—we call it prehabilitation—for weight-bearing workouts and sports, you're going to dramatically reduce your chance of injury," says Ellenbecker. Here are a couple of prehab exercises you can use to warm up before doing any lifting or work involving the shoulder. You don't even have to use weights. But if you do, make sure they're very light hand weights. The idea is to prepare the shoulder joints for activity, not overpower them with weights.

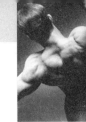

Side-Lying External Rotations

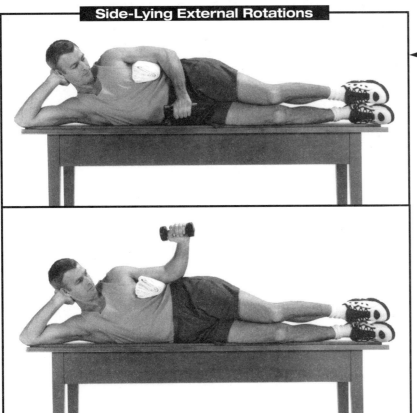

The Shoulder Joint

◄ **Side-Lying External Rotations**

This exercise helps tone and protect the rotator cuff.

Lie on your right side and prop your head up with your right arm. Place a small rolled up towel or pillow between your left arm and your body, halfway between your shoulder and elbow. Keep your left arm bent at 90 degrees—your left elbow should be close to your side. You can use either a light strap-on wrist weight or a light dumbbell.

Now raise your left arm slowly, until your hand is pointing straight up. Lower and repeat for 10 to 12 repetitions. Do three sets, then switch sides.

Prone Horizontal Abductions

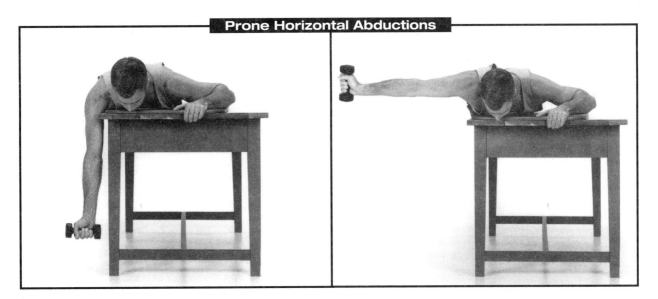

Prone Horizontal Abductions ▲

This is another great training exercise for shoulder mobility.

To do this exercise, lie on a table on your stomach, with your right arm hanging straight down off the edge toward the floor. You can use either a light strap-on wrist weight or a light dumbbell.

With the palm of your hand facing forward, raise your arm out to the side until it is parallel to the floor. Slowly lower your arm. Do three sets of 10 to 12 repetitions. Switch arms.

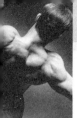
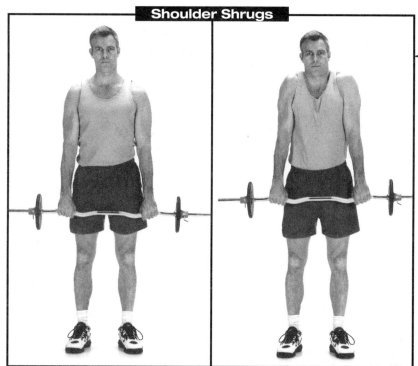

Shoulder Shrugs

Trapezius Muscles

◄ Shoulder Shrugs

Now you can start adding some weight to your shoulder workouts and work toward whatever your goals are, be they strength, size or tone. Helping to strengthen both shoulders and neck, this particular exercise is a great workout for the trapezius. And since it follows a very natural range of motion, it's very shoulder-friendly.

Start by standing upright, with your arms hanging loosely in front of you holding a lightly weighted barbell with a medium grip, palms facing your body. The barbell should be about upper-thigh level. Feet are shoulder-width apart, with shoulders back but drooped down as far as they naturally will go. Keep your chest out and lower back straight, with a slight forward lean.

Now lift the barbell up by raising both shoulders to the front of your body. At the highest point, rotate your shoulders toward your ears, then clench your shoulder muscles and roll them toward your back.

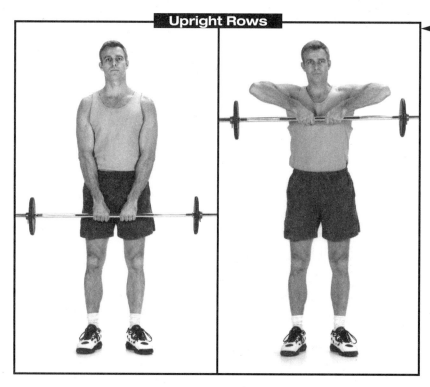

Upright Rows

◄ Upright Rows

This is a good exercise for both the trapezius and other muscles in the shoulders.

Stand upright holding a barbell in both hands, palms facing your body in a narrow grip, hands a few inches from the center of the barbell. Extend your arms down in front of you, holding the barbell at upper-thigh level. Your shoulders are slightly drooped forward, but your back is erect with a slight forward lean in the lower back.

Now lift the barbell up, pulling it toward your head until it's no higher than nipple level. "The old way of doing these was to bring the barbell up to your chin. But if you go that far up, you run the risk of injuring the shoulders rather than working them out," says Ellenbecker. Your elbows should be pointing out. Don't sway or rock for momentum. Hold the lift for a count of three, then lower.

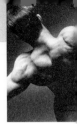

Deltoids

Side Lateral Raises ▶

These side raises work the lateral deltoids, the muscles on the side of your shoulders.

Stand upright, arms at your sides, holding a dumbbell in each hand, palms facing your body, elbows slightly bent. Keep your shoulders back, chest out and your lower back straight with a slight forward lean. Your feet should be shoulder-width apart.

Raise both dumbbells straight out from your sides until they're shoulder level. Pause, then lower. Keep your elbows slightly bent, and to avoid injury, don't let your arms leave the same plane as your torso.

Side Lateral Raises

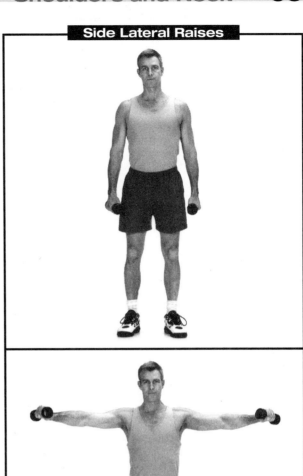

Alternating Front Lateral Raises

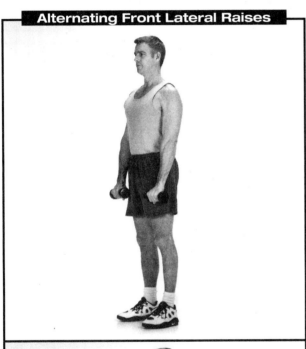

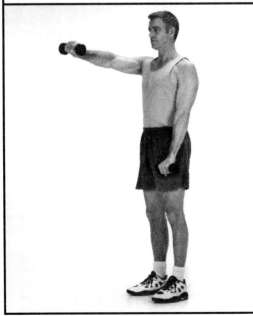

◀ Alternating Front Lateral Raises

Similar to the side raises, this lift works the deltoid muscles from a different angle.

As before, stand upright, with your arms in front holding a dumbbell in each hand, palms facing your body, elbows slightly bent. Keep your shoulders back, chest out and lower back straight with a slight forward lean. Your feet should be shoulder-width apart.

Raise one dumbbell toward the ceiling until it's shoulder level. Don't lock your elbow. Lower, raise the other arm. Repeat, alternating your reps.

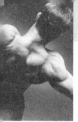

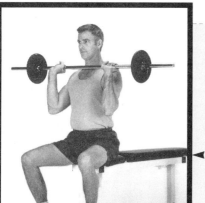

Ultimate Peak

It's a deceptively tricky exercise, but if you have the time and patience to do it right, you'll be head and shoulders above the average man. Well, you'll at least be shoulders above him.

The exercise in question is the military press, and like all things with the adjective "military," this is a tough, but relatively straightforward, lift that builds the deltoids muscles in the shoulders. Here's how to do it.

◄ Military Press

Sit at the end of a bench with your feet a little farther than shoulder-width apart. Hold a barbell in front of your shoulders with your palms facing up, hands shoulder-width apart and elbows pointing down. Your back is perpendicular to the ground, with your shoulders back, chest out and lower back slightly leaning forward.

Now slowly lift the barbell above your head until your arms are fully extended. Don't lock your elbows, and don't sway or rock your body to gain momentum.

For a variation, start with the barbell behind your neck and across your deltoids and trapezius. Your palms should be up, your hands shoulder-width apart. Lift the barbell behind your head.

Note: Many strength experts recommend wearing a weight belt while doing military presses, since the overhead lift puts a strain on the lower back as well as the shoulders.

Finally, if you feel any sharp pains while you're lifting—or feel pain in your shoulder joint after doing the workout, think about skipping this lift. "Muscle soreness is one thing," says Allen Kinley, assistant strength and conditioning coach at Texas A&M University in College Station. "But if you're feeling a sharp pain in your joint, your body is telling you to stop what you're doing."

Alternating Press with Dumbbells ►

This is another great exercise for the deltoids. Do this while sitting on a weight bench.

Grasping two dumbbells, straddle a bench with your legs slightly parted. Your feet should be firmly on the floor, your arms raised. Keep the dumbbells shoulder-width apart, shoulder level, palms facing each other. Your shoulders are back, chest out and there's a slight forward lean in your lower back. Keep your elbows unlocked.

Raise the left dumbbell up until your arm is straight, but don't lock your elbow. Lower, repeat with the other arm. Repeat, alternating your reps.

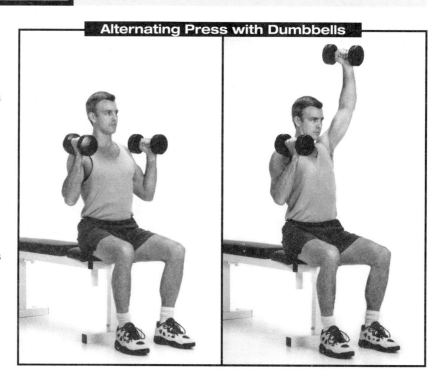

Alternating Press with Dumbbells

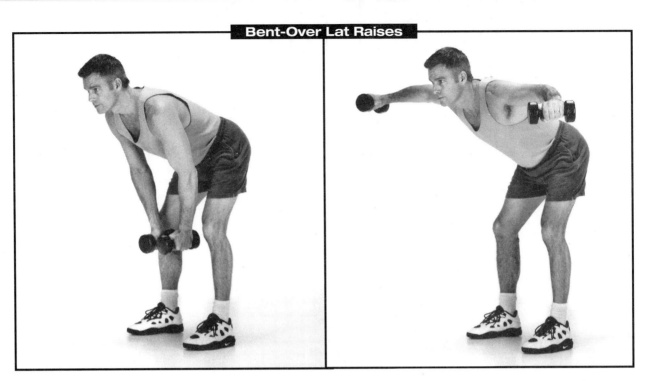

Bent-Over Lat Raises

Bent-Over Lat Raises ⏶

To work the deltoids at the back of your shoulders, bend over at your waist and hold a dumbbell in each hand. Your palms should face in toward each other, and your elbows should be slightly bent. Feet are wider than shoulder-width apart, and your back should be straight and roughly parallel to the floor.

Raise the dumbbells out toward your sides—as though you were flapping your arms. Raise your arms until they're parallel to the floor. Keep your back straight. Lower slowly.

FACT Many headaches are actually the result of tight muscles in the neck and shoulders. A quick cure? Lightly massage the neck muscles, suggests Egilius Spierings, M.D., Ph.D., a neurologist and headache specialist in private practice in Wellesley Hills, Massachusetts. Place your hands at the base of your head just behind your jaw and below your ear. Massage gently with your fingertips as you work down to the top of your shoulders. If that doesn't help, Dr. Spierings suggests using a heating pad placed on the back of your neck for a few minutes.

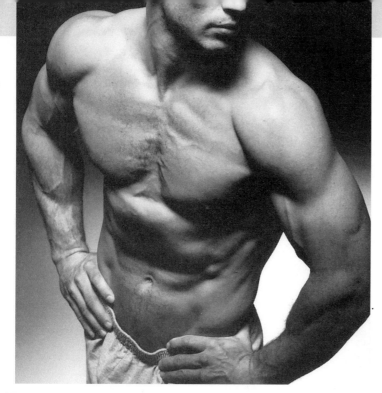

Chest

If weight lifters were to hold a popularity contest for their favorite exercises, the ones involving the chest would win—no contest.

"Chest exercises are absolutely the most popular kind of exercise around. When a guy hits the gym, they're the first thing he wants to do. Men love them," says Jeffrey Stout, Ph.D., assistant professor of exercise physiology at Creighton University in Omaha, Nebraska.

But love can be blind. Dr. Stout points out that most men work on chest muscles to improve their shape, to make them bigger, broader, more rounded. "That's bad. That means most guys are consequently working only a very small percentage of their chest muscles and completely ignoring others."

That may explain why months of countless bench presses don't seem to be getting you any closer to a chest you'll treasure. "You can't work out with the idea of having a great-looking chest. Focus instead on having a strong chest," says Dr. Stout. "Focus on working all the muscles, both in the sides and lower part of your chest. If you work toward that goal, then the well-chiseled look you've been after will come naturally."

Devising Chest Strategies

Part of the problem to building a well-rounded chest is that most guys don't know, muscle-wise, exactly what constitutes

the chest. For our purposes, we're talking about the area from your collarbone down to the soft center of your rib cage, and extending from armpit to armpit.

In this zone, the biggest, most obvious muscles are the pectoralis muscles—you know them as pecs, the breast muscles that lay across the upper half of the rib cage. Connected to your shoulders on either side, these muscles help out with any lifting or pushing activities you do.

Less visible, but of equal importance, are the subclavius and serratus muscles, which are under and to the sides of the pecs. These help to give your shoulders and arms greater maneuverability. The serratus, in particular, helps you to push and punch. These muscles also anchor and support the pecs in whatever activity they're doing. Working these unsung heroes can give your chest a fuller, more muscled look than doing straight pec exercises alone. It will also improve your overall upper-body strength.

"Those muscles under the pecs are the real workhorses in the chest—they give power to arm movements," says Dr. Stout. But because your arm and chest strength is closely linked, fully working the chest muscles can be a challenge. "You work your chest muscles through your arms—they have to do the lifting," says Dr. Stout. Which means it's easy to let your arms do the work and cheat your chest out of exercise. So as you approach the bench, pay attention to proper form when you do these exercises.

Take it slow. In particular, move slowly when lowering the weight, especially while doing presses. "That way, you're not as likely to injure your shoulder joints," says Allen Kinley, assistant strength and conditioning coach at Texas A&M University in College Station. Kinley adds that moving slowly through a lift prevents you from letting momentum do the work for you. "You're really cheating yourself out of a good workout" when you let momentum move the bar, he says. Plus, that sort of lifting tends to make you bounce the barbell off your chest, which will leave you the next day with a nice bruise and the feeling that you got punched in the chest.

Alternate wide and tight angles. Varying your grip on the weights will work the chest muscles from different angles. "You don't always have to lift with your

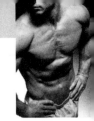

hands exactly shoulder-width apart on the bar. You can vary your routine with wide-grip presses and narrow-grip presses, where your hands are really close together in the center of the barbell," points out Dr. Stout. Varying your grip attacks the chest muscles from all sides. That way your arms aren't doing all the work.

Stay in control. The real trick to effective chest-building is not quantity, it's quality. Lifting heavy weights all the time can cause you to cheat. Use a moderate weight and do more reps instead. You'll still get good resistance from the weight, but it will be light enough that you can control the weight and do a slow rep—the key to building up muscle, says Dr. Stout.

Put someone on the spot. As a measure of safety, it's always a good idea to have someone spotting you—especially where chest exercises are concerned.

"Having a spotter will allow you to work out better during those times when you want to do a low number of reps with heavier weights," says Dr. Stout. "If you're by yourself, you're not as likely to use weights that will fatigue your muscles to the point of exhaustion," he points out.

Don't wreck your wrists. Cautionary note: Although one of the best chest exercises around is the push-up, there's a real danger that the exercise could give your wrists more of a workout than you intended.

"Consider that your wrists bear most of your body weight during push-ups done the traditional way with palms flat on the floor," says James Pedicano, M.D., a wrist and hand surgeon in private practice in Ridgewood, New Jersey. But Dr. Pedicano says you can take the pressure off your wrists by doing push-ups on your knuckles or by putting two octagonal dumbbells on the floor and gripping them.

"Either position forces you to make a fist, which straightens out your wrist, so all the force of the exercise isn't resting on the wrist," says Dr. Pedicano. Meanwhile, try these lifts.

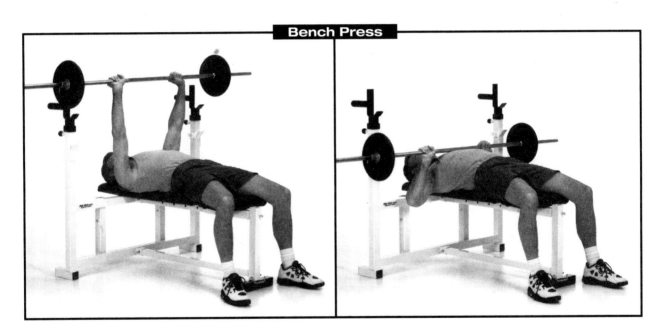

Bench Press

Bench Press ⬆

Lie on—what else?—a bench-press bench, with the barbell above your chest. Grasp the barbell with a medium grip (hands about shoulder-width apart) or slightly wider. Your palms should be facing your legs, and your feet should be resting flat on the ground. Your back is straight and against the bench.

Lower the barbell to your chest—right at nipple level. Your elbows should be pointed out while the rest of your body remains in position. Don't arch your back or bounce the bar off your chest. Raise to the starting position and repeat.

FACT Although obese chests have been measured at more than 120 inches across, the largest *muscular* chest belongs to Isaac Nesser of Greensburg, Pennsylvania, at 74¹/₁₆ inches.

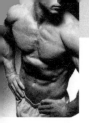

Narrow-Grip Bench Press ➤

Do a normal bench press with the proper form, but hold the barbell with a narrow grip. Your hands should be equidistant from the bar center, six to eight inches apart.

Note: Chances are you'll find this lift harder than the regular bench press, so decrease the weight for this exercise.

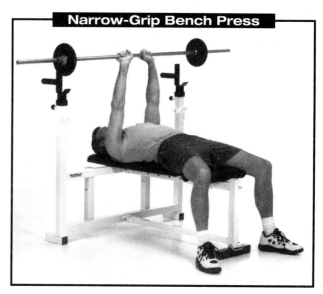

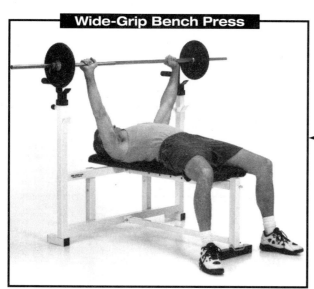

◄ Wide-Grip Bench Press

Do a normal bench press with the proper form, but now hold the barbell with a wide grip. Again, your hands should be equidistant from the bar center, a few inches wider than shoulder-width apart.

Note: As with the narrow-grip bench press, decrease the weight for this exercise.

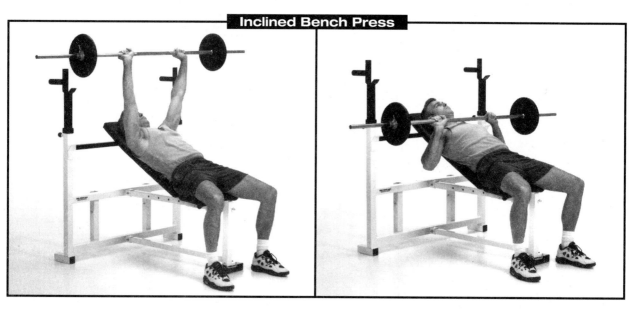

Inclined Bench Press ⬆

Lie on an inclined bench-press bench with the barbell above your body. Grasp the barbell with a medium grip or slightly wider. Your palms should face your legs, and your feet should be on the ground. Your back should be against the bench.

Lower the barbell to your chest, between your shoulders and nipple line. Your elbows should be pointing out, and the rest of your body should stay in proper form. Don't arch your back or bounce the bar off your chest.

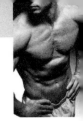

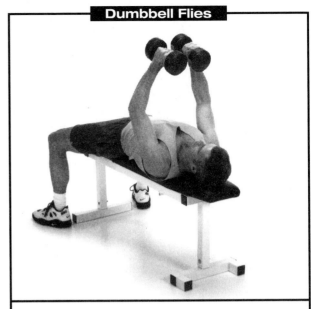

Dumbbell Flies ▶

    Lie on your back on a bench, with your legs parted and your feet firmly on the floor. Hold two dumbbells above you, palms facing each other. The dumbbells should be nearly touching each other above your chest. Your back should be straight and firm against the bench, and your elbows unlocked.

    Slowly lower the dumbbells out and away from each other in a semicircular motion. Keep your wrists locked. Lower until the dumbbells are at chest level. Your elbows should be bent at roughly a 45-degree angle, while your back should be straight. Raise to the starting position and repeat.

    Note: Watch out for your shoulder—it's going to try to sneak in and do the work in this exercise. "Really focus on doing this lift with your chest muscles," cautions Dr. Stout. "The more your shoulder gets into the lift, the greater the chance of injuring it."

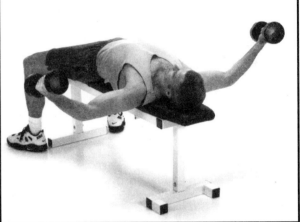

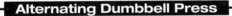

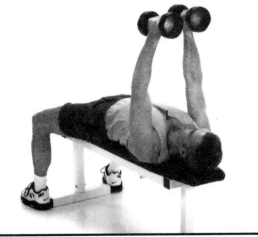

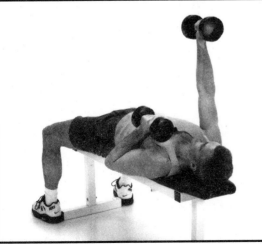

◀ Alternating Dumbbell Press

    Grasp two dumbbells and lie back on a bench with your legs slightly parted, feet firmly on the floor and your arms raised. Hold the dumbbells above you, palms facing each other. Your arms are extended, your back is straight and firm against the bench, and your elbows are unlocked.

    Lower the left dumbbell until it's even with your chest. Your elbow should be pointing to the ground. Raise to the starting position, then alternate with the right dumbbell. Repeat.

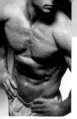
Dips ➤

Raise yourself off the ground and onto parallel dip bars. Your hands should be gripping the bar handles with your fingers on the outside, facing away from your body. Keep your elbows in close to your sides, and slightly bend your legs if your feet are dragging on the ground.

Lower yourself down to the point where your upper arms are parallel to the floor. Keep your elbows close to your sides, and bend your legs slightly if your feet are touching the ground. Raise, repeat. Do as many as you can while maintaining proper form.

Note: If you don't happen to have dip bars lying around the house, two benches or chairs will work just as well. Place your hands flat on the seats, and extend your feet behind you, then start dipping.

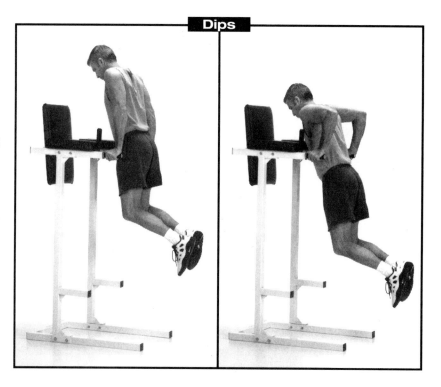

Dips

Push-Ups

Don't dismiss these as tired old standbys, good only when you're on the road and away from the club, or while you're waiting for that muscle-bound oaf to finish doing his super-sets.

"Push-ups are a great part of working out your upper body—not just the chest, but also the arms and shoulders," says Kinley. "It's certainly a good idea to make them a regular part of your workout."

And they don't have to be the old boring variety either. Push-up technology has advanced considerably over the centuries. Here's a sampling of different push-ups you can do. Since you're not using weights with these exercises, don't lock yourself in to a certain number of reps—just do as many as you can.

Push-Ups ➤

Lie face down on the floor, palms face down at shoulder level, fingers pointing forward. To accent your chest more, put your hands wider than shoulder-width apart; to hit the triceps and back more, bring your hands in closer, so your thumbs and index fingers touch to form a diamond pattern on the floor. The bottoms of your feet should be perpendicular to the floor. Your body weight is resting only on your palms and toes. Keep your legs and back straight.

Now push up until your arms are almost fully extended. Your elbows should be slightly bent, not locked. Lower yourself back to the floor—that's one.

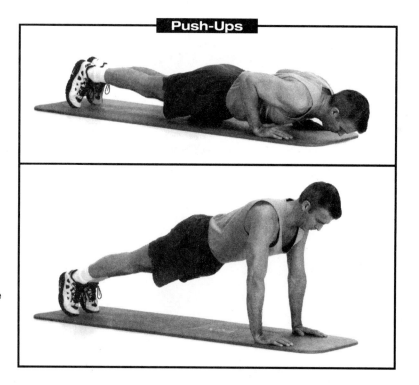

Push-Ups

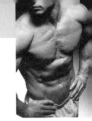

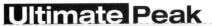

Ultimate Peak

So you've run the gauntlet of chest challenges and you're ready for some super exercises? Give these a try, but don't overdo it.

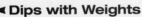

◄ Dips with Weights

Do dips as you normally would, but wear a special weight belt that has weight plates attached to a chain. Or you can hold a dumbbell between your feet for resistance.

◄ Push-Ups with Weights

Do a push-up with proper form, but have a partner place a weight plate squarely on your back for added resistance. The plate should be between your shoulder blades on your upper back. Dads: You can also do this with a toddler on your back for resistance.

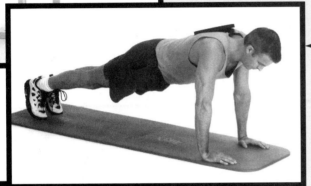

◄ Decline Bench Press

This is a risky exercise—"don't do it unless you have a friend to spot you," warns Jeffrey Stout, Ph.D., assistant professor of exercise physiology at Creighton University in Omaha, Nebraska. Lie on a decline bench with a barbell held above your body in preparation for the press. Grasp the barbell with a medium grip (hands about shoulder-width apart) or slightly wider. Palms are facing your legs, and your feet are hooked under the support bar, if there is one. Your back is straight and against the bench.

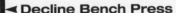

Lower the barbell to your nipple line, keeping your elbows pointed out. The rest of your body stays in proper starting form. Don't arch your back or bounce the bar off your chest. Raise, and repeat.

Note: Decline bench presses stress your chest from a different angle than standard presses, so decrease the weight.

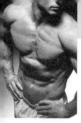

Decline Push-Ups

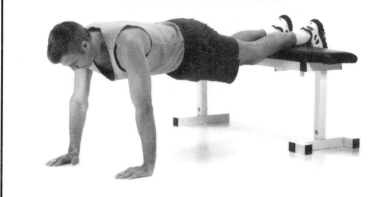

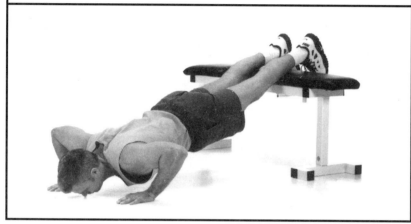

◄ **Decline Push-Ups**

Get in push-up position, but prop your feet up on a bench. Your hands should be roughly shoulder-width apart, and your back should be straight. Keep your elbows unlocked.

Lower yourself to the floor as far as you can, or until your nose touches the ground. Your back and hips should be straight, while your elbows should point out. Keep your feet on the bench.

Bent-Knee Push-Ups

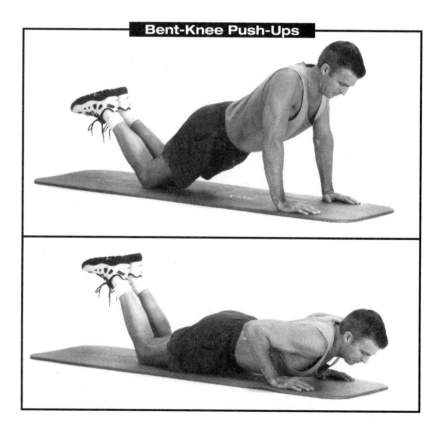

Bent-Knee Push-Ups ►

Don't dismiss these as a sissy's exercise. Assume the standard push-up position, except instead of having your legs out straight, keep your knees bent and your feet up off the ground. Sports trainers say a couple dozen reps on your knees can be a great warm-up before a workout, or as a prelude to tougher push-ups.

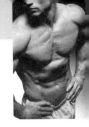

Inclined Push-Ups

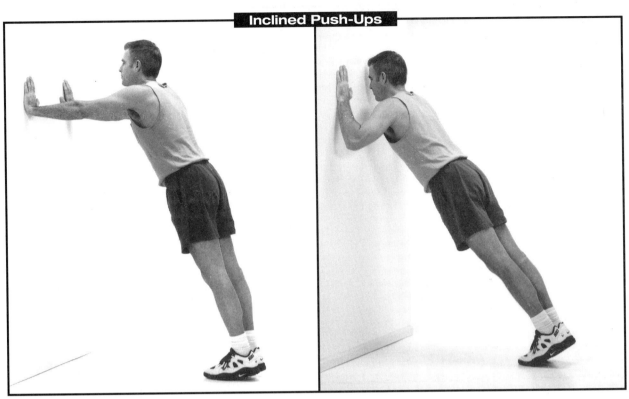

Inclined Push-Ups ⚠

Stand several feet back from a wall. Stick your arms straight ahead and lean forward, keeping your body straight, until your palms are flat against the wall. Your distance from the wall is correct if your heels are slightly raised. Do a push-up by bringing your forehead right up to the wall and then pushing back out. This push-up really targets the upper chest.

Man and Machine

Most physical training experts agree that the best way to really make progress improving your chest muscles is through free weights. "There just aren't that many machines that do as good a job working chest muscles as a good old barbell and a pair of dumbbells," says Jeffrey Stout, Ph.D., assistant professor of exercise physiology at Creighton University in Omaha, Nebraska.

If you have press machines at your gym, it's okay to use them, though. "You won't harm yourself using some of the machines that mimic exercises like the bench press," allows Dr. Stout. "But don't use them to the point of avoiding free-weight work. The free weights cause you to use more muscles to balance and steady the weight than a machine would. That's going to give you an extra workout."

One good chest exerciser, though, is the "pec-deck" machine. You sit in it, placing your arms behind two padded, rotating arms. Slowly, you lift the weight and bring your arms together. "It's an excellent exercise because it works the upper and inner pecs at the same time, kind of like dumbbell flies, only better," says John Porcari, Ph.D., executive director of the LaCrosse Exercise and Health Program and professor of exercise and sport science at the University of Wisconsin in LaCrosse.

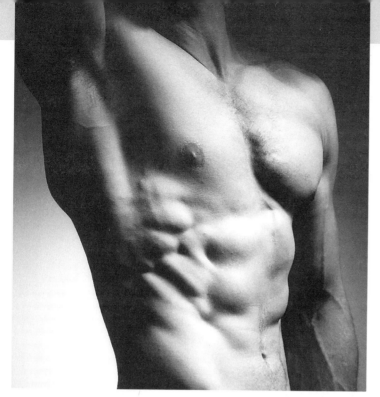

Abs

In the never-ending war against our potbellies, men are fighting a pretty powerful opponent—and it's not that overwhelming desire to dish yourself seconds at every meal, nor the underwhelming urge to get off the couch and flatten that spare tire. In the battle of the bulge, your main adversary is nature itself.

"It goes back to ancient times, when food was harder to find. Back then, our bodies adapted by storing fuel—in the form of fat cells—in the body. In men, that storage area was around the midsection. When food was scarce, your body could draw on the reserve," explains Doug Lentz, Pennsylvania state director of the National Strength and Conditioning Association and owner of the Chambersburg Sports Medicine and Rehabilitation Center in Pennsylvania.

In modern times, most men have no problem rustling up a meal or three, but we still eat—and our bodies still store excess fat—like an Ice Age was just around the corner. Consequently, Lentz says we get thicker and thicker around the middle, especially as we get older and our metabolisms slow down.

And that's nothing to belly-laugh about. Put simply, fat can kill you. When you eat fats, they can cause plaque to build up in the walls of your arteries, cutting off blood flow to your heart and leaving you with heart disease, the single biggest killer of men. Or, if you eat beyond what your body needs, your body

will store that excess fuel in the fat cells around your middle. When that spare tire inflates, it puts more pressure on your heart, which can cause high blood pressure and also lead to heart disease.

That's just page one in the catalog of woes. "Even though it's around your middle, excess fat does a number on your back," says Todd Ellenbecker, P.T., clinical director of Physiotherapy Associates Scottsdale Sports Clinic in Arizona. "The weight of it can really put a strain on lower-back muscles, and it's one of the reasons why so many men suffer lower-back pain."

Finally, with this type of fat, what doesn't kill you can certainly make you weaker, because the more fat we store in our guts, the less we tend to work the abdominal muscles. "And if those muscles get weak, it can cause a lot of problems," says Lentz.

There are only four major abdominal muscles, but this muscle quartet is one of the most vital in your body. Those abs—including the upper and lower abdominals and oblique muscles on either side of your abdomen—support the rest of your torso and lower back.

Abdominal muscles also help us move our legs and shift our hips. When you swing a bat, heft a box, kick a ball or shift your weight for more power, your abdominals are doing some of the work. The more fat you ladle on the belly, the more you'll expose other parts of your body to serious injury.

Cutting Out the Middle, Man

You have two obstacles, then, to looking good around your middle—belly fat and flabby abs. Don't confuse the two. "You might have very little fat around your middle, but that doesn't mean you have good abs. Those muscles could be weak. Conversely, some guys might develop strong abs from the work they do or games they play, but they'll wonder why they still have a potbelly," says Lentz.

The reason is that these guys are buying into the dubious exercise theory of spot-reducing. "It would be nice if it worked, but it doesn't," says Peter Lemon, Ph.D., professor of applied physiology at Kent State University in Ohio. Dr. Lemon studies the link between food and exercise. Too often, he says, men believe that doing a

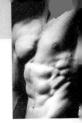

lot of abdominal exercise will somehow burn the fat—or spot-reduce it—in their abdominal area. "It'll never work. You might improve abdominal strength, but that alone won't get you the results you want," says Dr. Lemon.

No, ditching the gut and toning the abs requires two separate strategies, says Dr. Lemon. The first revolves around eating foods that are lower in fat and burning what excess fat you have, not with sit-ups and crunches, but with a different kind of exercise. Aerobic exercise.

"In most men, fat around the abdominals is the last thing their bodies burn off. Aerobic exercise is what gets your body to start burning it," says Lentz. That means at least 30 minutes, three to four times a week, of a low- to moderate-intensity exercise like speed-walking, cycling, stair-climbing or rowing.

That's not to say you should forgo your abdominal exercises. In fact, you should continue to do them. That way you'll strengthen the muscles underneath so that, once you shed the fat, you'll be able to show off those fab abs. Here's a bellyful of some of the best abs-strengtheners around. Unlike most resistance-training exercises, you should work the abs to exhaustion. In other words, do the exercise until you can't do it anymore. The only exception to this rule is if you do your abs exercises while holding dumbbells or a light weight plate. In that case, for the low-weight, high-rep principle, do 12 to 20 reps per set.

And in all cases, focus on good technique. Make sure you do all your abdominal exercises in a slow, controlled manner, Lentz says. Jerking, lunging or bouncing not only is bad technique but also could injure you.

Abdominals

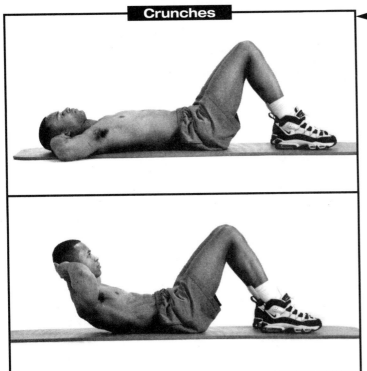

Crunches

◀ **Crunches**

One of the best exercises for your upper and lower abs, crunches are more effective than the sit-ups you may remember from junior-high gym class.

Start by lying flat on your back with your hands cupped near your ears or crossed over your chest—never pull on your neck during a crunch, because you could end up injuring your neck or upper back. Keep your feet together, flat on the floor and about six inches from your butt. Bend your knees at about a 45-degree angle, and keep your legs slightly apart.

Curl your upper torso up and in toward your knees until your shoulder blades are as high off the ground as you can get them. Only your shoulders should lift—not your lower back. Feel your abs contract, and hold the raise for a second. Lower to the starting position, then continue with your next rep without relaxing in between. As your abs get stronger, you can hold a light weight plate across your chest and do your crunches that way.

FACT It's okay to be hard on soft abs—exercise experts say the abdominals are among the few muscles in your body that you can work every day, says Doug Lentz, Pennsylvania state director of the National Strength and Conditioning Association and owner of the Chambersburg Sports Medicine and Rehabilitation Center in Pennsylvania. But, he adds, it is probably best if you can concentrate on different muscles on alternating days. On Monday, Wednesday and Friday, work on your crunches and vacuums. On Tuesday and Thursday, concentrate on the obliques.

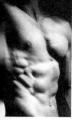

Crossover Crunches ➤

This crunch also works the obliques, which, Ellenbecker reminds us, are the side muscles that help shore up your back. Lie on your back with your feet flat and your knees at about a 45-degree angle. Keep your feet about hip-width apart and cup your hands behind your ears.

Raise your torso up, lifting your shoulders and shoulder blades off the ground. But instead of pausing at the top, slightly twist toward your left knee. Hold the contraction for a second, then lower to the starting position. Repeat, but this time twist to your right knee. Don't relax between reps.

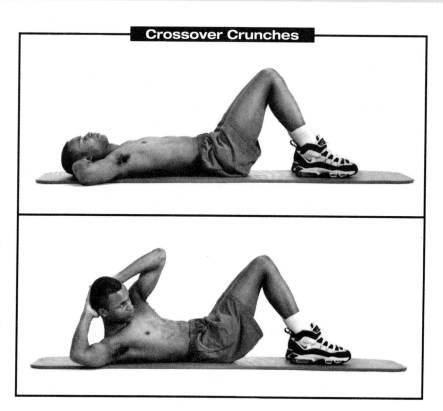

Crossover Crunches

Raised-Leg Crunches ➤

Lie on your back with your knees bent and your lower legs up on a bench or chair. Your thighs should be perpendicular to the floor, and your hands cupped behind your ears or folded across your chest.

Pull your torso up and in toward your knees, lifting your shoulders and shoulder blades off the floor. Hold the contraction for a second, then lower to the starting position. Repeat, but don't relax between reps. As you do the crunches, don't let your butt slide under the bench so that your thighs get bent toward your body.

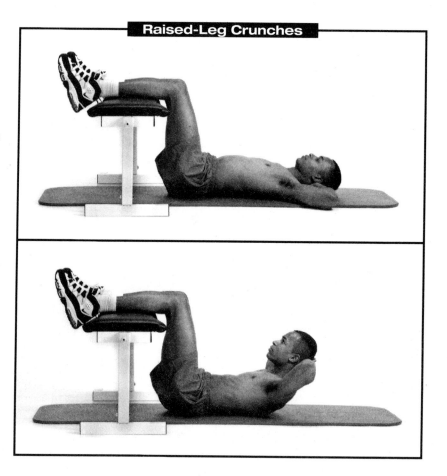

Raised-Leg Crunches

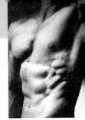

Frog-Leg Crunches ►

Another great cruncher for upper and lower abs. Lie flat on your back, this time with your knees spread and the soles of your feet together. Your knees should be as close to the floor as you comfortably can get them. Cup your hands behind your ears or fold them across your chest.

Keeping the rest of your body in place, lift your shoulder blades and upper back off the floor. At the same time, slightly curl your pelvis up and in, but don't lift your lower back off the floor. Concentrate on your ab contraction. Hold for a second, then lower to the starting position. Don't rest when you're done. Repeat your next rep, keeping your abs tight.

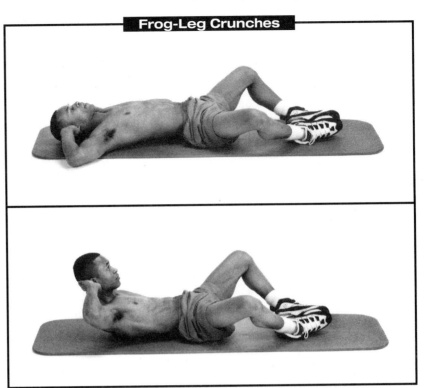

Frog-Leg Crunches

Hanging Single-Knee Raises ►

A fun exercise you can do while you're just hanging around.

Hang fully extended from a chin-up bar with your palms facing out and your hands a little wider than shoulder-width apart. Your feet should be lightly touching the floor.

Without swinging to pick up momentum, raise your right knee toward your left shoulder as far as you can, using your abs for power. Slightly thrust your pelvis forward to help, but don't rock. Hold for a second, then lower to the starting position and repeat with your left leg.

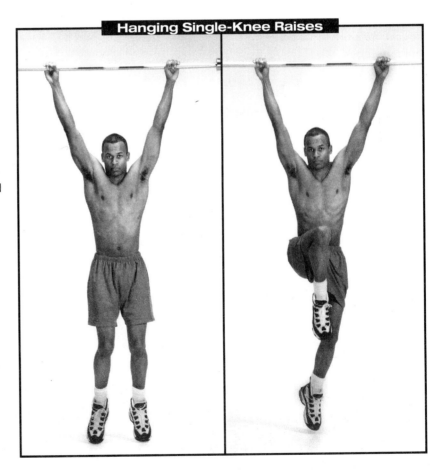

Hanging Single-Knee Raises

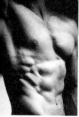

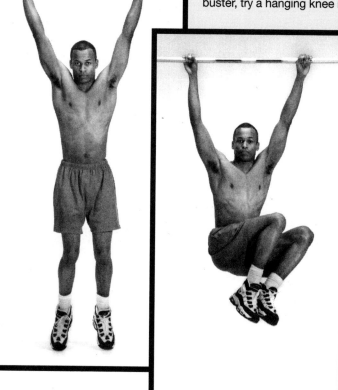

Ultimate Peak

As your abs get stronger, you may want to up the ante. For a great gut-buster, try a hanging knee raise crossover.

◄ Hanging Knee Raise Crossovers

Start by hanging fully extended from a chin-up bar with your hands a little wider than shoulder-width apart. Your palms should be facing outward and your feet lightly touching the ground.

Now, keeping your legs together, slowly lift your knees up toward your left shoulder as high as you can. Slightly thrust your pelvis forward, but don't rock or sway for momentum. Hold for a second at the top, then lower and repeat on your right side. Don't rest between reps. Keep your abs tight.

For an even tougher variation, lift your legs instead of just your knees. Keep your feet together, and lift toward your left shoulder as high as you can. You'll need to slightly tilt your pelvis forward. Lower, then repeat on the right side.

Vacuums ►

If you've ever tried to suck in your gut at the beach, you're already familiar with the basics of this exercise.

Sit in a kneeling position with your feet crossed behind you and your hands on your hips or thighs. Keep your upper body upright. Breathe out, then immediately suck your stomach up and in as far as it will go. Hold for five seconds. Do two to three sets of ten reps. You can also do this exercise from a standing position.

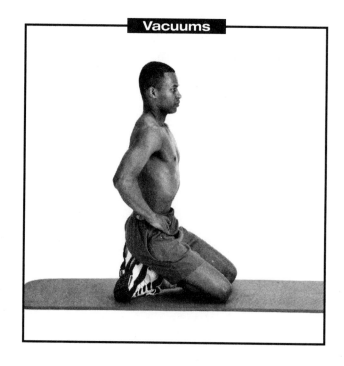

Vacuums

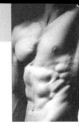

Raised-Leg Knee-Ins

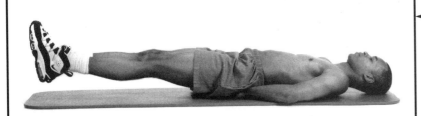

◄ **Raised-Leg Knee-Ins**

Lie on your back on the floor. Your arms should be close to your sides, with your hands palm-down and just under your butt. Press the small of your back against the floor and extend your legs outward with your heels about three inches above the floor.

Using your abdominal muscles and keeping your lower back against the floor, lift your left knee, keeping your right leg hovering above the floor. Hold, then straighten your leg to the starting position and repeat the movement with the other leg. Keep your abs taut throughout the exercise.

V-Spread Toe Touches

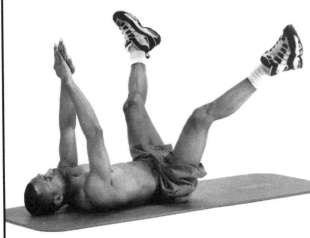

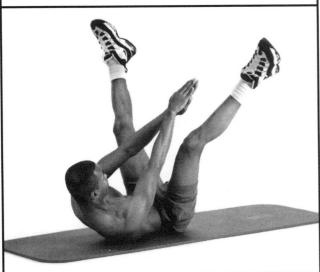

◄ **V-Spread Toe Touches**

Lie flat on your back with your legs straight up in a V-position. Don't lock your knees, and raise your arms to the ceiling.

Curl your shoulder blades up and reach toward your right foot with both hands. Hold for a second, concentrating on your abs, then lower to the starting position. Repeat, this time reaching for the left foot. Don't pause at the lower position. Keep your abs tight.

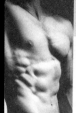

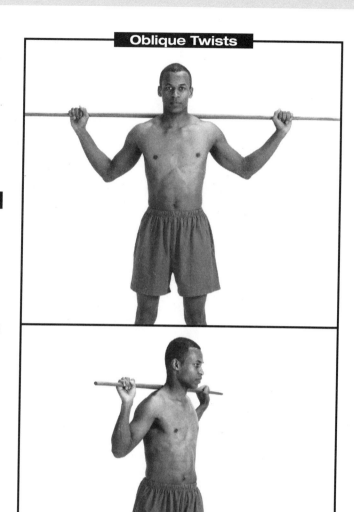

Oblique Twists

Obliques

Oblique Twists ▶

These next few exercises work the side, or oblique, muscles of your abdominal area.

Stand upright with your feet about shoulder-width apart, hips facing forward and your knees unlocked. Hold a broomstick across your shoulders, behind your neck so it's resting on your trapezius and upper deltoid muscles. Your hands should be grasping the ends or outer portions of the broomstick.

Keeping your hips still and facing forward, twist to your left as far as you can go. Then come back to the starting position. Pause for a second, then twist in the opposite direction. Keep a slow, steady pace and concentrate on working your obliques.

Man and Machine

Abs aren't just tough to work out—they're also tough to design machines for.

"If you have an exercise mat and a place to stretch out to do your crunches, you don't need much more than that," says Doug Lentz, Pennsylvania state director of the National Strength and Conditioning Association and owner of the Chambersburg Sports Medicine and Rehabilitation Center in Pennsylvania. However, he does allow that oblique machines "can target those muscles pretty well." You work the machine by sitting down, then folding your arms around a metal, rotating arm at your side. Then, you slowly turn from one side to the other, rotating the metal arm, which lifts the weights. When you've finished one side, the machine allows you to turn around and work the other side.

But one abdominal machine you might want to avoid is the crunch machine. You sit in an elevated chair, grasp handles overhead, lock your feet under a bar and bend inward, pulling the top weight with your arms and the bottom weight with your feet, until your elbows are touching your knees. This machine can injure your back more than it exercises your gut, warns Paula Watson, P.T., a physical therapist for the Texas Back Institute in Dallas.

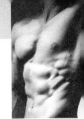

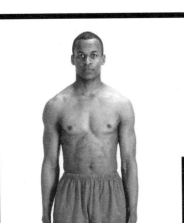

Ultimate Peak

To boost your obliques, grab a couple of dumbbells and do some sidebends. Here's how.

◄ Sidebends with Dumbbells

Stand upright with a dumbbell in each hand. Your feet should be about shoulder-width apart, and your arms should be resting at your sides with your palms facing in.

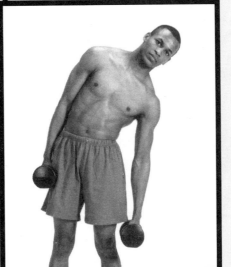

Bend to one side, allowing the dumbbell to drop down your leg until you feel your obliques working. Keep your body facing front in the same plane—don't turn your torso into the sidebend. Once you've gone as low as you can, slowly bring yourself upright to the starting position and repeat. Don't rest between reps. Keep your abs and obliques contracted. When you're done with one side, work the other.

Oblique Crunches

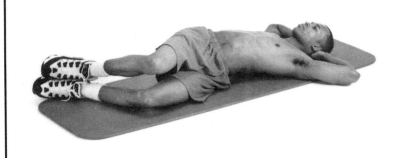

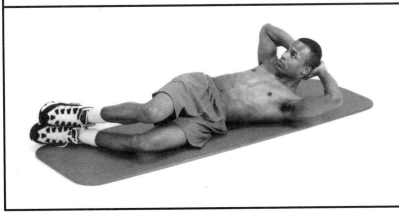

◄ Oblique Crunches

Lie flat on your back with your knees bent and your hands cupped behind your ears. Now let your legs fall as far as they can to your left side, so that your upper body is now flat on the floor and your lower body is on its side.

Keeping your shoulders as parallel to the floor as possible, lift your upper body up until your shoulder blades clear the ground. Concentrate on the oblique contraction and hold the crunch for a second. Lower to the starting position and do your next rep. Don't rest between crunches—keep your abs tight. After one set on your left side, switch to your right and continue.

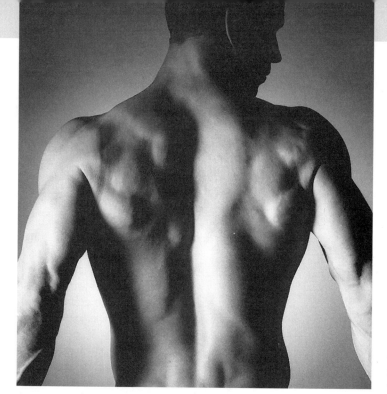

Back

Your back is your personal tower of power. That stack of bony disks is the key to your strength and mobility. As important as the spine, though, are all the muscles wrapped around it—muscles that let us stoop and scoop, twist and turn, or stand tall when it's time to be counted.

But the back is also one of life's great trouble spots. Roughly 80 percent of American men suffer some type of back pain—that's active guys and couch potatoes alike. Except in the most serious of cases, that pain comes from any of the half-dozen muscle groups that support the upper, middle and lower back.

"Most men would not have that kind of back pain if they had a specific back exercise program," says Doug Lentz, Pennsylvania state director of the National Strength and Conditioning Association and owner of the Chambersburg Sports Medicine and Rehabilitation Center in Pennsylvania. And he's not just talking about weight training to keep back muscles strong. Your back muscles already carry a heavy load every moment of the day—your body weight. This means they're pretty tight from a life of lifting. "So it's just as important to do stretching and flexibility exercises to loosen the back muscles up and take some of the stress and tension out of them," says Lentz.

Back to the Future

It's hard to say which of your back muscles is the most important. "They're all necessary for certain functions and motions," says Lentz. The topmost muscles allow you to move your neck, and they work in concert with your shoulder muscles to help you lift. Mid-back muscles like the erector spinae allow you to bend over and stand back up. Lower-back muscles, like the quadratus, work together with the oblique abdominal muscles, helping to support your spine and giving you greater range of movement. If any one of these muscle areas is weaker than the others, it can lead to serious back pain and leave you open to a muscle pull or worse. "The stronger and more flexible your back is, the better you'll feel," says Lentz. "You'll stand straighter, you'll breathe better and you'll have more power with less pain." So here are some specific tips to work all of your dorsal muscles. Get your back into them.

Work the abs for your back. One of the best ways to strengthen your lower back is not necessarily to pump up the muscles behind you, but the ones in front and at your sides—specifically, your abs.

"When I see men with back problems and I evaluate their workout routine, often I see that their problem is they're not getting enough of a lower-abdominal workout," says Paula Watson, P.T., a physical therapist for the Texas Back Institute in Dallas. As Watson explains, abs support the back whenever you lift, twist, bend or stand up straight.

So make sure you do plenty of abs work as part of your back workout. Basic crunches are good, but focus on exercises that also work the lower abs, obliques and the quadratus, like frog-leg crunches or oblique twists. (See Abs on page 76.)

Sit back. When your workout is done, be sure to take a load off that back.

"After back exercises it's really important to do a cooldown, something that's going to relax the back," says Watson. That cooldown can be as simple as lying flat on your back on an exercise mat for five minutes. "Just lie there in a comfortable position, practice some deep breathing and stretch your arms and legs out," says Watson. "It helps the back tremendously and keeps you from feeling sore afterwards."

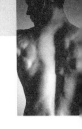

Work on flex time. But before you do any back exercises—heck, before you do *any* exercises—be sure to spend ten minutes warming up and then ten minutes stretching, especially stretching your legs. "For instance, if your hamstrings are too tight, they can limit the range of motion in your back and make it especially hard to bend over," says Watson. The more you warm up and stretch, the more flexible and responsive your muscles will be.

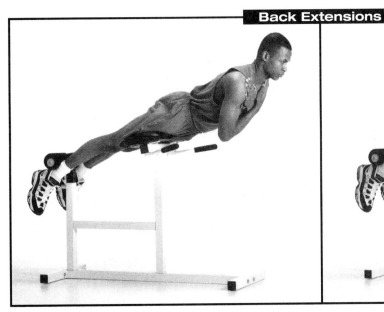

Back Stretches

◄ **Back Stretches**

Lying flat on your back, lift one knee to your chest, then lift the other, keeping your lower back on the floor all the while. Your hands should be behind your knees, sandwiched between your upper and lower legs. Hold the stretch for 30 seconds, then release. You may use your hands to support your legs; the idea is to stretch your back, not exercise your thighs. For an added stretch, try to touch your forehead to your knees.

Back Extensions

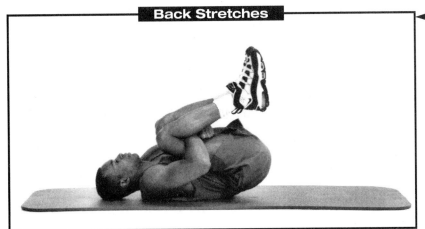
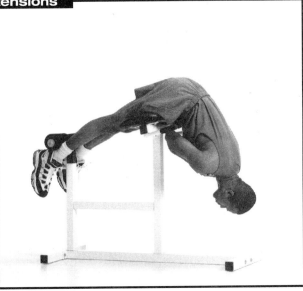

Back Extensions ▲

Here's a great all-back exercise, especially for your erector muscles. Position yourself in a back extension machine with your ankles locked behind the padded bars and your groin area and upper thighs resting on the padded platform. Your hips should be over the edge of the platform, and your body held straight so it is at a roughly 20-degree angle to the floor. Fold your arms across your chest.

Bend over at the waist, with your upper torso lowered to a point a few inches above perpendicular to the floor. Your arms should still be crossed over your chest and the rest of your body should stay in the starting position. Raise to the starting position, repeat. Do as many as you comfortably can, working up to no more than three sets of 20 reps. If you need more of a challenge, do the back extension holding a weight in your arms.

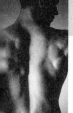

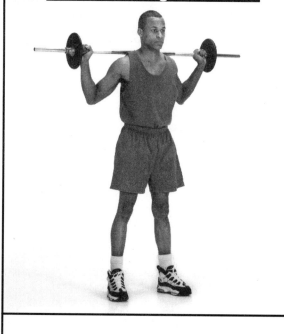

Good-Morning Exercises

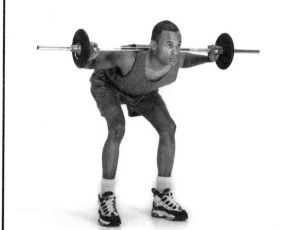

◄ Good-Morning Exercises

To work your lower back, stand with your legs shoulder-width apart, holding a barbell with very light weights across your shoulders and behind your neck. Hold your hands wider than shoulder-width apart but within the weights, with your palms facing out. Keep your upper body upright, shoulders back, chest out, and your lower back straight with a slight forward lean.

Keeping your back level, slowly bend over at the waist until your body is roughly at a 90-degree angle and parallel to the floor or as far as you can go while still maintaining proper form. Keep your head up and back straight. Keep your legs straight and knees unlocked.

Only do as many of these as you can while maintaining proper form. If your back starts to round or if you feel any pain, stop. You may wish to start with an unweighted barbell. Work up to no more than three sets of 8 to 12 reps.

Rumanian Dead Lifts

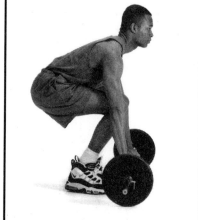

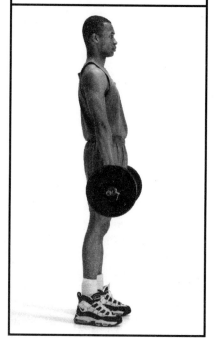

Rumanian Dead Lifts ►

This is a modified version of the old stiff-legged dead lift, which Lentz says was too hard on the lower back. If your hamstrings are tight, start with an un-weighted barbell or broomstick until you are flexible enough to do this with proper form. Then, work with a lightly weighted barbell.

Stand upright with the barbell in front of you, your legs shoulder-width apart. Keeping your shoulders back and chest out, push your butt back and bend your knees as you reach for the barbell. Grasp it with both hands, palms facing in, shoulder-width apart.

Moving only from the hips, and keeping your butt pushed back to maintain your balance, pull the barbell up the front of your legs to your thighs. Slowly lower the barbell as far as you can while maintaining proper form. How to tell if your form is good? Stand sideways next to a mirror and observe yourself doing the exercise. If your shoulders or back begin to round at any point as you lower the bar, stop and return to the upright position. Unless you are quite flexible, you probably will not be returning the barbell to the floor between reps. Only do as many of these lifts as you can while maintaining proper form. If you can't sustain a straight back, stop. Work up to no more than three sets of 8 to 12 reps.

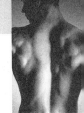

Ultimate Peak

No one wants you to do backbreaking work for a stronger spine. But if you have been doing a regular routine of back exercises, you might want to move to a higher level by adding these to your workout.

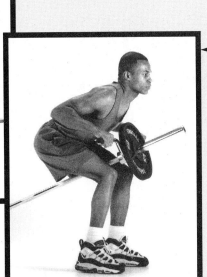

◄ T-Rows

Straddle a T-bar rowing machine with your feet firmly on the ground. Using a narrow grip, hold the T-bar slightly off the ground so your back is relatively straight and not hunched. Bend your legs slightly and keep your upper body as straight as possible, but bent over at the waist.

Lift the T-bar up toward your body as you would in a normal bent-over row. Bring the weight up as high as you can, or until it touches your lower chest. There will be a little more up-and-down movement of your upper body, but don't sway or rock to gain momentum. Your elbows should be pointing up and slightly out as you lift.

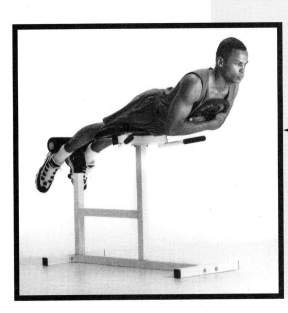

◄ Back Extensions with Weights

This is the same exercise as the standard back extension, only this time hold a weight plate to your chest by crossing your arms over it. Start with light weight, then add more as your muscles get stronger. Work up to three sets of 8 to 12 reps.

FACT The backbone we pride ourselves on having and showing in times of adversity is a figment of our imagination. In fact, what we think of as the backbone is really a series of small bones—33 to be exact.

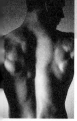
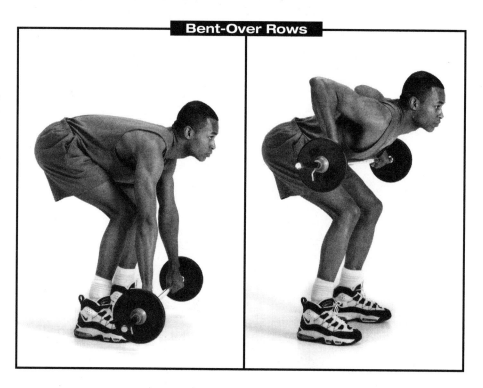

Bent-Over Rows

Bent-Over Rows ➤

To work your upper back, stand bent over at your waist, back straight, hands gripping a barbell palms down in a wide grip. Your feet are shoulder-width apart. Keep your legs straight and your knees unlocked.

Keeping your back straight, pull the barbell in toward your body so the bar is touching your lower chest. Your elbows should be pointing up toward the ceiling.

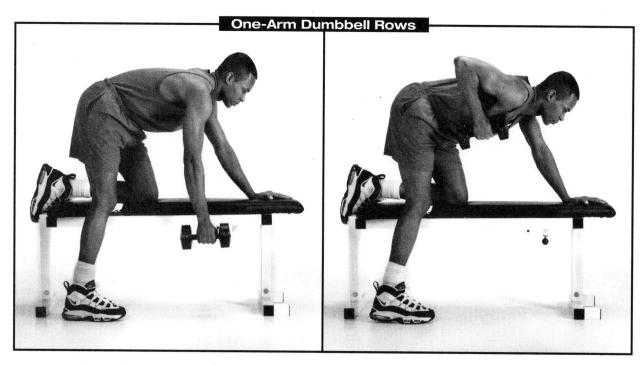

One-Arm Dumbbell Rows

One-Arm Dumbbell Rows ⋀

Stand partly over a bench, with your body weight resting on your bent left leg and left hand, both of which should be on the center of the padded portion of the bench. With your right foot firmly on the floor, hold a dumbbell in your right hand. Keep your back straight; your eyes should be facing the ground. Extend your right arm down toward the ground, elbow unlocked.

Pull the weight up and in toward your torso. Raise it as high as you can, bringing it in to your lower-chest muscles. Your right elbow should be pointing up toward the ceiling as you lift.

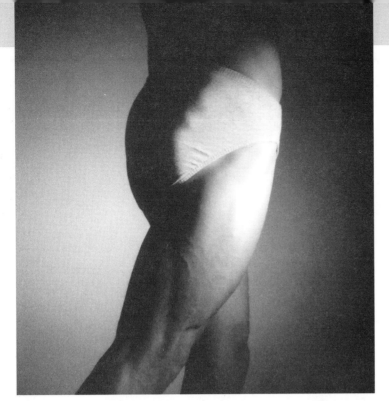

Buttocks

When it comes to a firm butt, most men are usually interested in those of the opposite sex, not their own. When we exercise, the butt muscles—or, to be more precise, the gluteal muscles—often get moved to the rear of the workout, and that's if they get worked at all.

But your glutes are not the kind of muscles you want to leave behind in your ongoing quest for powerful fitness. In the end, good glutes do more than give us a place to sit or a way to attract women—they actually help us to be more graceful and powerful in physical endeavors. At the gym, on the field, in your life, having a stronger rear end gives you important physiological advantages.

How to Be a Butthead

There are three main muscles to the butt. The largest and closest to the surface is the gluteus maximus. It forms the bulk of a buttock's mass. Beneath it is the gluteus medius, another thick muscle, though not as big as the gluteus maximus. It is a popular place for doctors to inject shots into. The third muscle is—you guessed it—the gluteus minimus, and it is the smallest and deepest of the three.

"The glutes are really important for your mobility—especially around the hips. Plus, they let you rotate and extend your legs," explains Doug Lentz, Pennsylvania state director of the

National Strength and Conditioning Association and owner of the Chambersburg Sports Medicine and Rehabilitation Center in Pennsylvania. These muscles—known as the gluteus maximus, gluteus medius and the gluteus minimus—hang on the upper part of your pelvic bone, forming a kind of hindquarter headquarters for explosive power. Plus, by stabilizing the pelvis and offering a strong foundation for your back, good glutes can help alleviate lower-back pain.

Because butt muscles are so closely involved with leg movement, many exercises you do for the legs also are great for the glutes, says Tom Jackson, P.T., a physical therapist at ARC Physical Therapy in Anaheim Hills, California. "Lunges, squats, leg presses—these exercises that we think of as good primarily for the thigh muscles also happen to work the gluteal muscles effectively," he says.

In addition to those leg exercises, you can target the glutes even more with the following toning routines—just consider them the means to a good end.

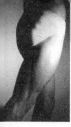

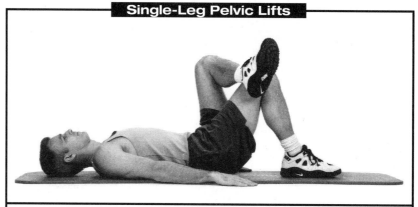

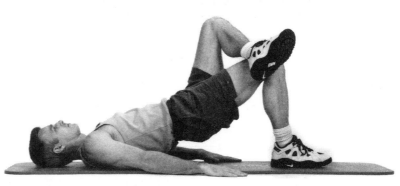

Single-Leg Pelvic Lifts ➤

Lie on your back with your right knee bent, foot flat on the floor. Cross your left leg over your right so your left ankle is resting a few inches above the knee of your right leg. Your arms should be at your sides, with your hands palms-down on the floor.

Now slowly and deliberately lift your pelvis up toward the ceiling. As you lift, clench your butt muscles together. Keep lifting until your back is straight—but not arched. Lower, then repeat. Work up to a maximum of three sets of 20 reps.

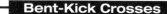

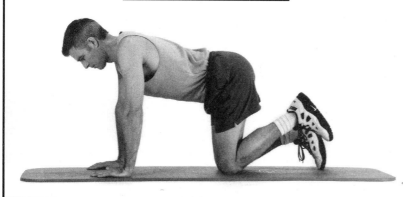

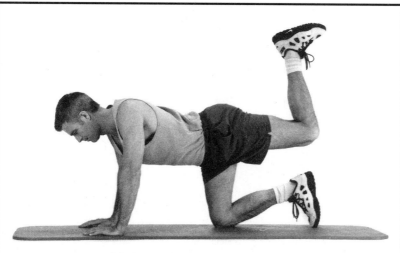

◄ Bent-Kick Crosses

To work the glutes with this exercise, get down on your hands and knees. Now raise one leg a few inches off the floor—bend it at about a 90-degree angle. This is your starting position.

Next, push your leg up and back, forcing your heel to the ceiling. Feel your glutes contract as you push up. *Note:* Don't let your thigh go beyond a position parallel to the floor. And as you're doing the exercise, make sure your leg stays bent at a 90-degree angle. Work up to a maximum of three sets of 20 reps for each leg.

Ultimate Peak

Exercises for the glutes are tough enough when you're lifting just your body weight. But when you start adding resistance weights to a lift, then you're talking about a serious butt-burner.

Bent-Kick Crosses with Ankle Weights

Try doing a bent-kick cross with some light ankle weights. When you do regular bent-kick crosses, you're giving your glutes a good workout because the position isolates them and you're working against gravity to push your leg up. Adding weights ups the intensity, but do so with caution. "You don't want to add too much weight before you're ready," says Doug Lentz, Pennsylvania state director of the National Strength and Conditioning Association and owner of the Chambersburg Sports Medicine and Rehabilitation Center in Pennsylvania. Also, as with any weighted lift, be sure to do the lift slowly and smoothly. "Don't jerk through the motion, especially when you have weight on an extremity," says Lentz. "If you swing around a lot or do the lift improperly, the momentum of that weight is increased and it could cause some damage."

Raised-Leg Curls ▶

Get down on all fours on the floor wearing an ankle weight on your left foot. Raise your left leg to about butt level and extend it straight, away from your body and roughly parallel to the floor.

Curl your heel toward your butt until your lower leg is perpendicular to the floor. Keep your thigh parallel to the ground. Your thigh shouldn't move much—all the movement is done below the knee. Don't sway your body or arch your back, and concentrate on the contraction in your butt. Do one to three sets of 8 to 12 reps for each leg. If this exercise gets too easy, you can progress to using a leg curl machine or the Rumanian dead lift, suggests Lentz.

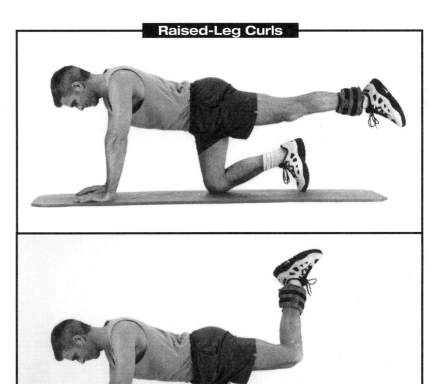

Raised-Leg Curls

FACT Anthropologists see our butts as a milestone in human evolution, created when early man began to stand and walk upright. Our glutes adapted to this new posture by expanding and becoming more rounded, forming the familiar protuberant human butt.

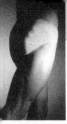

Jump Squats ►

This exercise is a cousin to the squats you do for leg strength, only it has a slightly more dynamic component to really get your butt muscles working. Start by standing with your feet slightly more than shoulder-width apart, with your arms crossed in front of you. Keep your head up and back straight, and squat until your thighs are almost parallel to the floor.

Now jump straight up. But don't let your lower legs power this jump—concentrate on getting the force from your butt, thighs and hips. Return to the squat position and repeat. When you reach the point where doing a set of, say, 20 reps becomes easy, try it holding five-pound dumbbells at your sides.

Jump Squats

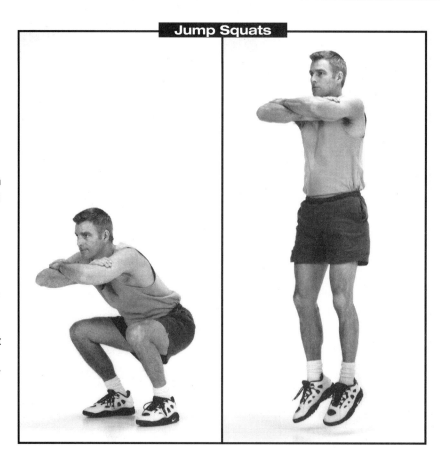

Narrow Dumbbell Squats

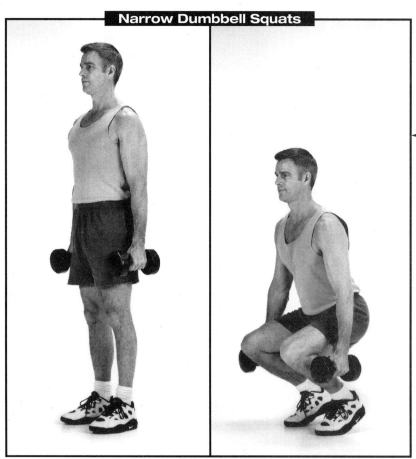

◄ Narrow Dumbbell Squats

For this modified squat, you'll need two dumbbells. Hold one in each hand, arms at your sides, palms facing your body. Stand with your feet only a few inches apart.

Squat down until your thighs are parallel to the floor. Don't bounce. As you come back up, flex your quadriceps and your butt muscles as much as you can. Keep your back straight throughout, and don't lean forward.

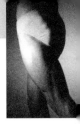

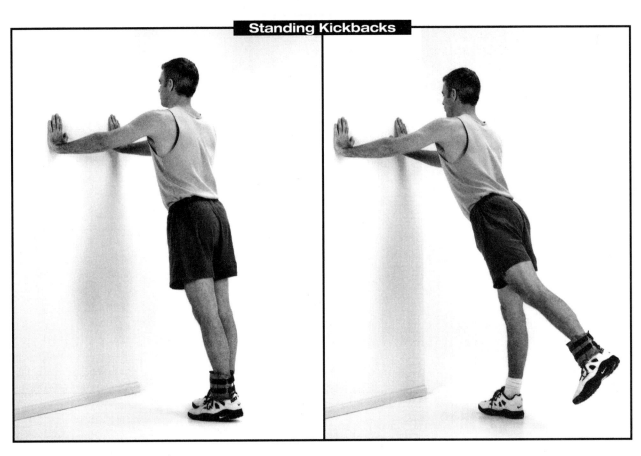

Standing Kickbacks ⬥

With an ankle weight on one leg, stand facing a wall, leaning slightly forward so your whole body is in a straight line. Your weight should be shifted to the unweighted leg. Place one or both hands lightly on the wall, just for balance.

Now slowly move the weighted leg back as far as you can, feeling the contraction in your butt. The knee of your weighted leg should be slightly bent. Don't arch your back or overextend your leg. Hold for a few seconds before lowering. When you've done about ten reps, switch the weight to the other leg and repeat the lift again.

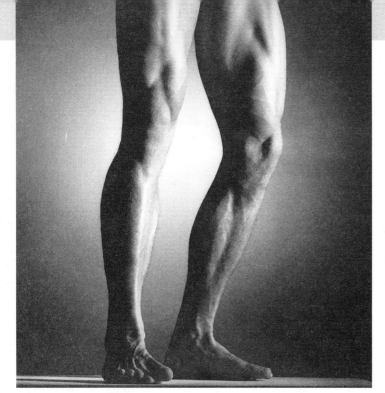

Legs

You hate doing leg exercises. It's okay to admit it. The plain truth of it is that most men resent doing any leg work, whether it's on the job or in the gym. Oh, running or stair-climbing is all well and good, but when it comes time to do the lifts and curls so necessary to toning your thighs and calves . . . well, let's just say it's not as much fun as a good bench press or biceps curl.

"Guys hate it, hate it, hate it—they always leave leg exercises until the end of the workout—and then conveniently forget to do them. Their excuse is that they get a good leg workout from playing sports or using the treadmill," says Doug Lentz, Pennsylvania state director of the National Strength and Conditioning Association and owner of the Chambersburg Sports Medicine and Rehabilitation Center in Pennsylvania. "That stuff is fun. Leg exercises feel too much like work."

How to Be a Leg Man

Don't kid yourself—leg exercises are hard work. But if you want to beat your opponents and succeed in your goal of total-body fitness, you can't cut off your legs.

"It almost goes without saying that your legs are the key to almost every sport you play. They're vital for your speed, your

jumping power, your stamina—the list goes on and on," says Tom Jackson, P.T., a physical therapist at ARC Physical Therapy in Anaheim Hills, California.

Some of the most powerful muscles in our bodies reside in the space between the hips and the ankles. On the front of your thighs, you have the quadriceps, the workhorses of the legs. Whether you're running, jumping or pushing, your quads are right in the thick of it, channeling the power of your lower body.

On the inside and outside of your thighs, you have adductor and abductor muscles, respectively. These muscles run all the way up to the hip and help you close your legs or move them out to the side.

Meanwhile, on the back side of your thighs are the hamstrings, the cords of muscle that work opposite the quadriceps. Everything the quads get you into, the hams get you out of. When you coil for a leap, the hamstrings help spring you forward; when you swing your leg back for a kick, the quads help you put that extra snap on the ball. Working together, your hams and quads also serve another vital function— they stabilize and protect your knees.

Moving down to the lower part of your legs, you have the calves. Your stability and balance absolutely depend on these muscles, since your calves help you maneuver and position your feet. They also stabilize your ankles. Finally, on the front of your lower leg, there lie the tibialis and other shin muscles. You've noticed these muscles if you've ever had a case of shinsplints. But they do more than make you feel stiff after a hard run; they support your arches and also help you raise your foot.

As Lentz points out, the advantages to a consistent leg regimen are manifest in two important ways. "These muscles are a large part of what makes you fast and powerful. To put it simply, the more you do leg lifts and similar exercises, the better your speed and explosiveness will be." So stop pulling your own leg and start getting serious about shaping the muscles that will enable you to run faster and jump higher. Here's how.

Put your legs first. If you're constantly rationalizing your way out of legwork, Lentz says to make leg exercises the first stop on your exercise circuit. "It's like doing chores on a Saturday—get the hardest ones done first and enjoy the rest of the day. Also, most exercise specialists suggest doing your large muscle, multi-joint exercises first." In the case of fitness training, shift your workout routine so you save the routines you enjoy—like chest exercises—until the very end. "Now you have something to work toward," says Lentz.

Warm up without wearing out. The other problem with letting stair-climbing, cycling and running serve as your warm-up exercises is that men have a tendency to overdo these warm-ups and end up wearing their legs out. "Do that, and you won't feel like doing any specific weight training with your legs, which is bad," says Lentz. Remember, a warm-up is light exercise intended to get your blood pumping, not the first leg of an Ironman competition. Keep your warm-up time to ten minutes, and if you warm up on a machine, put it at a moderate setting. If you run to warm up, keep your running to a light jog, not a hard sprint.

Stretch your legs a bit. Few muscles are tighter than the ones in our legs. The hips, thighs and calves are all in the constant business of keeping us the upright men we are, which means they can get pretty tightly wound from the constant stress of carrying us around. You can make exercising easier on your leg muscles by taking a few minutes to stretch them before and after your workout. "Make it part of your warm-up—after you've done the initial warming up part. You never want to stretch a cold muscle," says Jackson. Be sure to do stretches for the hamstrings and quads. And when you do a modified hurdler stretch, pull your foot and toes toward you, which will stretch the calf, too.

Don't lock yourself out. When you do your leg lifts, make them slow and smooth. "And don't lock your knees when you're pushing out or lifting up. You want your knees to be slightly flexed, just shy of full extension," says Lentz. Never mind that locking your knees out while lifting weights can cause serious knee injuries—it's also cheating your leg muscles out of a workout because the knees are holding the weight your muscles were supposed to be handling.

Upper Legs

Leg Press ►

"This is one of the best all-around leg exercises," says Jackson, and with good reason, since the leg press works most of the upper-leg muscles, especially the quadriceps, the muscles on top of the thighs, which help you leap and sprint.

To do this exercise, you'll need a leg press machine—sit in it with your feet on the foot plate in front of you (make sure the seat is adjusted so your knees are bent at about a 90-degree angle or slightly less). Grasp the handlebars at your sides and hold your upper body upright, but relaxed.

Now push forward on the foot plates and straighten your legs until they're almost fully extended in front of you. Keep your knees slightly flexed—not locked. Your upper body should remain upright and relaxed, and your hands should hold the handlebars for support.

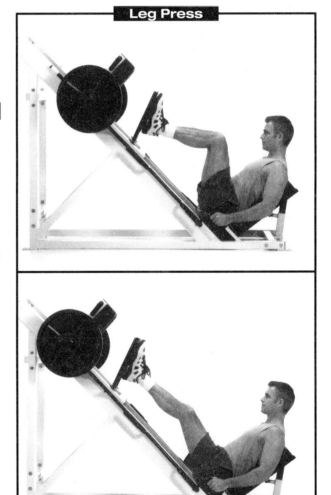

Leg Press

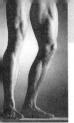

Dumbbell Lunges ►

A great hip and leg exercise. Start by standing upright with a dumbbell in each hand. Your arms should be fully extended at your sides, and your palms should be facing in. Your feet should be about hip-width apart, torso upright.

Step forward with your left leg farther than you would in a normal step. Your upper body should remain upright and slightly forward. Your left leg should be bent at a 90-degree angle; your knee shouldn't be out beyond your toes. Your back leg should be bent at the knee. Your rear foot should remain in the same position—it's okay if the heel is raised slightly, though. Once you've done 10 to 12 reps, switch legs, or you can alternate feet if you prefer. If you are a beginner and want to be particularly careful, you can start off without using weights. Make sure that you are comfortable moving through the full range of motion before you pick up the dumbbells.

Dumbbell Lunges

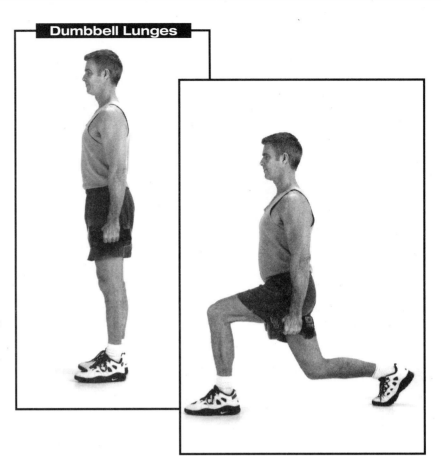

Squats

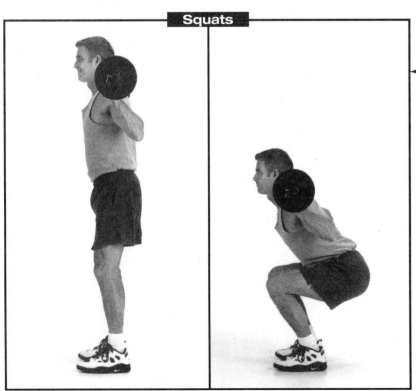

◄ Squats

This barbell exercise works not only the quads but also the hamstrings, the muscles on the backsides of your thighs. Hold the barbell with your palms facing forward and place it behind your neck—it should be even across your upper shoulder muscles. Stand up straight with your feet hip-width apart, toes forward and slightly out. Bend your knees slightly, and lean slightly forward.

Now squat down as though you're about to sit in a chair. Your thighs should be parallel to the floor. Keep your feet flat. Rise to the starting position.

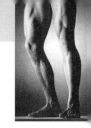

Dumbbell Step-Ups and Step-Downs

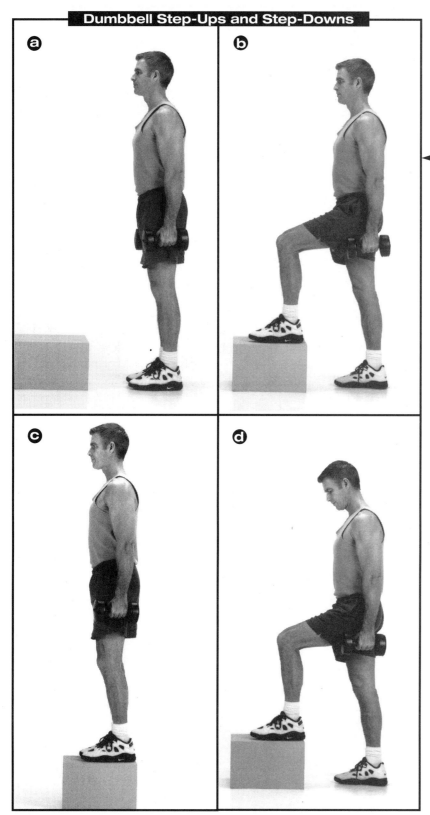

◄ Dumbbell Step-Ups and Step-Downs

ⓐ Hold a dumbbell in each hand, palms facing your body, arms extended down at your sides. Stand upright, with your shoulders back and chest out. You should be standing about one step away from a sturdy box that's roughly 12 to 18 inches high. It's best to do this on a nonslip floor so the box doesn't shift.

ⓑ Step forward with your left foot, placing it in the center of the box as you step. Keep the dumbbells at your sides; your upper body should still be straight and upright.

ⓒ Complete the step so that you're standing on top of the box, feet together in the center. The dumbbells should be hanging at your sides, and your body should be upright.

ⓓ Step backward so the foot of your right leg is at about the starting position. The step will be slightly longer than an average step. Bring the other foot back to the starting position. Repeat, this time leading off with your right leg. Do up to three sets of 8 to 15 reps.

FACT Some men are so desperate to have good legs without doing any work that they're willing to get calf implants. For around $6,500 to $8,000, a plastic surgeon cuts open your legs and inserts plastic sheaths that make each leg look fuller and stronger.

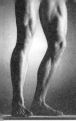

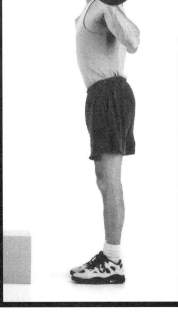

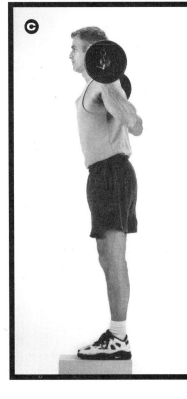

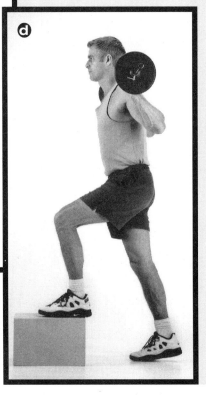

Ultimate Peak

If you want to make your legs go the extra mile, be a barbell barbarian and try this exercise. This is quite similar to the dumbbell step-ups and step-downs in the chapter, but it uses a barbell instead. It's much more challenging, however, because it tests your balance and shoulders as well as your legs' lifting muscles.

◄ Barbell Step-Ups and Step-Downs

ⓐ Hold a barbell with a moderate weight—something you could easily lift 10 to 15 times—behind your neck, evenly across your shoulders. Your palms should be facing out. Stand upright, with your shoulders back and chest out, with a slight forward lean in your lower back. Stand about a step away from a sturdy box that's roughly 12 to 18 inches high and sitting on a nonslip surface.

ⓑ Step forward with your left foot, placing it in the center of the box. Keep your body erect, with the barbell in position behind your neck.

ⓒ Shift your weight to your left leg as you step the rest of the way onto the box. When you've completed the step, both feet should be together in the center.

ⓓ Step backward so the foot of your right leg is at about the starting position. Bring your other foot back to the starting position. Now repeat, this time leading off with your right leg. Do up to three sets of 8 to 15 reps. As this gets easier, you can increase the weight or the number of reps.

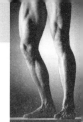

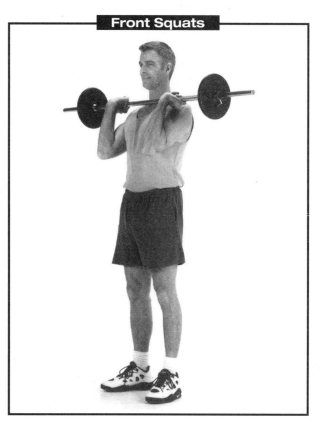

Front Squats

Front Squats ►

Do this squat with the same technique as a traditional squat, except grasp the bar palms-up, hands shoulder-width apart. Your elbows should be pointing forward as the barbell rests across your upper chest.

Leg Extensions

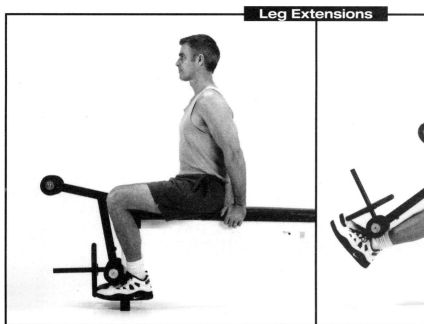

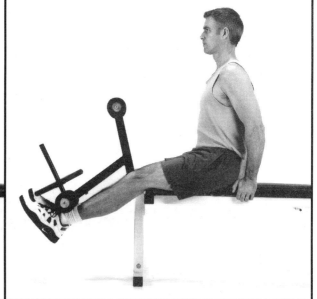

Leg Extensions ▲

For the leg extension, sit in an extension machine, with your legs behind the padded lifting bars and your hands grasping the bench or, if available, the machine's handles at the sides of your body. Your knees should be bent at 90 degrees or slightly more, with your toes pointing in front of you.

Straighten your legs by lifting with your ankles and contracting your quads. Don't lock your knees at full extension. Your toes should be pointing up and slightly out. To work out the muscles even more, do the lift using only one leg at a time.

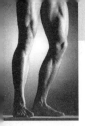

Leg Curls ►

Curls burn your hamstrings and your calves. Lie on a leg curl machine, with your ankles hooked behind the lifting pads and your knees just over the bench's edge. Hold onto the bench or the machine's handlebars, if available, for support. Your legs should be fully extended with some flex at the knee. Your toes should be pointing down.

Keep your pelvis pressed against the bench and raise your heels up toward your butt so that your legs bend to about a 90-degree angle. Keep your feet pointing out away from your body.

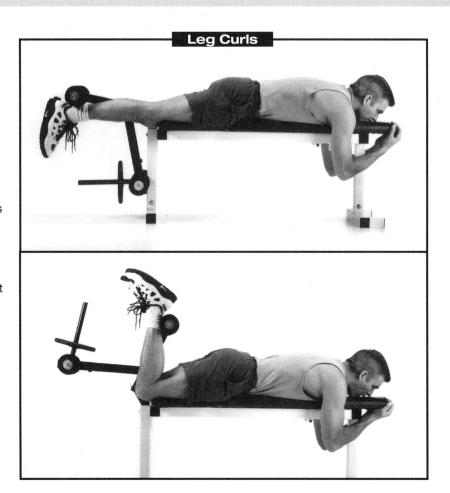

Leg Curls

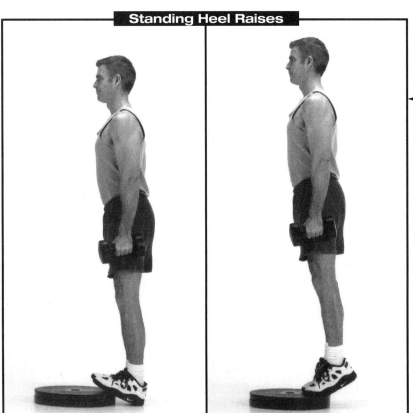

Standing Heel Raises

Lower Legs

◄ Standing Heel Raises

If you want to raise prize calves, stand with a dumbbell in each hand. Your feet should be hip-width apart, with your toes on a platform, weight or block a couple of inches off the ground. Your heels should be on the floor, with your arms extended at your sides. Put your weight on the balls of your feet so you're leaning forward slightly.

Rise all the way up onto your toes. Feel the contraction in your calves and pause briefly at the top. Your arms should remain in position, though your body will probably be more upright. Lower. Do one to three sets of 8 to 15 reps.

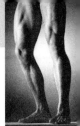

Seated Toe Raises

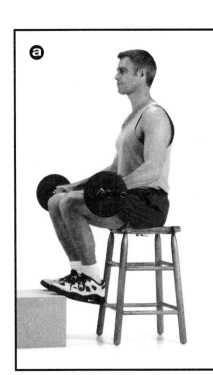 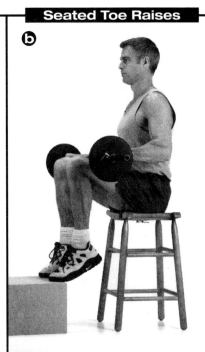 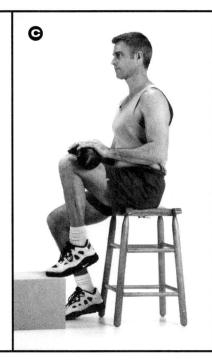

Seated Toe Raises ▲

ⓐ Another calf-carver, this raise is begun by sitting down, with the balls of your feet on a raised platform or footstool about a foot away from your seat. Your heels should be off the platform. Hold a barbell on your upper legs, a few inches away from your knees.

ⓑ Now slowly and deliberately raise up your toes as high as possible. Hold for a moment, then relax and re-peat. Your hands should only be steadying the barbell in

your lap—don't let them carry any of the weight. Do two to three sets of 20 to 30 reps.

ⓒ *Note:* If you have dumbbells, you can do these exercises one leg at a time. Use your hands to rest the dumbbell on your thigh a few inches away from the knee and repeat the lift as above. Switch legs when you've completed your set.

Man and Machine

Nowadays, many experts are shying away from two popular machine exercises—leg extensions and leg curls.

"They don't approximate any activity that you do in everyday life. But they're not exactly bad for you, if you do them correctly," says Doug Lentz, Pennsylvania state director of the National Strength and Conditioning Association and owner of the Chambersburg Sports Medicine and Rehabilitation Center in Pennsylvania. The operative term here is "correctly," especially where the leg extension machine is concerned. "If your knee is too far back or too far

forward from the edge of the seat, you can cause problems," Lentz warns.

Still, if your goal is to have upper legs with that extra bit of definition, and if you're careful, you can put these sculpting machines at the end of your workout.

Meanwhile, don't shy away from leg-working machines entirely. If you do, you'll miss one of the best leg exercises going—the leg press. "Now that's one I do recommend," says Lentz. "It's safe, it's simple and it really lets you put a lot of leg muscles through their paces."

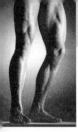
Toe Raises with Seated Leg Press Machine ➤

Sit in a leg press machine and push against the plate with your feet until your legs are fully extended.

Press forward with your toes and the balls of your feet, pushing the foot pad forward a few inches. Feel your calf muscles contract. Hold the press a moment, then relax. To work your main calf muscles, keep your feet straight. To work your outer calves, point your toes in, with your heels out. To work your inner calves, change that position to toes out and heels in. When you are done, carefully return the plate to its original position.

An important note: Leg press machines vary considerably in design. If the plates on your machine permit, do this exercise with your heels extending below the bottom edge of the plate so that just the balls of your feet are touching. This will permit you to move your foot through its full range of motion as you do the exercise. However, many machines have large plates that prohibit hanging your heels; in this case, your foot extension will be less.

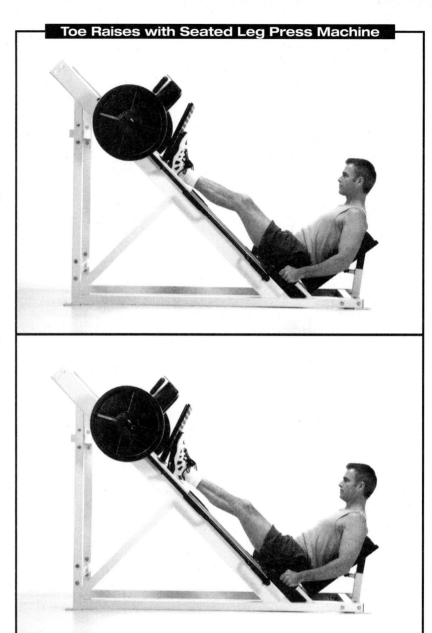

Toe Raises with Seated Leg Press Machine

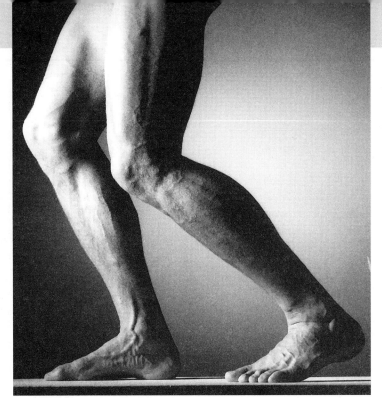

Leg Joints

Leg joints—hips, knees and ankles—get dished some of the hardest physical punishment in a man's life. Did you know just the simple act of walking up a flight of stairs puts hundreds of pounds of pressure on the knees and ankles—with each step?

"When they exercise their legs, most people don't really do it with the idea of strengthening their hip or knee joints," says Dan Hamner, M.D., director of sports medicine and rehabilitation for the New York State Athletic Association and visiting professor of rehabilitation at New York Hospital in New York City. But you'll sure notice those joints when they're bent out of shape or feel like they're grinding themselves into powder with every move you make.

You can start right now to do leg lifts and stretching exercises that will not simply build muscle, but build *balanced* muscle, creating a solid yet supple latticework that will support the joints, keeping them where they belong, and keeping you where you belong—in the game, not sidelined with a bad hip or a bum knee. Here's a quick look at each of the major leg joints, along with some ways you can keep them from getting out of joint.

Getting Hip to Leg Joints

But first let's look at what your leg joints do. Hips are the pivotal structure on a man's body—literally. When we swing a bat or a racquet, throw a punch, or block an opponent from shooting a basketball, we get much of our power from our hips. "The muscles that cross the hip joint are very strong to begin with, but they can get very tight on you," says Dr. Hamner. "You don't need to just strengthen these muscles; you need to stretch them. A lot."

Knees, meanwhile, are the most commonly injured joint on men. We blow them out doing squats the wrong way; we tear them up on the basketball court; we ruin them in football games.

"On the lower body, it seems like knees take all the punishment when we're physically active. They have to deal with the impact of our own body weight as well as the pressure of stopping and starting, making fast turns. And if you get hit—someone tackles you or falls on you—then you have someone else's body weight and momentum to deal with," says Todd Ellenbecker, P.T., clinical director of Physiotherapy Associates Scottsdale Sports Clinic in Arizona. With the knees, your emphasis should be on strengthening the muscles nearby—especially the quadriceps and hamstrings. "The stronger the surrounding muscles are, the more they'll absorb shock and shore up the knee," says Ellenbecker.

Ankles are the last of the major leg joints, and they're almost as frequently wracked up as the knee. The ankle joint is a pivotal but delicate area, where your leg and foot bones are connected to the main ankle bone. It's a center of power in terms of your speed and mobility as well as your balance. Ironically, many of the ills that befall the ankle are problems we bring on ourselves.

"Wearing the wrong shoe for an activity, putting yourself off-balance by improper form—those are just a couple of ways you can really injure your ankle—and believe me, I see a lot of sprained ankles among athletic men," says Dr. Hamner.

But you don't have to be one of those men. Here, we recommend several ways to keep your joints strong and flexible. Don't treat these like strength-building exercises and try to jam on as much weight as you can. Your joints won't like that. Follow the specific number of reps we list and use light weights. Plus, with a few additional tricks, you can keep the stress on your leg joints to a minimum.

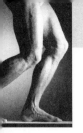

Be a gait keeper. If you've been getting twinges in your hips when you run or when you do exercises like lunges, the problem may not be your hip joint after all.

"Sometimes hip problems, especially tightness, come indirectly from walking on the outside edge of your feet," says Dr. Hamner. That's called supination. To see if you do it, check the soles of your shoes: If the outer edge of the forefoot is worn more than any other part of the shoe, chances are you're a supinator. "It's not a serious problem unless you do a lot of running and neglect to stretch the short rotator muscles around the hip," says Dr. Hamner.

A sports medicine doctor can check your gait by having you run on a treadmill. If that isn't possible, an experienced podiatrist can check your walking gait and determine if you need special insoles to correct the problem. Or you can shop around a good athletic shoe store. "Many shoes today are designed for people who walk on the inner or outer edge of their feet. If you can get yourself a pair, you'll be saving yourself some trouble down the line," says Dr. Hamner.

Do it right. When you're in crouching positions, such as during a squat or while you're in a tuck for sports like skiing, try to keep your thighs parallel to the floor. If you go down any lower and then try to come back up, you can risk putting too much strain on the knee, says Michael Bemben, Ph.D., assistant professor of health and sport sciences at the University of Oklahoma in Norman. "You especially want to avoid anything where you're doing deep, ballistic knee bends—that really hyperflexes the knees and stretches the ligaments around them too much," says Dr. Bemben.

Do some sole-searching. Make sure you're wearing the right shoe for the right sport. "Cross-trainers are good, especially for weight training," explains Tom Brunick, director of the Athlete's Foot WearTest Center at North Central College in Naperville, Illinois, and a technical editor for *Runner's World* magazine. As Brunick explains, cross-trainers are designed to help protect the foot and ankle, giving them more support. "The base of support that's built into the design of the shoe is especially important when you're doing side-to-side motions, as you

will in a lot of sports. It helps stabilize the foot and keeps you on balance."

One note: If you run, buy a running shoe, not a cross-trainer. "Because of the impact running has on joints, you really need a shoe designed with a lot of cushioning and support for the straight-ahead motion of running," says Brunick. Running shoes are specially designed to support those needs.

Strengthen with sport. Different sports that can strengthen and tighten the muscles around the knee are actually good, not bad, say the experts.

"If you don't overdo it, it's actually very good to do some exercise that works the muscles around the knee—the quads, the hamstrings. The stronger they are, the better they'll support the knee," says Dr. Bemben. Cycling, in-line skating and stair-climbing are some good examples of knee strengtheners.

Get a leg under you. Although a shoe can certainly help you in the ankle-support department, it can't do all the work. You can help ankle strength and stability by doing balance exercises.

"There's a simple exercise you can do—I call it the stork leg," says Dr. Hamner. "All you do is just stand on one leg and balance on it. Do it for as long as you can." As you get better, shift your weight on the leg you're standing, shifting first to the inside of the foot, then to the outer edge of the foot. Or, as you're standing, swing your free leg in front of the leg you're standing on, bring it back to your side, then swing it back behind your leg, keeping your balance all the while.

Other ankle strengtheners are knock-kneed and bowlegged heel raises. These are similar to the standing heel raises mentioned in the Legs chapter on page 94, except you don't use weights. For the bowlegged heel raises, splay your feet outward. When you raise your heels, roll to the inside part of your forefoot. For knock-kneed heel raises, start with your feet splayed inward. When you lift your heels, roll to the outside of your forefoot. Do two sets of 50 reps. For variety, Dr. Hamner suggests doing these one leg at a time. Stand about 18 inches away from a wall and support yourself against the wall with your hands. Wrap the toes of your free leg around the back of your working leg and do two sets of 20 reps.

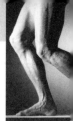

Hips

Hip Abductors

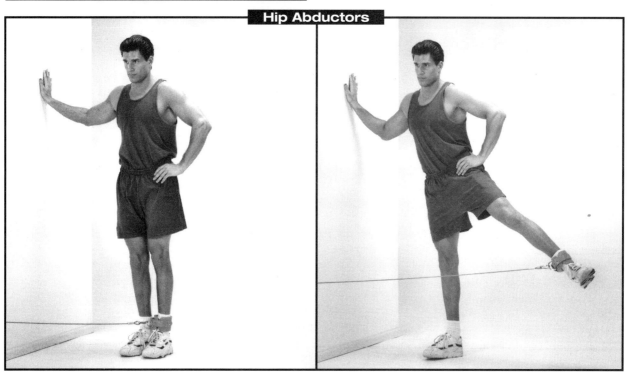

Hip Abductors ▲

This exercise strengthens and stretches your abductor muscles—the ones responsible for moving your leg out to the side. You'll need some kind of low-lying pulley mechanism for this exercise. Some gyms have pulley machines just for this exercise; others have wall-mounted units. You could even use an elastic cord in a pinch. Stand straight, legs together, with your right side facing the pulley. The ankle strap should be around your left ankle. Stand back so that the line attached to the ankle strap is taut.

Raise your left leg out to the side as far as possible, keeping your back straight. Don't bend your knee or swing from side to side. Lower your leg to the starting position. Use a light weight and do 12 to 20 reps, then switch legs.

Hip Flexions

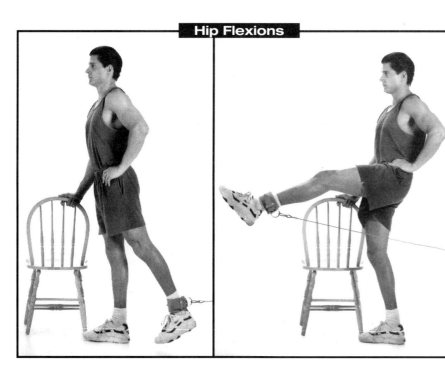

◄ Hip Flexions

Another pulley-machine exercise, this one works your hip flexors. These muscles let you swing your leg forward and are essential for kicking and running. Stand facing away from the pulley, with the ankle strap on your left ankle. Grab a support in front of you, something waist-high so you won't have to bend over.

Raise your left leg in front of you until your thigh is parallel to the floor. Keep your leg and back straight; don't bend forward or backward. Use a light weight, do 12 to 20 reps and then switch legs.

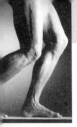

Knees

Inside Leg Lifts ►

This lift strengthens the muscles on the inside of your thigh, which helps reinforce proper kneecap alignment.

Start by lying on your left side, with your left leg outstretched, right leg bent and right foot flat on the floor behind your left leg. Support your head with your left hand; use your right hand for balance.

Now slowly lift your left leg off the floor, raising it toward the ceiling as high as possible. Hold at the top of the lift, then lower. Do 10 to 12 reps, then switch legs. To make the exercise slightly more difficult, strap on some 2½- to 5-pound ankle weights.

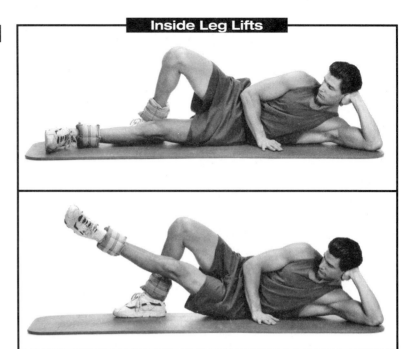

Inside Leg Lifts

Outside Leg Lifts ►

This is an exercise that helps create proper kneecap alignment, but it's also good for the hip joint, since it works muscles on the outside of the hip.

Lie on your right side with both of your legs outstretched; support your head with your right arm.

Lift your left leg up and back slowly. Keep your knee straight, but let your toes drop a bit so your heel is pointing toward the ceiling. Raise the leg about 18 inches, hold for a moment, then lower. Do 10 to 12 reps, then switch sides. As with the inside leg lift, you can add ankle weights to make the lifts more challenging.

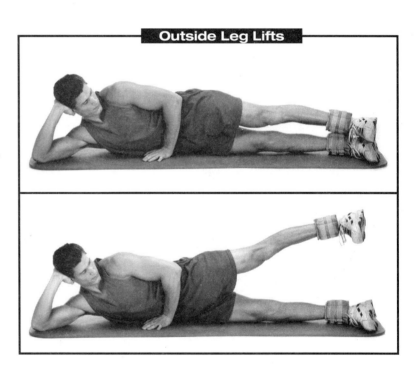

Outside Leg Lifts

FACT You may be able to reduce your risk of ankle sprains simply by wearing high-top athletic shoes. In one study, high-tops were shown to provide a third more protection against ankle sprains than low-tops.

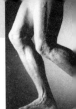

Soothing Your Joints

Got a bum knee? Cramped hips? Achy ankles? Even the strongest leg joints may deal you a few aches and pains every now and again. But you can get quick pain relief using these simple techniques.

• For nagging knees: If you've strained a knee ligament, you can avoid future pain by gently stretching it. After the knee stops hurting, try this: Stand, putting one hand against a wall for support. Slowly bending your knee, reach down and grab the toes of the injured leg with your opposite hand. Pull on your foot until the heel is close to your butt. Tighten the buttock of the leg you are lifting. The muscles will be a little sore, but stop if you feel any sharp pains. Hold for 20 seconds, then relax. Repeat, this time pulling your leg a bit further back. Do both knees.

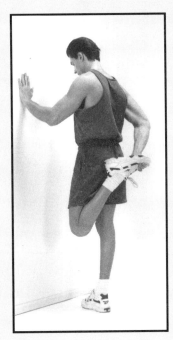

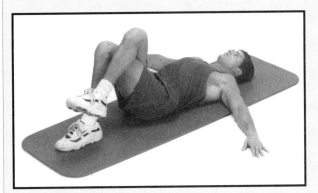

• For looser hips: If your hips feel like they're seizing up every time you start to make a break for the basket, try a secretary stretch. It works the short rotator muscles around your hip. Lie on your back with your knees up and together and your feet flat on the floor. Put your right leg over your left leg.

Now use your right leg to pull your left leg toward the floor, until you start to feel a good stretch in the left hip. Keep your upper back, head and shoulders flat on the floor. Don't touch the floor with your left knee; just pull it down to a level that feels appropriate. You might wish to extend your right arm for balance. Repeat on the other side.

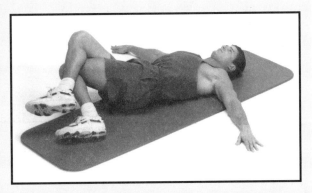

• For a sprained ankle: After you've elevated and iced the ankle, the best thing you can do for it is to gradually get back on your feet again, says Dan Hamner, M.D., director of sports medicine and rehabilitation for the New York State Athletic Association and visiting professor of rehabilitation at New York Hospital in New York City. "I'm not saying get up and run on it. But once your doctor has determined it's just a sprain, after a day or so, you do want to start getting back to your regular walking pattern." Dr. Hamner suggests trying to put a little weight on the injured leg. "You'll get the muscles contracting, and that's going to help with any swelling." But be sure to care for the injured joint, too. "A couple times a day, you'll still want to get it elevated and put some ice on it for about 15 minutes or so at a time."

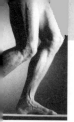

Freehand Squats

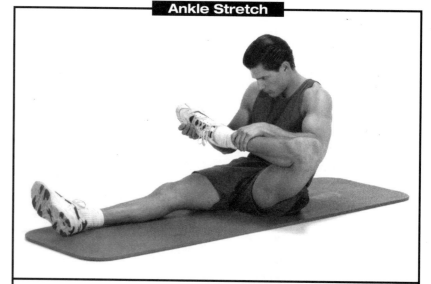

◄ Freehand Squats

This exercise is similar to the squat you'd use with free weights, but doing it without weights allows you to focus on the motion of the exercise, without putting too much pressure on the knees.

Stand with your feet flat on the floor, shoulder-width apart. Fold your arms in front of your chest. Keeping your back straight, slowly bend your knees until your thighs are parallel to the floor. Hold, then slowly return to the starting position. Do up to 20 reps, or until you start to feel a burn in your quads, the top muscles of your thigh (they help support the ligaments of your knee). Stop if you feel any knee pain. If you are having balance trouble doing this exercise, hold an unweighted dowel or broomstick behind you across your shoulders.

Ankles

Ankle Stretch ►

Help keep your ankle supple with this stretch. Sit on the floor and bend one leg up to you so you're grasping your lower leg with one hand and holding your foot with the other.

Now rotate your ankle clockwise and counter-clockwise, like a pendulum. Do 10 to 20 swings, then switch legs.

Ankle Stretch

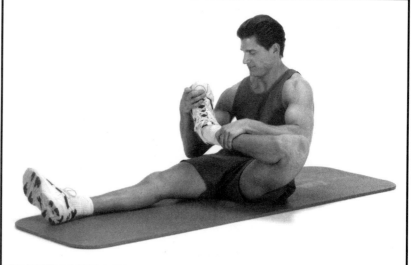

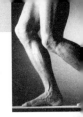

Side Ankle Lifts

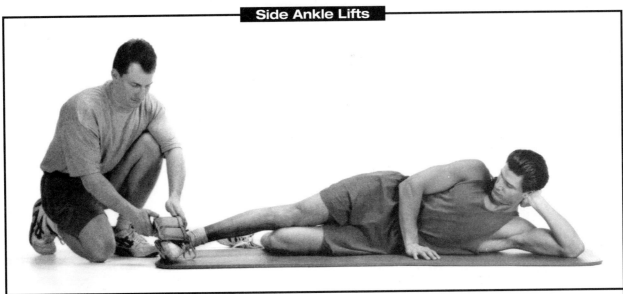

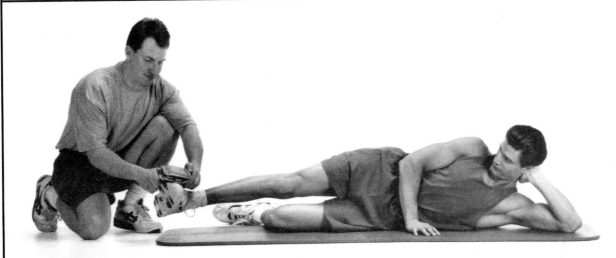

Side Ankle Lifts ▲

This lift works the stabilizing muscles on your ankle. Lie on your left side with your right leg straight and your left leg bent—your knees should be together with your left foot behind you.

Now rotate your foot to the right—the little toe should be pointing toward the ceiling. Your heel will lift some as you do this, but the important part of the exercise is the rotation of the foot, not the lift. Pause for a moment, then lower the foot. Do at least 30 to 50 of these, then switch legs.

Note: For more resistance, have a partner place a light ankle weight across the edge of your foot. He'll need to hold it in place as you do the exercise.

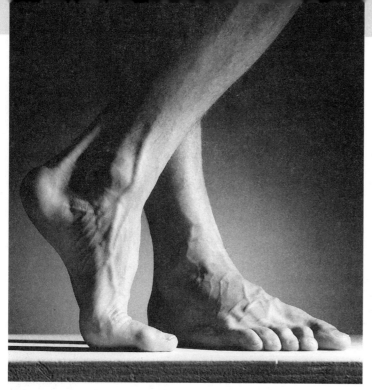

Feet

In the course of the average day—filled with all the usual running, walking, stair-climbing and foot-tapping—the average man's feet absorb roughly three million pounds of pressure. It's a wonder our feet don't fail us more often than they do.

The pounding rises dramatically when you throw in a little physical activity. Running tacks on an additional 500 pounds of pressure with each stride. Other exercise can put even more pressure on your feet, creating times that will try any man's soles.

"If you're playing any sport where you have to use your feet—and that's pretty much all of them—it starts to become obvious what a good idea it is to work on the foot muscles as well as the muscles that help you move the foot, like the calf and shin muscles," says Allen Kinley, assistant strength and conditioning coach at Texas A&M University in College Station. The reasons are simple, says Kinley: First and foremost, you'll keep those muscles stronger and the ankle joint limber.

The foot is a complex network of 26 bones, 56 ligaments and 38 muscles. That's a lot of moving parts, which could explain why 87 percent of us suffer from foot pain during our lives.

Now, toe strength is not a trivial thing, particularly if you do a lot of hiking or climbing. Toes help you keep your balance by constantly bending and shifting to adjust your weight. They also play a key role in pushing your body forward. Want to see how important they are? Curl them up tightly and try to walk. It's not easy. Our point: It is not at all goofy to take a few minutes to build up toe strength and dexterity.

Keeping Your Dogs from Barking

"The muscles around the foot are notoriously tight—we're always putting a tremendous amount of pressure on them, even when we're just walking," says Dan Hamner, M.D., director of sports medicine and rehabilitation for the New York State Athletic Association and visiting professor of rehabilitation at New York Hospital in New York City. The more you can stretch and work these muscles, adds Dr. Hamner, the less sore and more on balance you'll be. Bonus: You're also less likely to suffer the nagging foot cramps you've probably felt from time to time, usually when you're doing something like pushing the limits of your morning run. So if you don't want your feet to fail you now—or ever—try these feats of strength.

Foot Stretches ►

Before you put your feet through their paces—whether it's a pick-up basketball game or a 10-K run—be sure to warm up those muscles first. "Do a brief warm-up activity, such as slow jogging, and follow that up with some stretching—especially if you're about to go running," says Dr. Hamner. Then try a modified hurdler's stretch: Sit on the floor, put your left leg out straight in front of you; bend your right leg so the bottom of your right foot is resting against the inside of your left thigh. Now bend forward from your hips, stretching your arms out as far as you can toward your left ankle. For an even better stretch, if you are flexible enough, use one hand to pull the toes of your outstretched leg toward your knee. Hold the stretch for 20 seconds, then switch legs.

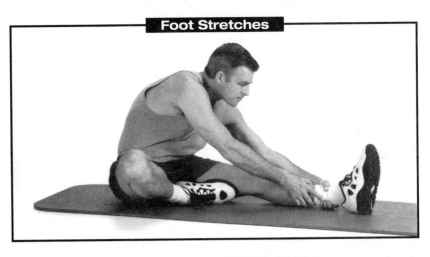

Foot Stretches

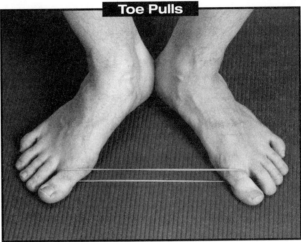

Toe Pulls

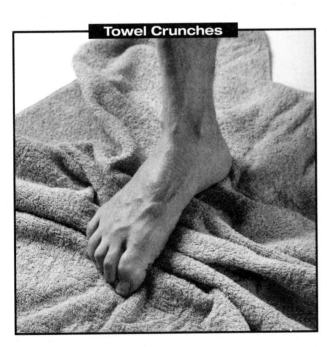

Towel Crunches

Towel Crunches ▲

Take off your shoes and socks and sit on a chair. Spread a towel across the floor and, grasping one end with your toes, crunch it under your feet—essentially, you're making fists with your toes. Use the muscles in the bottom of your feet and in your toes as well. Keep your heel on the floor at all times. Repeat with your other foot.

Toe Pulls ▲

All you need for these exercises is a rubber band. With your feet flat on the floor, side by side, place one thick rubber band around your big toes and pivot at your heels to move your feet away from each other, out to the sides. Hold for five seconds. Do ten reps.

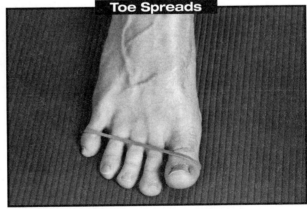

Toe Spreads

Toe Spreads ▲

Put a rubber band around all the toes of one foot and spread them. Do ten reps of five seconds each. Repeat on the other side.

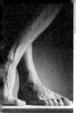

Weighted Foot Flexes ▶

Sit on a table so your feet are dangling in the air. You should be wearing ankle weights wrapped around your feet, near the base of your toes. Your upper body should be upright, arms resting at your sides, and your toes should be pointing down to the floor in a natural, un-flexed position.

Raise your toes up toward your shins as high as possible. The rest of your body should stay the same, but your weighted toes should be lifted up and in, so you feel the contraction in the muscles along your shin. Re-turn to the starting position and repeat.

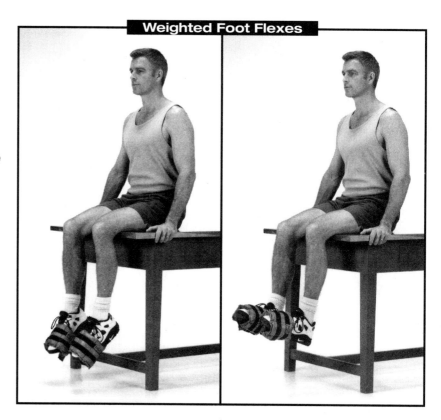

Weighted Foot Flexes

Toe Raises ▶

Stand upright with your toes over the ledge of a platform, weight or block. Hold on to a wall with one hand for balance, if you need to. Your toes should be extended as far out over the edge as you can, but main-tain your posture and balance and keep your heels on the step or block.

Pull your toes in toward your shins as far as you can. The rest of your body should remain upright, and you should feel the contraction around your shins. Hold for a second, then lower and repeat. Do up to three sets of 12 to 20 reps.

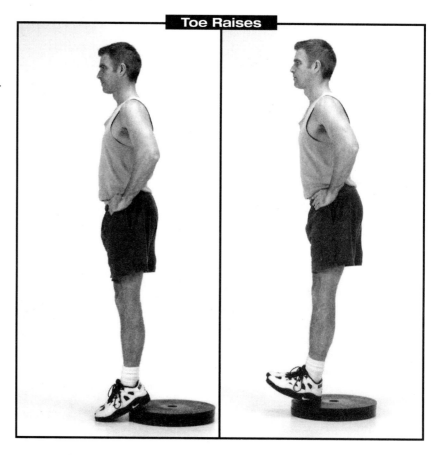

Toe Raises

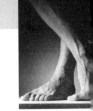

Bowlegged Toe Raises

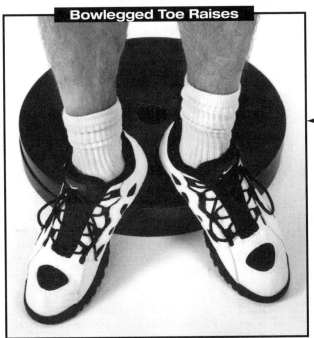

◄ Bowlegged Toe Raises

Do toe raises as you normally would, but start with your feet splayed outward with your body weight focused on the outsides of your feet in a bowlegged position. This stresses the muscles slightly differently than in the standard position.

Knock-Kneed Toe Raises

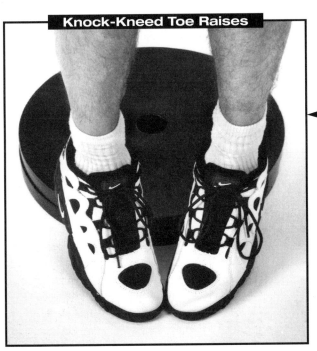

◄ Knock-Kneed Toe Raises

Do standard toe raises as you normally would, but start with your feet splayed inward with your body weight focused on the insides of your feet in a knock-kneed position. This will stress the muscles slightly differently than in the standard position.

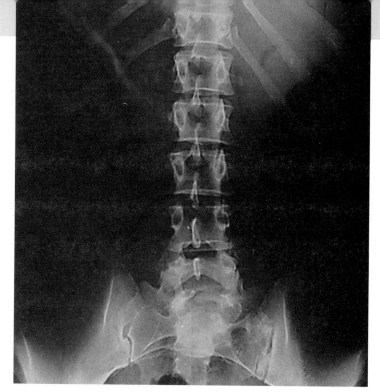

Bones

Fat lot of good muscles will do you without the bones to back them up. Bones—in the form of your skeleton—are the support structure for your whole body, of course, but they're also the surface upon which muscles rely.

When you do something physical, your muscles dig in their heels and pull, using whatever bones they're attached to as a means of support. The stronger those bones are, the stronger you'll be, because you're giving your muscles a more solid platform to do their thing.

Growing up, you were probably told that drinking lots of milk was the one thing you could do to make sure your bones would be strong and healthy. But, fortunately, you can do better than that.

"I don't think that most men really think much about their bones—if they're exercising, they're really concentrating more on their muscles," explains Todd Ellenbecker, P.T., clinical director of Physiotherapy Associates Scottsdale Sports Clinic in Arizona.

That's because we can see our muscles. Bones are more of an out-of-sight-out-of-mind proposition. Nevertheless, you'd do well to start boning up on your bones. And you should realize that the sooner you start, the stronger your bones will be—and the stronger you'll be for the rest of your life.

Bone Meals

Although we recognize the idea of equality between men and women, when it comes to bones, guys have a tactical advantage in the battle of the sexes—our skeletons tend to be bigger, stronger and less likely to deteriorate as we get older. The reason can be summed up in one word: testosterone.

"Testosterone keeps bones strong," says Michael Bemben, Ph.D., assistant professor of health and sport sciences at the University of Oklahoma in Norman. And studies have shown that men who suffered serious fractures, such as breaking a hip bone, had extremely low levels of testosterone.

"But there's more to strong bones than hormones," says Dr. Bemben. All the testosterone in the world isn't going to keep your bones firm unless you're getting plenty of the raw material you need to make bones in the first place. Nutrition is vital for keeping your skeleton in top shape, he says. Without the proper elements getting to your bones, they'll become brittle and soft. You won't be able to lift as much weight or take much punishment in sports. So here are a few nutrition tips to keep your bones healthy.

Call for calcium. Bones do not live on sunshine alone. You also need calcium, an important tool your body uses to make more bone tissue. Nutrition experts recommend about 1,000 milligrams of calcium per day.

As a kid, you probably got plenty of calcium from drinking milk; that's a strategy that will still work for you as an adult—one eight-ounce glass will give you more than 300 milligrams. If you can't or don't drink milk, try salmon, sardines, low-fat yogurt, low-fat cheese or pinto beans—not all at the same time, of course.

Worship the sun. Although you've heard plenty about the dangers of staying out in the sun, some exposure is absolutely necessary for stronger bones. Sunlight helps our bodies produce vitamin D, one of the most essential factors for good calcium absorption, says Dr. Bemben. Don't go overboard—too much sunlight is the leading cause of skin cancer. Instead, stay out of direct sunlight, especially between the hours of 10 A.M. and 2 P.M., when the sun's rays are most harmful.

Boning Up with Weights

When physical trainers tell you weight training is a great body-builder, they're not just talking about muscle, they're also talking about bone.

"Just like muscle, bones are living tissue. They have an ongoing metabolism, and weight training can affect them," says Dr. Bemben. "When you do any kind of activity where your bones have to bear weight, they're going to be stimulated, and newer, stronger bone cells are formed."

Although a regular weight-training regimen will give your bones plenty of exercise, there are some areas of the skeleton that could use more attention than others. Here are some specific ways to work those areas.

Get your back up. Your back has to support a lot of weight. So to strengthen your back properly, you'll need to focus on exercises that put weight on your back in a controlled manner, Dr. Bemben says. "You don't want to put so much weight on that you'll injure your back, certainly, but you can focus on exercises where your back has to support a lot of your body weight, such as walking or jogging." Some overhead weight-training exercises will also strengthen the back bones, including lat pull-downs, overhead triceps extensions and military presses.

Put your wrists through the wringer. The ulna, an area just above the wrist, is often susceptible to damage and weakness, says Dr. Bemben. You can help combat that tendency with wrist exercises like wrist rolls (see page 56). "More important, be careful how you land when you fall," says Ellenbecker. "If you land on your hand or wrist abruptly, you can snap it." When you fall, try to tuck in your chin and roll over your shoulder—this distributes the force of the impact so it's not all in the wrist.

Put your hips into it. As you get older, your hips become an increasingly common area for breaks, says Dr. Bemben. You can nip hip weakness in the bud by doing plenty of leg exercises that work the hips, such as seated leg presses.

Pull your own weight. Finally, doing an exercise that lets your skeleton carry your own body weight is often all you need to keep bones strong.

"For example, swimming may be a great aerobic exercise, but it's not so good for your bones, because they don't have to bear any weight," points out Dr. Bemben. Instead, do some running, or even walking. "Your bones will have to carry your whole body weight, and that's good exercise for them."

FACT Astronauts can lose significant amounts of bone mass while in space. "Without gravity acting on the skeletal system, the bones become incredibly wasted," says Michael Bemben, Ph.D., assistant professor of health and sport sciences at the University of Oklahoma in Norman.

Part Four
Workouts for Every Scenario

Basic Fitness

- **There is no such thing as a one-size-fits-all workout program. No matter how simple your fitness goals, you must make some choices about the types and intensity of exercise you will do, based on health, lifestyle and personal preferences.**

- **That said, effective exercise routines are structured similarly: warm-up, stretching, weight training, aerobic exercise, cooldown, stretching.**

- **To be truly fit, plan on at least three 90-minute workout sessions a week. However, research shows that as few as three 30-minute sessions a week will positively influence your health.**

- **Consider a periodization program of strength training to get the best of all worlds: strength, size, stamina.**

Let's say you don't have any fitness goals other than to be generally healthy and energized. You don't play a sport; you don't face any unusual physical demands; your body doesn't have any particular quirks that need fixing. All you want is to live well, and you're willing to give three or four hours a week to exercise in order to achieve that.

Hey, it's a terrific goal—pure, unpretentious, reasonable. And in our hearts, we wish we could tell you there is a golden formula that will work perfectly for you and the rest of the 90-some million men in America. But the thing is, a one-size-fits-all workout program just doesn't exist. A thousand guys, a thousand different exercise programs—that's the reality. Why is that? Your age, your weight, your genetics, your previous exercise history, your lifestyle, where you live, your exercise preferences *all* dictate in some way what is the right exercise for you.

So if you are to get fit, you have no choice but to make some choices about exercise goals and desires. Our goal here is to keep the number of choices down to as few as possible.

The next 34 chapters each outline specific exercise and training needs for specific sports, lifestyles or goals. The point of this book is to let you pick and choose from each of these chapters for your own needs. But if all you want is to be generally fit, we'll make it as easy as we can.

In this chapter we'll outline what it takes to obtain a basic level of fitness. In the next chapter we'll detail a "universal" weight-lifting regimen—we call it the Core Routine—that covers every part of your body that you need to exercise. From there, it's up to you.

The Basic Fitness Template

A fitness routine should be simply but solidly structured. As a general rule, you should be working out at least three days a week, with a rest day between each workout to give your muscles time to recover and, more important, get stronger. Monday, Wednesday and Friday is the most common schedule, says John Graham, director of the Human Performance Center at the Allentown Sports Medicine and Human Performance Center in Pennsylvania. But do whatever works best for you.

The ideal basic workout takes about 90 minutes. That's 4½ hours a week at the gym. On those three workout days, you should do:

- A ten-minute warm-up. Do a light aerobic activity to get blood flowing through your muscles. Walking, stair-climbing, doing jumping jacks, whatever, as long as it's not overly strenuous.
- Five minutes of stretches. Do both your upper and lower body. Hold each stretch for 20 to 30 seconds. You should get in eight to ten stretches during the five minutes.
- Thirty minutes of weight training. This is the centerpiece of your workout, essential to gaining strength and stamina.
- Thirty minutes of aerobic activity. This is key to a healthy heart and lungs as well as weight control.
- A five-minute cooldown. Just like the warm-up, but this is to slowly adjust your body back to its regular levels.
- Five minutes of stretches. These can be the same as above, or you can substitute. Just be sure to hit all the main muscle groups.

Your Key Decisions

So, what choices must you make? We'll tell you.

- Pick an aerobic activity. Running, walking, bicycling, swimming, stair-climbing, rowing—it's up to you.
- Pick your stretches. We make that easy for you: Consult Flexibility on page 32 for a good seven-stretch, full-body routine. You needn't look further.
- Pick your weight exercises. Again, we make that easy for you. The next chapter lays out a perfect weight-lifting regimen we call the Core Routine. These seven lifts will serve the needs of your entire body.
- Decide how much of each weight lift to do. That's the toughest one. For an answer, you'll need a little science.

Do you want muscles capable of short surges of great strength? Or do you want muscles that purr and rumble steadily like a well-oiled V-8 engine, minute after minute. That's what muscular stamina is.

The science behind achieving strength and/or stamina applies to most types of physical training, says Ken Sprague, coach and strength trainer, owner and operator of the original Gold's Gym and author of *Sports Strength*. We covered it lightly in the Weight Lifting chapter. We'll review now.

- For sheer strength, put in lots of heavy effort for short periods. Do a series of all-out bursts.
- For muscular stamina and tone, stick with medium efforts for longer periods.
- For a balance, build a program that mixes it up.

(There's a fourth category, body shaping, in which you pump up muscles by doing as many as 15 reps with little rest in between. But this is not the stuff of a general health program. Plus, it takes a much larger time commitment. Still interested? See Body Shaping on page 126.)

Some people want or need extreme strength or extreme stamina. Four-time Mr. Universe Bill Pearl listed a few examples in his book *Getting Stronger*.

Among those who need pure strength, according to Pearl:

- Power lifters
- Olympic lifters
- Football linemen
- Shot-putters

Among those who need great endurance:

- Swimmers
- Rowers
- Cyclists
- Distance runners

Most athletes, Pearl notes, need a combination of both strength and endurance. He calls the combination general conditioning. And that's what most of us want: a reasonable level of strength, plus the endurance to end our days with energy in reserve. Here's how to achieve any of these goals.

To Build Strength

You'll find hundreds of gems of practical advice for building strength—no matter what your lifestyle—in the many chapters that follow. But the science of strength training has a few basic tenets. Understanding what they are will help you develop your muscular system to its highest fitness level. Graham suggests the following:

Lift heavy weights. As you've learned, low reps of fairly heavy weights are what build strength the fastest. Specifically, to build strength, you should lift as follows:

- Do three to five sets of each exercise per workout.
- Do three to eight reps per set.
- Use fairly heavy weights, defined as 75 to 85 percent of your one-rep maximum.

Know the role of rest. Lifting weights alone will not build strength. Strength grows while you're resting. That's why we recommend weight training every other day. Those rest days allow your muscles time to recover from the overload of the day before. And when they recover, they grow back stronger than before.

When you're in the low-rep, high-weight world of strength building, remember that you need to rest more between sets, too. According to Tom Baechle, Ed.D., chair of the exercise science department at Creighton University in Omaha, Nebraska, you should take a breather of two to five minutes between sets. Do not scrimp on rest between sets.

To Build Stamina

Muscular endurance, on the other hand, is all about *not* resting. It's about lifting and lifting and lifting until you can't do any more. With this type of training, you need to follow the toning principles we've mentioned in the Weight Lifting and Aerobic Exercise chapters, says Sprague. Toning—that is, building lean muscle mass—is the secret to building stamina, since it requires you to do high repetitions of low weights. The longer you do that, the more you'll extend the time that your muscles, and your body, can endure in any activity. Here's your basic plan for endurance training, according to Sprague.

Lift high, stay low. Here are the specifics of your lifting routine.

- Do two to three sets of each exercise per workout.
- Do 12 to 20 reps per each set.
- Use light weights, defined as 50 to 60 percent of your one-rep max.

Keep recovery time short. Another key element to building stamina is to restrict your rest periods between sets. In this case, we're recommending 20 to 30 seconds—just enough time to let you catch your breath, but not enough that your muscles get used to working for a shorter period of time.

Participate in endurance activities. Building stamina goes beyond weight training. Stamina and endurance should be the key descriptors of most every activity you do. So if you're trying to build stamina for your muscles, you need to get out of the gym and focus on endurance activities, Sprague says. Running, long-distance cycling and full-court basketball are all great endurance sports and, consequently, great endurance builders.

Combining Your Power

For most men, of course, the ideal always lies in the middle. To achieve a balance of both strength and endurance training, Pearl recommends a hybrid of the strength and stamina principles. Here are the basics.

Shoot for the middle ground. When you lift, Pearl suggests the following:

- Do three to five sets per workout.
- Do 8 to 12 reps per set, with 10 being optimal.

- Use moderate weights, defined as 70 to 80 percent of your max.

Build periodized power. To ensure that you continually make progress, get your workout on a periodization schedule. Different fitness trainers and physiologists offer different periodization programs, but the concept remains the same: By constantly mixing up the intensity of your workout, you keep your muscles constantly on edge, always adapting. If you stick with the same intensity for any length of time, your muscles catch on and quit adapting as efficiently, and thus you progress much more slowly, if at all.

Schedules vary. Some trainers recommend three cycles; some recommend more.

All periodization programs feature an active-rest phase, a period in which you do little or no weight training at all, but instead use the bulk of your training time for other fitness activities, such as sports or aerobics. Sprague recommends the active-rest period be the same length as the other cycles.

To give you an example of how periodization can shake up a workout and work out your body in more and varied ways, here's a five-cycle periodization program developed by Sprague. Each cycle could be as short as a week or as long as a month, he says, but the length is up to you to determine. When you've gone through all five phases, start over again.

Muscular endurance phase	2–3 sets	12–20 reps (light weights)
Bodybuilding phase	3–5 sets	8–12 reps (moderate weights)
Strength phase	3–5 sets	3–8 reps (moderate to heavy weights)

Then, to step beyond the basic principles, Sprague recommends the following:

"Peak" phase	1–3 sets	1–3 reps (heavy weights)
Active-rest phase		(cross-train, play racquet sports, basketball, etc.)

By incorporating elements of these phases and principles into any workout schedule, you'll be building the most well-rounded body possible and training yourself to handle any physical situation. In short, you'll be the picture of fitness.

The Core Routine

Peak Points

- **There are seven primary muscle groups in the body. A good weight-lifting routine hits each group.**

- **Use the Core Routine as a foundation on which to build a complete workout; don't assume that these seven exercises will strengthen every muscle.**

- **Use free weights rather than machines if you have to make a choice. But if both are available, rotate between them for more well-rounded strengthening.**

Everyone knows it's ridiculous to build a house from the roof down. You have to start with the foundation and work your way up. So it is with building a better body.

You may see other guys in the gym doing advanced exercises—heck, you probably do a few of them yourself. You won't be able to do many of those exercises consistently or safely, though, if you haven't been following a core weight-lifting routine.

By "core," we mean a basic resistance regimen that provides a balanced, healthy level of physical fitness. We mean exercises that prepare your body for more challenging activities, such as your favorite sports. By "core," we mean the foundation of your physical fitness routine.

Meeting the Core Requirements

Although the warm-up, stretching, aerobic exercise and cooldown are all essential elements of a core routine, for our purposes here, we're focusing on the core of your core—weight training.

For basic muscle-training, there are only seven major muscle areas you need to hit with weights. If you must choose between free weights and machines, you probably should go with free weights. But if you have access to both, then by all means use both.

"Mixing machine and free-weight lifts isn't a bad idea. It

keeps the routine varied," says John Graham, director of the Human Performance Center at the Allentown Sports Medicine and Human Performance Center in Pennsylvania. Variety is important, even within a consistent routine. The more you can vary the work your muscles do, the better-trained those muscles will be to perform whatever tasks you require.

Although the core routine lists some essential exercises for fitness, they're not the only exercises you should do. "They're good as a base, as a starting point," says Graham. But depending on your lifestyle or favorite activities, you'll need to add other exercises to this workout for a complete—and completely customized—personal fitness regimen.

You'll find hundreds of suggestions for those other exercises in the chapters that follow. But first, here's your core routine. For maximum versatility, we've provided machine-weight alternatives for each free-weight exercise we recommend. Although the free-weight versions of these exercises are described elsewhere in the book, take a moment to review the following positioning tips. They'll help you to do each exercise more safely and effectively.

Reference Points

Legs

Free Weight: Squats ►

When you squat down, make sure you stop when your thighs are parallel to the floor. Go any lower and you risk injuring your knees—or falling on your butt.

Machine: Leg Press

Sit with your back against the back of the seat, placing your feet flat on the plate with your legs bent 90 degrees or less and your arms holding the handrails. Exhaling, push the pedals until your legs are fully extended, but your knees are not locked. Inhaling, slowly return your legs to a 90-degree position. Don't let the weight come back too fast, warns Barney Groves, Ph.D., associate professor of physical education at Virginia Commonwealth University in Richmond.

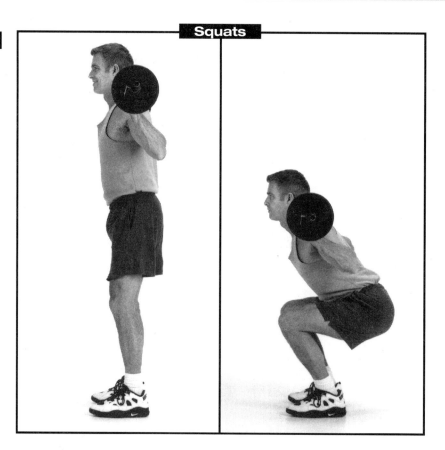

Squats

Chest

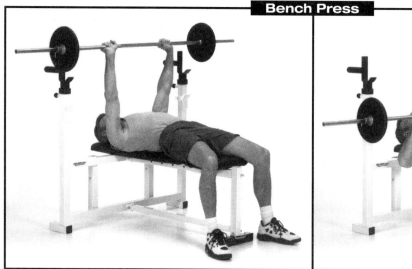

Bench Press

Free Weight: Bench Press ▲

As you do this lift, remember your four contact points—feet, butt, shoulders and head. Your feet should be planted firmly on the floor—everything else should be flat on the bench for an effective, injury-free lift.

When lowering a barbell, pause at the bottom of the movement, letting the weight lightly touch your chest. Never let the weight down so quickly that your chest springs the bar back up, as some lifters do. Dr. Groves says that's a good way to damage your sternum.

Machine: Bench Press

Lie on the bench like you would if you were using a barbell. Grip the handles above your head with your hands slightly more than shoulder-width apart. Make sure your head is at least two inches away from the weight stack. Exhaling, lift until your elbows are fully extended. Inhaling, return to the starting position and repeat until the set is completed.

Back

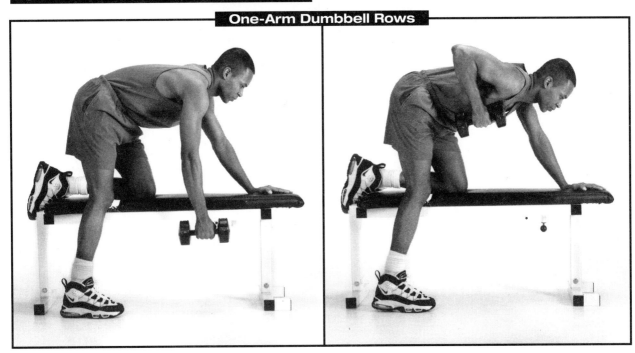

One-Arm Dumbbell Rows

Free Weight: One-Arm Dumbbell Rows ▲

This exercise works the back without much risk of throwing it out. Just remember to keep your back straight and one foot flat on the floor. Although it seems like your arm is doing all the work, don't overcompensate and try to get more of your back behind the lift. You'll likely injure yourself.

Machine: Seated Rows

Sit on the floor and grasp the handles at the end of the cable, keeping your upper body straight and your knees slightly flexed. Exhaling, pull the bar to your chest with your arms, avoiding any torso motion. Inhaling, return toward the starting position until your elbows are fully extended.

Shoulders

Free Weight: Alternating Press with Dumbbells ►

Although you generally want to keep your back straight with over-head lifts (especially on difficult lifts like the military press), it's okay to keep a slight forward lean in your lower back when you do this lift. Just make sure your shoulders are back and your chest is out.

Machine: Lateral Raises

Sit in the seat; put your chest against the front pad and position yourself so the arm pads are resting just above your elbows. Lift your arms, raising your elbows up to shoulder level, then lower and repeat.

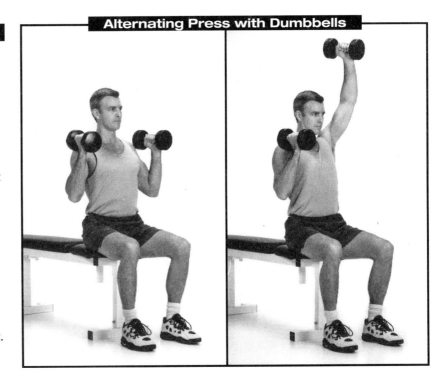

Alternating Press with Dumbbells

Biceps

Concentration Curls

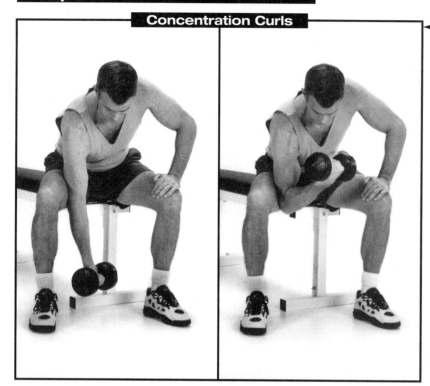

◀ Free Weight: Concentration Curls

This lift really targets the biceps. But as you lean forward for the curl, remember to keep your back straight. Brace your elbow against your thigh and lean on your free hand if you need support. Do this curl slowly and focus on your biceps—don't let your shoulder sneak in and do the work.

Machine: Biceps Curls

Adjust the seat so that your elbows are slightly lower than your shoulders. With your chest against the front pad, place your elbows on the top pad and grasp the handles with an underhand grip. Exhaling, curl upward as far as possible. Inhaling, return to the starting position. Keep your butt firmly planted on the seat; keep your head up and avoid letting your shoulders come forward to help.

Triceps

Overhead Triceps Extensions

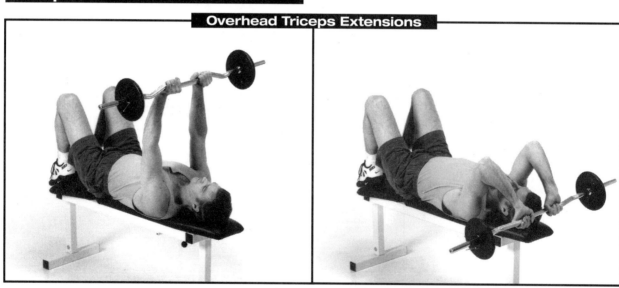

Free Weight: Overhead Triceps Extensions ▲

This behind-the-head lift is a little tricky because it's easy to let your elbows bow out as you lower the bar. In that position, you're not isolating your triceps anymore. Remember to keep your elbows pointed toward the ceiling and close to your ears. If you have trouble doing that, the weight is probably too heavy.

Machine: Cable Push-Downs

Standing with your feet shoulder-width apart, grasp the push-down bar with an overhand grip, hands six to ten inches apart. Adjust the cable so the bar is at chest height. This is your starting position. Exhaling and keeping your upper arms squeezed against your ribs, extend your forearms until the bar touches your thighs. Avoid moving your upper arms and torso. While inhaling, return the bar to chest height. To truly isolate your triceps, remember to hold your elbows close to the sides of your belly.

Abdominals

Free Weight: Crunches ►

In this case, the "free weight" you'll be using will be your very own body. Remember that with any crunches, the trick is to work your abdominal and oblique muscles, not wreck your back. Make sure you do these on an exercise mat, and keep your lower back flat on the floor.

Machine: Abdominal Curl Machine

This is one of the only ways to use weights to exercise your abs in isolation. Sit in an abdominal curl machine with your upper chest and shoulders behind the torso pad and your feet securely hooked under the foot rollers. Depending on the machine, either grasp the handgrips or rest your arms across your body under the pad. By contracting your abs, push your body forward to a position halfway between the starting position and parallel to the floor. (Don't cheat by pulling at the pad with your arms or bearing in with your shoulders and back.) Hold for a moment, then return to the starting position. Abs generally can handle more reps than other muscles, so Graham recommends three sets of 20 reps, with a weight level set at 50 to 60 percent of your one-rep maximum.

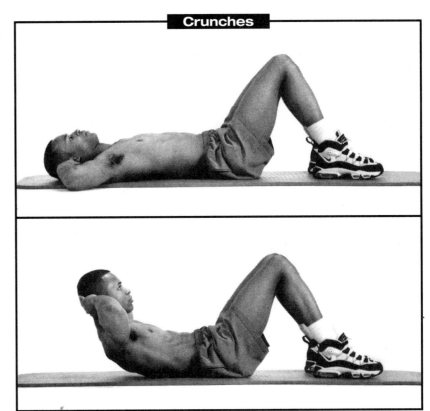

Crunches

Body Shaping

Peak Points

- Shaping your body means building mass, which requires being patient while results accrue over weeks and months. It also means spending more time in the gym. Have you got what it takes?

- Being able to lift the same large amount of weight with each set isn't your goal: Continually stressing, or pumping, your muscles is.

- You pump up by doing multiple exercises for each major muscle group, doing 12 to 15 repetitions per set, performing at least three sets of each exercise and allowing only about 45 seconds of recovery between sets.

It happens to a lot of us. We try out a sport, we invest a moderate amount of dedication, we get a modicum of results—and we want *more*. We work harder and begin to see real changes in ourselves, and suddenly the Significant Other begins complaining that we're spending too much time with our new passion.

With resistance training, this only happens to some of us. That's understandable, since on the face of things, lifting weights doesn't seem nearly as much fun as sports like biking, running or in-line skating. It takes a special kind of dedication to move beyond the resistance training that's required for fitness and into the realm of training that will really sculpt, shape and transform your body into something wholly new. This is the dedication of the man who can see beyond the pain or pleasure of the moment and project into the future.

This is also the dedication of the man who has at least a little time to spare. Any activity you're enthusiastic about takes time, but adding size and definition to your muscles demands both a high degree of consistency and a large volume of effort. In this beginner program, you don't necessarily have to exercise

more days than we are recommending for most everyone (three days a week), but you will have to do more in the gym when you're there.

The Principles of Pump

Most of what we know about building muscle mass comes from observation: Researchers, athletes and coaches have noticed that lifting weights in certain ways tends to produce certain types of results. Beyond that, physiologists don't really un-

Reference Points

derstand what makes muscles get bigger, which may be fine, since most of us don't really care.

What we do know boils down to this: To get big, you have to get pumped. All the principles of bodybuilding feed into this one idea: It's important to keep nearly continuous stress on muscles, congesting them with blood and between-tissue (interstitial) fluid.

You know this feeling. It's the one you have after a weight workout, when your muscles feel firmer and actually look bigger. It's the feeling that makes you think we ain't kidding when we say you'll get results fast. These results are temporary, unfortunately, but they give you a preview of coming attractions. Over time, the pumped feeling becomes permanent; the pump itself seems to play a major role in this. "Whether it's increased delivery of protein or direct stimulation of muscle cells or something else, we don't know," says Wayne Westcott, Ph.D., strength-training consultant to the national YMCA and senior fitness director for the South Shore YMCA in Quincy, Massachusetts. "But it appears that for some people, the pump itself actually promotes muscle growth."

Said another way, "A really good body-shaping program requires a certain amount of burn," says Barney Groves, Ph.D., associate professor of physical education at Virginia Commonwealth University in Richmond. Each of the following principles forms a cornerstone for any body-shaping program.

Hit muscles with multiple exercises. Ever notice how guys who are really built, who really spend a lot of time in the gym—how their each and every muscle seems to stand at attention, sharply defined like an illustration from an anatomy text? You won't get that look from doing just one exercise for a given area of the body. Rather, you need to do a number of different exercises for each muscle group. That way, you'll call more muscles into play, exact effort from areas that otherwise get off easy and keep up the pump for major muscles that are used repeatedly.

Do lots of repetitions. If you want strength, defined as the ability to lift something one time, train in a way that prepares you for just that kind of movement—by exerting force against a heavy resistance only three to five times. For shape and size, however, all you're really after is the pump. And to get that, you need to lift the weight more times. Bodybuilders occasionally do as many as 20 reps per each set of an exercise. But most bodybuilding routines run more in the 12- to 15-rep range. Start with 12 reps of each exercise and progress to 15, Dr. Groves suggests. When you can do more than 15, add enough weight to reduce you to 12 reps again.

Do lots of sets. For fitness, we've shown how it's possible to get most of what you need with just one set. But to promote muscle growth, you'll need to do more. Multiple sets stimulate muscles repeatedly, keep

blood flowing and pump muscles up. The number of sets you do is something you can increase gradually. If you're currently doing only one set, a beginning bodybuilding program requires at least two to three sets. From there, you can build up to three to five. (Competitive bodybuilders might do as many as 15 sets of a given exercise.) One reason multiple sets may be important, research suggests, is that greater training volume increases the amount of testosterone the body produces—and testosterone fuels muscle growth. "It's generally agreed that testosterone flow starts to kick in at around six or seven sets," Dr. Groves says.

Keep rests short. With strength programs, rests are long. They need to be if you want to be able to keep lifting heavy weights: The long recovery allows blood flow to return to normal, wastes to be cleared out, energy to be replenished and fatigue to dissipate. "If I rest three to five minutes, my muscles return to 95 to 98 percent of what they were before the workout," Dr. Groves says. "If I'm bodybuilding, I don't want that. I want to keep on pumping." With bodybuilding it doesn't matter if you can't lift as much weight from one set to the next. In fact, it's assumed that you'll be lifting less as your workout progresses—exactly the opposite of some strength programs. What's important is that muscles are continually being fatigued. For body shaping, rests generally range from 30 to 60 seconds. "Allow no more than 90 seconds," Dr. Groves says, "and 45 seconds is ideal."

The Beginner's Workout

If you're already doing weight workouts regularly, stick to your schedule but replace your old routine with the one that follows. You can do this workout three times a week and get excellent body-shaping results. The main difference between this and the Core Routine on page 121 is that for every major muscle, we've listed several exercises, not just one. In many instances, the extra exercises are from the Achieving a Peak Body section of this book—or we've simply teamed both the machine and free-weight exercises already listed in the Core Routine.

This brings up a point: It's possible to design a multiple-exercise program using free weights alone, but most of the trainers, coaches and physiologists we've consulted prescribe a certain number of exercises using machines. What this means is that you'll probably want to join a gym. If you're seriously interested in bodybuilding, no doubt you're way ahead of us on that score. Gyms not only provide an important variety of equipment but they're also a source of trainers to guide your efforts and people who can spot you when doing difficult or dangerous moves.

First, let's teach you a few exercises we want you to include that aren't elsewhere in the book. Then we'll show you the entire routine.

Lat Pull-Downs ►

This is a popular machine exercise. Here's how to use the machine correctly.

Sit at a lat pull-down machine. (Unless it doesn't have a seat, in which case kneel underneath it.) Reach overhead and grasp the pull-down bar with your hands positioned wider than shoulder-width apart. Hold onto the bar with your arms extended. Your palms should be facing away from your body, your upper back straight and your eyes forward.

Keeping your back straight, pull the bar down in front to touch your upper chest, then extend your arms upward again.

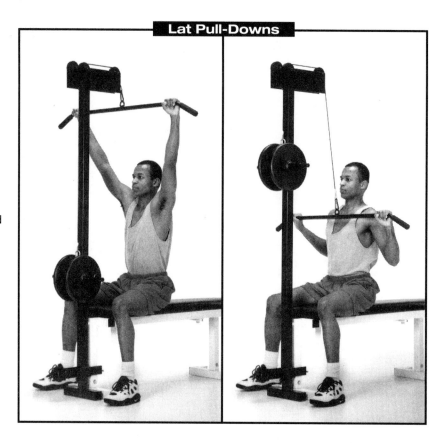

Lat Pull-Downs

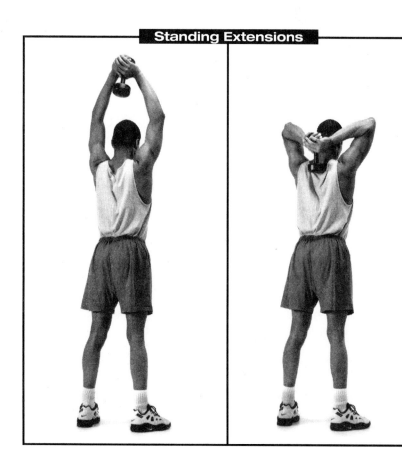

Standing Extensions

◄ Standing Extensions

This exercise helps to build your triceps. Standing with your feet about shoulder-width apart, grasp a dumbbell with both hands and hold it carefully above your head.

Keeping your elbows pointed toward the ceiling, slowly lower the dumbbell behind your head as far as you can, or until it touches the back of your shoulders. Slowly raise the dumbbell back above your head.

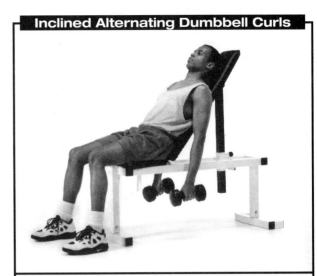

Inclined Alternating Dumbbell Curls

Inclined Alternating Dumbbell Curls ➤

Lie on an inclined bench with dumbbells on the floor beside you, parallel to the bench. Grasp the dumbbells, palms facing inward.

Keeping your upper arm stationary, curl the barbell in your right hand toward your shoulder, rotating it a quarter turn as you lift so your palm is facing your shoulder at the top of the lift. Then lower the weight again so your right arm is extended toward the floor. Repeat with the other arm.

Inclined Alternating Dumbbell Curls, Palm Down

Do this right after you finish your regular inclined alternating dumbbell curls. Do the same exercise with the same dumbbells (or lighter ones if those prove difficult)—only this time, rotate your hand so that your palm faces away from your shoulder at the top of the lift.

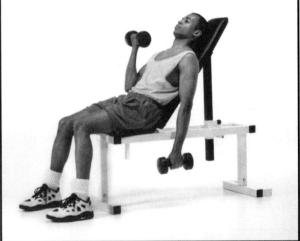

The Program

Do at least three sets of each of the following exercises. If this seems a lot more time-intensive than what you usually do, it is. But bear in mind that you're probably also cutting your minutes in recovery between sets by at least half, thereby making up for some of the time now devoted to extra exercises.

Shoulders
- Alternating press with dumbbells
- Lateral raises
- Upright rows

Chest
- Bench press
- Inclined bench press
- Dumbbell flies

Back
- One-arm dumbbell rows
- Seated rows
- Lat pull-downs

Biceps
- Preacher curls
- Inclined alternating dumbbell curls
- Inclined alternating dumbbell curls, palm down

Triceps
- One-arm triceps pull-downs
- Overhead triceps extensions
- Standing extensions

Legs
- Squats
- Leg extensions
- Leg curls

Abdominals/obliques
- Reverse curls
- Oblique crunches

Advanced Shaping

Peak Points

- **Your workout needs to be more intense: more exercises, more sets, more days in the gym.**

- **Because your workout is more intense, you need to allow more time for recovery—at least two days' rest between bouts for any given muscle group.**

- **To maintain intensity and also get enough rest, you should split your routine so that you do different parts of your workout on different days.**

We'll be honest: If you've reached the point where you're ready for advanced body shaping, you probably don't need us anymore. You've been hanging out in the gym, getting tips from other lifters, reading the muscle mags—or, at minimum, you've absorbed everything we've told you in the Weight Lifting and Body Shaping for Beginners chapters.

On the other hand, if you simply want to move to the next level, it isn't necessary to become wrapped up in the muscle subculture, with its oiled bodies, bikini briefs, power pills, tanning booths and competitive spirit. Nor do you need to pay attention to the dubious theories, pseudoscientific product promotions and other assorted weight-lifting hucksterisms that claim to provide an edge over some other guy.

At its most fundamental, advanced body shaping is nothing more than stepping up the application of knowledge you already have. To recap: "You need a lot of repetitions, a lot of sets and a lot of different exercises for each muscle," says Barney Groves, Ph.D., associate professor of physical education at Virginia Commonwealth University in Richmond and a competitive lifter who has taught weight training for more than 30 years. "An advanced routine is more of the same," he says. "I sometimes do 15 to 20 different sets for one muscle group."

You may already be doing the *quantities* that Dr. Groves suggests, but to get the most outcome, you'll have to increase the *intensity* of your training program as well. Think of advanced body shaping as a layering process: As you move to the next level, you add intensity and complexity, which, at this point, will require some adjustments to your routine.

Stepping Up the Program

Here's what you need to do to take your body-shaping routine to the next level.

Train more. You'll first be adding another layer of exercises to those you're already doing, following the principle that the more you hit a muscle in different ways, the more muscle fibers will be called into play. In the workout that follows, we're adding at least one exercise for each major area of the body to the routine established in the Body Shaping for Beginners chapter. Second, you'll be increasing the number of sets you do of each exercise. Assuming you're already doing at least two sets, you should now increase to at least three or four sets per exercise. "It really does make for a time commitment," says Jeff Chandler, Ed.D., chair of the research committee of the National Strength and Conditioning Association, and director of research at Lexington Clinic Sports Medicine Center in Lexington, Kentucky. We'll deal with that in a moment.

Allow more recovery. Because you're stressing each muscle group with a high degree of intensity, you'll need to give your muscles more rest between workouts. As a rule, serious bodybuilders avoid training the same muscles more than twice a week. Unless you're blessed with superior genetics, a training volume greater than that undercuts your gains because your muscles don't get adequate time to rebuild between bouts of exercise—which is essential for bulking up and shaping your body. When you hit muscles again too soon, you feel drained, which prevents you from working with an all-out effort. With high-intensity training, there should be at least two days' rest between each bout for a given muscle group.

Split your routine. If you're both training more and resting more, something needs to give. Let's say you intend to follow your standard routine, trying to cram all your exercises into a single workout. This will be difficult because it's time-consuming and, with the kind of effort we're talking about, downright grueling. Plus, if you build in two days of recovery between workouts, you're only in the gym about twice a week. Somehow, going from three days of exercise a week to two just doesn't *feel* right.

To make all these considerations work together, it's necessary to expand your workout into what's called a split routine. With a split routine, instead of doing your entire workout each time you exercise, you break it into sections so that you're working out four to six days a week, but doing different parts of

How to Be a Hit Man

Think of your most intense workout ever. You were really struggling on those last repetitions, right?

But tell the truth: If your life depended on it, you probably could have done just one more. Or maybe two, or three—but finally you would reach a point where further effort was utterly impossible. That's the difference between working to *pre-fatigue* (or tiredness, which is what you normally do) and working to *failure*.

Working to failure is the cornerstone of a controversial technique known as High Intensity Training, or HIT. The idea is that by working to failure during one or two sets (which is all your body can take), you build strength and size as well as—if not better than—you would by doing many sets working to fatigue. Practitioners of the HIT method are so intent on completely exhausting their muscles that they work beyond their capabilities, using spotters to help lift on those last agonizing repetitions.

About a third of the NFL's teams and several college basketball teams use some modification of a HIT program, according to Jeff Chandler, Ed.D., chair of the research committee of the National Strength and Conditioning Association, and director of research at Lexington Clinic Sports Medicine Center in Lexington, Kentucky.

Does HIT work? There are many testimonials that indicate that HIT workouts can be effective, but there is currently little research to back them up. "The majority of the research currently available indicates that the volume of work performed—the number of sets times the number of repetitions—is more directly related to increased strength and mass than single sets," explains Dr. Chandler. He allows that a great deal is still not understood about resistance training, but sees two flaws in a strict HIT approach.

First, Dr. Chandler says, constant training to failure means you need more recovery time, which dictates fewer workouts. It's tougher to make progress when you're working out less, he says. And second, training to failure may increase your risk of overuse injuries—like the repetitive use that causes tennis elbow—and traumatic injury that may occur when fatigue causes technique to break down.

But never say never. "When you really get down to what people are doing, some HIT guys are using multiple sets and some multiple-set guys occasionally train to failure. Variety is a plus," Dr. Chandler says.

your routine on different days.

One way to structure a split routine is to do the upper body one day and the lower body the day after. Or, since most exercises you do are in the upper body, you could more evenly distribute the load by doing a three-day cycle.

The program outlined here uses a three-way split, in which you work the back, biceps and forearms on Monday and Thursday, the chest, triceps and shoulders on Tuesday and Friday, and the abdominals and legs on Wednesdays and Saturdays. Sunday is the only day off, but each muscle group has at least two days' recovery before being specifically worked again. There's nothing magic about one kind of routine over another. What works best will be the routine that most easily fits into your schedule.

Stick to your diet. Before getting to the particulars, a word about nutrition. A lot of bodybuilders maintain that because protein provides the raw material for muscle growth, you need to eat more protein to grow bigger muscles. "Proper diet is important,"

Dr. Groves concurs, "but getting more protein and less carbohydrate isn't part of it." The typical American diet already provides two to three times more protein than you need—more than enough surplus to supply whatever extra demands your growing muscles may cause. Ideally, protein should comprise 10 to 15 percent of your diet, with carbohydrates accounting for 60 percent and fat 25 to 30 percent.

The Advanced Workout

Most of the exercises described in this workout are the same as those in the beginner's workout from the last chapter, although, as we've noted, each major muscle group has at least one new exercise. Most of these are drawn from other chapters in this book, but two—the dead lift and the "nose-breaker" extension—are moves we've avoided recommending elsewhere because the injury potential is higher for these exercises than for others that work the same muscles. Being an advanced lifter, you should be able to do them safely. Here they are.

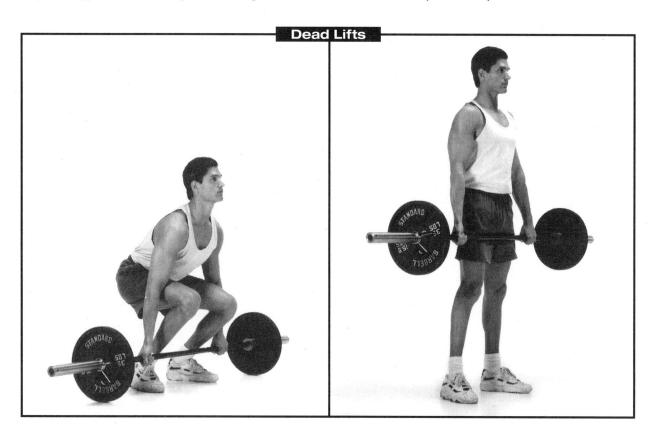

Dead Lifts

Dead Lifts ▲

Earlier we described the Rumanian dead lift, which is a slightly altered version of this more traditional exercise. The difference? This one puts more tension on your back.

Stand with your feet shoulder-width apart, with a barbell on the floor in front of you (the bar should be over your feet and close to your shins). Keeping your back straight, your head up and your shoulders directly over or

a little ahead of the bar, squat down and grasp the bar with your arms extended and positioned just outside your knees. One palm should face out, the other palm in.

Stand up holding the bar, raising it straight up off the floor, using your thighs and back, keeping your arms extended and back straight. Once upright, lower the weight back to the floor again.

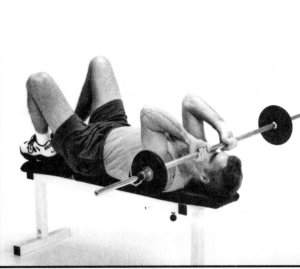

Nose-Breaker Extensions

Nose-Breaker Extensions ▲

Lying on a bench, lift a barbell from the rack or have a spotter hand it to you. Extend your arms straight above your head, hands close together on the bar, palms out.

Keeping your upper arms straight, with your elbows pointed toward the ceiling, lower the bar until it touches your forehead. (This position puts a lot of stress on the forearms. You may wish to use a lighter weight for this version of the overhead extension. You should also use a spotter to help balance or "save" the bar, or this move may live up to its name.)

The Program

This is an advanced workout. Attempt it only if you're able to perform the exercises with good technique and are already conditioned enough to withstand the repeated stresses involved. Don't attempt this workout until you've mastered the beginner's workout in the previous chapter.

Mondays and Thursdays

Back
- One-arm dumbbell rows
- Seated rows
- Lat pull-downs
- Dead lifts

Biceps
- Preacher curls
- Inclined alternating dumbbell curls
- Inclined alternating dumbbell curls, palm down
- Concentration curls

Forearms
- Wrist rolls

Tuesdays and Fridays

Chest
- Bench press
- Inclined bench press
- Dumbbell flies
- Dips

Triceps
- One-arm triceps pull-downs
- Overhead triceps extensions
- Standing extensions
- Nose-breaker extensions

Shoulders
- Alternating press with dumbbells
- Side lateral raises
- Upright rows
- Military press

Wednesdays and Saturdays

Abdominals/obliques
- Reverse curls
- Oblique crunches
- Raised-leg crunches

Legs
- Squats
- Leg extensions
- Leg curls
- Dumbbell lunges
- Standing heel raises

Ridding Fat

If asked why we exercise, some of us might point to our biceps and say we want to look stronger, more chiseled, and be more apt to turn heads at the beach. But most of us would instead probably point to our bellies and say we want to look less bloated, less flaccid, less likely to be mistaken for a landlocked whale at the beach. Both answers, however, depend on one thing: ridding the body of fat.

The two major components of fitness—strength and endurance—have a direct bearing on how much fat hangs on the body. Without lean muscle (which displaces fat), there is no strength. Without aerobic fitness (which burns fat), there is no endurance. Sounds pretty simple: "I exercise, therefore I am lean."

But even a slightly pudgy person realizes that fighting fat is never easy or fast—which in many minds are the same thing. "The biggest mistake people make is thinking they will lose a tremendous amount of weight with exercise in the first several weeks," says Peggy Norwood-Keating, director of fitness programs at the Duke University Diet and Fitness Center in Durham, North Carolina. "If they do," she adds, "they're probably overtraining."

This isn't meant to be a downer. It's meant to be realistic and practical. If you're primed for quick and easy solutions,

you're setting yourself up to be suckered by nutritional nonsense in the form of "revolutionary" fad diets or hardware hucksterism in the form of worthless gadgets hawked on some infomercials, says Norwood-Keating. You'll end up poorer and smarter, but not consistently thinner. Dieting, in particular, has become a dirty word in serious weight-loss circles as research finds that rapid drops in poundage almost never last, and that on-again-off-again flab fluctuations are inherently unhealthy. We assume you'd rather hear (and we'd certainly rather tell you) about achieving actual results in ways that really work.

A quick, but important, aside: As a field of science, nothing is completely certain in weight loss—but greater certainty exists than you might expect if you've been paying attention to news stories, says James Hill, Ph.D., associate director at the Center for Human Nutrition at the University of Colorado Health Sciences Center in Denver. News organizations love reporting stories that seem to turn conventional wisdom on its head. This can get awfully (and unnecessarily) confusing.

A now-classic example is the 1995 front-page headline in *The New York Times* suggesting that eating pasta makes you fat. This assertion wasn't based on a study, but on a mishmash of concepts that individually were valid but together didn't add up to what the headline said they did. "I think (the writer) got the story wrong," says Dr. Hill, who was quoted in the article. Even studies often reach surprising or contradictory conclusions. Truth, however, generally lies where the heaviest weight of evidence falls—and that's probably with the tried and true.

Focusing on Fundamentals

It's easy to get wrapped up in the minutiae of weight loss—how many calories you must burn to lose a pound, the relative badness of saturated versus unsaturated fat, the mathematical equation for converting grams of fat into calories. Getting hung up on this stuff is like being a sports geek who would rather cite statistics than pick up the ball and play the game. Here's all you really need to know to get the job done.

Appreciate calories. The word "calories" is a technical term, not a bridge-club topic. A calorie is a unit of energy. Think of weight loss as a systems engineering problem: Food brings energy in; movement and body operation use it up. To lose weight, you have to burn more energy than you take in, says David Levitsky, Ph.D., professor of nutrition and psychology at Cornell University in Ithaca, New York.

There's been a lot of talk in recent years about what kind of calorie on the supply side is most important. One idea that's been bandied about is that taking in too much fat is much more damaging than taking in too much carbohydrate. That's because (we're told) calories of fat are stored more efficiently as flab than calories of carbohydrate are. This is true, but not very significant, according to Dr. Levitsky, whose research is sometimes cited on this issue. In other words, that's getting lost in the minutiae again.

The big picture is this: Fat is an issue because it has more calories per gram than carbohydrates do—nearly twice as many, in fact. That means you can eat roughly twice as much beans, pasta, cereal and potato than you can bacon, hamburger, cookies and ice cream to get the same number of calories. But make no mistake: Even if calories of carbohydrate are somehow "better" than calories of fat, you'll still gain weight on carbs if you eat more of them than your body uses.

Manage your eating. Let's say you're the manager of a major utility and one quadrant of your power grid is getting overloaded with more energy than it can safely store. Do you cut the flow to your entire service area so that everywhere lights are dimming and computers are fritzing? No, you target the problem and selectively reduce the energy that's caus-

ing it. Likewise, if you're trying to get rid of a pot-belly, it makes no sense to drastically deplete your entire body's power supply. "You lose lean muscle mass as well as fat if you simply restrict calories, and that will work against you," says Norwood-Keating. "You really need to eat sufficient calories to sustain both exercise and your resting metabolic rate."

The general recommendation for a well-balanced diet, says Norwood-Keating, is one that provides 60 percent carbohydrate, 25 to 30 percent fat and 10 to 15 percent protein. Beyond that, there are a couple of less important but helpful ways to redistribute energy flow and regulate peak consumption, according to experts.

• Eat early, not late. Most obese people get from half to three-quarters of their calories after 6 P.M. This is a mistake, since the body seems to be more efficient at storing fat during the night, says Jay Kenney, R.D., Ph.D., nutrition research specialist at the Pritikin Longevity Center in Santa Monica, California.

• Eat often. Large meals cause a surge of the hormone insulin, which makes the body hold onto its fat stores (probably as an eons-old way of warding off starvation). Eating many smaller meals throughout the day keeps insulin levels down and fat-burning potential up, even when you eat the same number of calories, says Thomas Wolever, M.D., Ph.D., associate professor of nutritional sciences at the University of Toronto.

Burn energy with aerobic exercise. To use up more calories than you take in, activity is essential. Aerobic exercise is particularly important for actual weight loss, however, because it's the type of exercise that will tap into fat stores while you do it. We covered the main components of this type of exercise—intensity, duration and frequency—in Aerobic Exercise on page 27. But here again, it's important to keep focused on the basics.

"There's a misperception I see all the time that if you lower the intensity, you'll burn more fat," says Norwood-Keating. "It drives me nuts." This notion (which may even form the basis for easy-does-it "fat-burning" classes at your gym) is based on findings that lower-intensity activity burns a higher percentage of fat calories (compared to carbohydrate and protein) than higher-intensity exercise. But note: The percentage of burned calories that are fat is higher, not the total amount of calories. And what you want to do is burn more calories. "Within a set amount of time, higher intensity exercise will still burn more calories, even though the percentage that's fat will be less," says Norwood-Keating.

Consider the telltale results from one study at The Cooper Institute for Aerobics Research in Dallas. Three groups walked three miles a day. One group walked the distance fast (in 12-minute miles), one at a moderate pace (15-minute miles) and one at a slow pace (20-minute miles). The slowest group burned the most fat, which seems to imply that low-intensity exercise is superior for fat burning. But the slow group also exercised the longest. If the fast group had kept on going for the hour that the slow group was walking, they would have burned more calories.

Rev your metabolism with resistance. Losing fat means changing body composition, and nothing goes more to the heart of body composition than resistance training, says Norwood-Keating. This is not just a matter of making muscles bigger or leaner (although that certainly helps). It's also a matter of creating more lean tissue, which takes more energy to sustain than fat does. From a power utility point of view, fat is a blighted factory building with a darkened parking lot. Muscle is the same building blazing with interior light and humming with heavy industrial machinery. Developing your muscles "enhances your burn capacity by giving you a higher metabolic rate," Norwood-Keating says. The more lean muscle you have, the more calories you burn even when you're inactive.

Work the gut. It's a weight-loss truism that spot-reduction is impossible: You can't do a single exercise (sit-ups) to reduce fat in a single part of the body (the gut). Still, it's important for a number of reasons to work the abdominal muscles if you want to lose weight (or look like you have), explains Norwood-Keating. First, abdominal exercise is part of any overall strength-training routine. Beyond that, firming up the abs lends greater structural support to the back and torso, which improves posture. Plus, stronger gut muscles do a better job of holding the stomach in.

The Fight-Fat Workout

Aerobic exercise versus resistance training: It's really not an either/or proposition. You need to do both regularly, says Norwood-Keating. She advises her clients to work both elements into their routine, with the time divided 50-50. An hour-long workout can easily contain a 30-minute aerobic routine and two sets at each station of our Core Routine (see page 121). If you're out of shape or are heavy enough that a sustained aerobic workout is quite taxing, Norwood-Keating recommends that you start with a 10- to 12-minute aerobic warm-up, do your weight routine, then finish with a 10- to 12-minute aerobic cooldown. (Remember: Even split aerobic exercise has tremendous benefits.)

For specific muscle exercises, you don't need to look much further than the Core Routine, which hits all the major muscle groups and will help make you firmer and leaner. There are, however, a number of abdominal exercises that would be worth adding to your routine. Some of them you can do anywhere, anytime, such as vacuums. Here are some other abs exercises our experts suggest.

The Meaning of "Lite"

In addition to the fallacy that you can't overstuff yourself with calories of carbohydrate, there's also the erroneous notion that you can eat as much as you want of anything labeled low-fat, nonfat or "lite." In truth, some products with low-fat or lite labeling still contain significant amounts of fat. Confusion over the meaning of these terms prompted the Food and Drug Administration to issue regulations on their use. When making food decisions, be aware of what the following terms actually tell you.

• "Low" means that the product falls under a legal limit for whatever claim is being made. To be "low-calorie," a product must have 40 calories or less per serving. To be "low-fat," it must have three grams or less per serving. To be "low-cholesterol," it must have less than 20 milligrams per serving.

The bottom line is that these products don't have a lot of the bad stuff, but they do have some. Note the serving size (now required to be reasonable, but still typically on the small side) and watch your intake.

• "Free" signifies an actual absence of the stuff—or at least so little of it that it hardly counts. It's the "healthiest" term, but taste may be an issue.

• "Reduced" means this particular product has 25 percent less fat, calories, sugar or whatever is being claimed than it used to have, or than a similar product (often with the same name) does. Its real meaning to you depends entirely on how bad the original is.

• "Lean" is a meat term meaning the cut has less than ten grams of total fat, four grams of saturated fat and 95 milligrams of cholesterol per serving.

• "Extra-lean" is twice as good as lean on the fat scale: It must have less than five grams of total fat and two grams of saturated fat—but is still allowed 95 milligrams of cholesterol per serving.

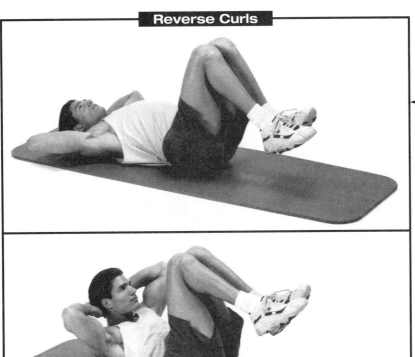

Reverse Curls

◀ Reverse Curls

Lie on your back, with your thighs at about a 90-degree angle to the floor and your knees bent and touching each other. Your feet should be positioned together loosely by your butt, and your hands should be behind your head. This is your starting position.

With your hands behind your head, raise your chest toward your knees while simultaneously bringing your knees toward your chest. Return to the starting position. With this and the following exercises, remember to exhale as you come up and inhale as you lower yourself back down.

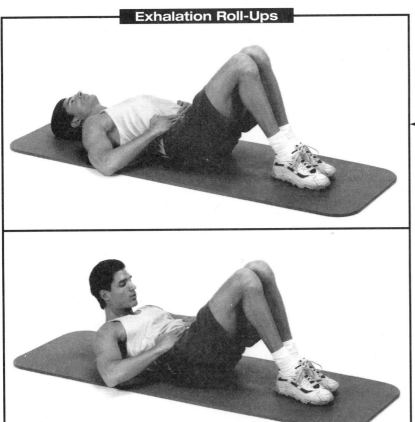

Exhalation Roll-Ups

◀ Exhalation Roll-Ups

Lie on your back with your knees bent and your feet flat on the floor about two feet from your butt. Place your hands on your stomach, with your index fingers pointing toward your navel.

Roll your shoulders and upper back off the floor. At the top of the motion, gently exhale, pushing the air out so that your stomach tightens. Pause for two seconds, roll back down to the starting position and breathe in. Do five to six repetitions.

Reverse Trunk Rotations ▶

To hit the abdominals, the obliques and muscles along the spine and lower back, try this exercise.

Lie on your back with your arms extended straight and perpendicular to your sides. Your knees should be bent and together, and your feet together, tucked close to your butt.

Keeping your shoulders and arms in contact with the floor, drop your bent knees to the right side, so that the outside of your right leg touches the floor. Raise your knees again, pass through the starting position and drop your knees to the left. Do two sets of 8 to 12 repetitions.

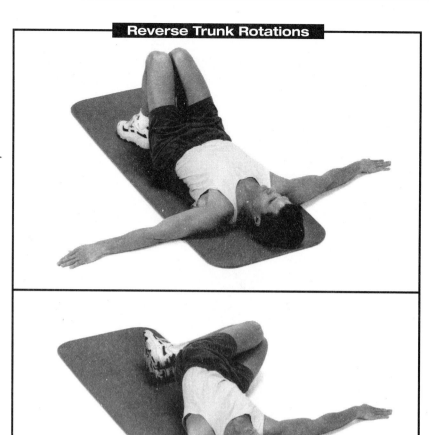

Reverse Trunk Rotations

The Inactive Man

Peak Points

- **Re-examine your feelings about physical exertion. Adjust your attitudes.**

- **Find an activity you like and begin to incorporate it into your daily and weekly routine.**

- **Look to build a more active lifestyle around the activity you enjoy most.**

- **Start slowly, gently, with just a couple minutes of exertion. Progressively work your way up to 10, 15, 20, 30 minutes or more for each exercise session.**

Got two minutes? Let's talk. Mind if we walk while we do this?

You ache too much, okay? You stress out easily and run a constant risk of injuring yourself. Your health's not that great—you're more prone to colds and flus and infections than you should be. You don't sizzle with energy. You don't seem lithe and limber. In fact, face it, you're really pretty physically weak. Most of the time people know better than to ask you to help them move the piano or lift the fridge. You look like you respect yourself some, but you aren't in very good shape.

Do you mind if we ask why?

What's holding you back?

What's keeping you from seeking your peak potential, your top form, your optimum health, your natural energy, your sharpest image?

Your body, after all, is a machine. If it isn't worked regularly and kept tuned, it rusts, malfunctions and falls apart.

You know this. But thinking about exercise makes you cringe, makes you tired, recalls pain. That's why we asked if you have two minutes. Because that's all it takes to start exercising and completely change your outlook and prognosis.

No pain, no gain? Hogwash, says Charles Swencionis, Ph.D., head of the health psychology program at Yeshiva University in New York City and co-author of *The Lazy Person's Guide to Fitness*.

If you're hurting after exercise, then you've injured your-

self, he says. Injuries—and their resulting pain—are one of the greatest reasons people fall off the exercise wagon. So, Dr. Swencionis says, it's important you avoid overdoing it, particularly at first.

So your first day exercising, Dr. Swencionis says, allow no more than two minutes of concentrated activity. Then add 30 seconds each day until you're up to a respectable 20, 30, 40 or more minutes.

But we're not going to start you off actually *exercising* on your first day in our program. You're going to like this. Your first assignment is to watch TV. Watch lots of it. Watch it in the evenings. Watch it all weekend. See, we want you to do something you're good at. There is a catch. You can watch all the TV you want as long as you're watching ESPN or sports and workout activities on other networks or videos.

That's the beginning of Level One.

Level One Program

Learn about exercise. Read about it—ways to do it, benefits of it. Socialize with fit, active friends and talk about their regimens. Rent videos showing active people, watch sports and games on television—these are all things that will get you thinking about exercise, a good first step, says Dr. Swencionis. "Rent and watch videos of the

Reference Points

Chapters

sports that people do in your town, and find one you like," he says.

Complain and gripe. That's right, bellyache about it. Carry on about why you don't exercise, about what happened when you did, how sore you felt. This is actually a positive process, says Dr. Swencionis, because it gets you thinking about exercise, your lifestyle and your needs, and, yeah, your pitifully weak excuses.

Clarify your values. Do it on paper. List how you feel about exercise. Is it good, bad, fun, only for bodybuilders? List all the positives and negatives you can think of about exercise, generally, and about specific forms of exercise.

Then, says Dr. Swencionis, examine the list item by item and ask where each idea came from and whether it's true in your life now or is a holdover from some ancient experience. As a more experienced person now, would you change the statement somehow? If so, rewrite it so it is valid now. And then, he says, rate it from one to ten on how important of a value it is.

This process, he says, can help you find useful ways to approach exercise.

Plus, he says, look at your history. Maybe once you loved to exercise, play sports and so on, but life changed and something had to give, and now you're in absolutely terrible physical condition. That's a great reason to get moving again.

If that's you, Covert Bailey, a popular fitness writer and author of *Smart Exercise*, says he'd ask you, "How come you fell out of the club, man? Look around you, there's mountains to climb, roller-blading . . . . It's hard to believe all the new sports around now that weren't when I was a kid."

State your reasons. "Different people have different reasons for exercising," says Dr. Swencionis. "Some do it to look nicer, some to feel more healthy, some to have more energy, some to lose fat, some to be stronger, some to live longer and more vibrantly."

Exercise can do all those things. "Aerobic exercise, combined with a low-fat diet, lowers high blood pressure, lowers cholesterol and controls diabetes," he says. "Just a loss of 10 to 15 pounds can mean you can decrease or even stop taking drugs for these conditions with your doctor's approval. Aerobic exercise increases your sense of well-being and lessens tendencies toward depression and anxiety. Building muscles in the right places—in the back, the abdomen and sides—can heal a bad back or greatly reduce the amount of trouble it gives you."

Bailey asks, "Want to die at age 70 in a wheelchair, or do you want to be having fun with the rest of us?" The choice, he says, is up to you.

Find your reasons for exercising and write them down on paper, where you can refer to them again

Just Do It

Everybody needs a little motivation to exercise at times. Here are some proven helpers.

Tell everybody. If you talk about your exercise program with your friends and family, you'll make it more a part of your life. It shows you're adopting a new image of which you are proud. And you can expect friends to rib you if you fall off the exercise wagon after talking it up. That kind of peer pressure can really help, says Charles Swencionis, Ph.D., head of the health psychology program at Yeshiva University in New York City and co-author of *The Lazy Person's Guide to Fitness*.

Find friends to exercise with. Research suggests that people who exercise together may be more likely to stick with it than are Lone Rangers, says Jonathan Robison, Ph.D., an exercise physiologist, nutritionist and executive co-director of the Michigan Center for Preventive Medicine in Lansing.

Besides, Dr. Robison says, "Studies show that people who feel connected with other people and with groups are healthier than those who do not feel connected. So if you find a physical activity that is enjoyable and that you can do socially with other people you enjoy being with, what more could you want? When talking health and wellness, those two things are really, really important."

Join a gym you can't miss. Is it on the way to or from work? Is it close enough to the office that you can drop in at lunchtime or walk to it after leaving the office? Making it convenient, and making it obvious—that is, you see it every day, want to or not—encourages you to make use of it, says Dr. Swencionis.

Keep a log. People who record their daily exercise tend to stick with the program more religiously than those who do not.

Get outdoors. "Studies show that feeling a connection with nature has physiological as well as psychological benefits," says Dr. Robison. We feel better, he says, when we see the sky, the ground, wild animals and the scenery rolling by than when, for example, we're pumping away on a stationary cycle in the basement. Most people, he says, would prefer to save the indoor equipment for days when it's raining or has snowed three feet.

and again over the next few months.

Use your imagination. Imagine the benefits of exercise—a slimmer, firmer you moving lithely with flexible, pain-free joints. This helps psyche you up, says Dr. Swencionis.

Your imagination can do even more, he says. Once you learn an exercise, if you will visualize yourself doing it perfectly, second by second, inch by inch, you'll discover an amazing physical benefit. "Visualization rehearses the motor pathways so the actual movement, when tried, is easier," he says.

Take notes. Any time you see someone enjoying an activity that looks like it might be fun, write it down so you don't forget. Then, when you get bored, you have another activity to explore.

Level Two Program

We're actually going to take the plunge. We're going to force ourselves to move. As Bailey says, "Get out and go. Find something fun and do it. Make sure it's fun because, if it isn't fun, you won't do it very long."

Run, says Bailey. If you can't run, walk. If you can't walk, crawl. If you can't crawl, roll. The idea, he says, is to get moving.

"The proper exercise for starting out is whichever exercise you'll enjoy and do," says Dr. Swencionis. "It's more beneficial than the perfect exercise that you won't do."

He adds, "There must be some kind of physical movement that you enjoy. Swimming? Walking? Shuffleboard? Softball? Roller-skating? Bicycling?"

"When you find one you like—or several you like, start out slowly. First, get your heart rate up some by running in place." You want it beating faster than normal, but not so fast that you can't comfortably carry on a conversation, he says. Once the heartbeat is up and blood is flowing through your muscles, do some stretching, says Dr. Swencionis. "Stretching before exercise improves performance," he says. "Stretching after exercise decreases the pain and soreness some people experience."

Once you feel limbered up, he says, exercise for just a few minutes your first day.

Start slowly. Very slowly. Very gently. A big mistake many people make is to start enthusiastically and overdo it—get exhausted, get hurt, get great new reasons and evidence why exercise is not for them. And starting slowly and gently doesn't just apply to the first time you start exercising, but to every time you start something new, every time you add weight or a new move to your routine, according to Dr. Swencionis. Start gently. Give yourself plenty of time to stretch and build new muscle.

Just give it 30 seconds. That's right. Start your exercise program with a two-minute workout, then add 30 seconds a day until you're up to 20 minutes, a half-hour or hour, wherever you want to be. One minute may seem, well, minute, but it's a start, says Dr. Swencionis. And if you add 30 seconds a day, you'll be enjoying the benefits of an impressive 15-

Ten Fun Activities You Might Try

Not sure how to get moving again? Here are some great first activities recommended by our experts to put you back on the road to fitness.

- Pre-breakfast bike ride
- Post-dinner neighborhood walk
- Lunchtime stair-walking (up and down) at work
- Morning calisthenics
- Living-room stretching routine
- Driveway basketball shooting
- Solo tennis against garage door or wall
- Roller-blading around the block with the kids
- Early evening nature walk
- Wiffle golf-ball hitting in the backyard

minute conditioning routine before a month is up. That's real progress. If you miss exercise for more than three days at any point, subtract 30 seconds for each day missed and start over from there, he says.

Come on, you say. I'm all pumped up about this. What do you mean "give it 30 seconds"? Listen to Dr. Swencionis: "Most people jump in too fast. They start by doing a half-hour or hour even of high- to moderate-intensity exercise and then injure themselves, or have pain from muscle and joint soreness even if they aren't actually injured. They feel sore and give it up. We have to avoid that. Start with no more than a couple minutes and then increase by 30 seconds a day."

Go for the gusto, but not for the burn. You don't have to hurt yourself to get fit. Really, says Dr. Swencionis. All you have to do is add a little effort to your routine each time, and you *will* build muscle, increase metabolism, burn fat, get stronger. You must repeat the routine at least every three days or else your body begins to lose conditioning, he says.

Pick a time. Morning, noon, evening, midnight, whenever you can work out regularly, says Dr. Swencionis. For some people, certain times of the day feel better than others for exercise. Find your time during Level Two and mentally and physically mark it off on your calendar as *your* exercise time.

Believe in your ability to change. Monitor the stories you're telling yourself about your exercise program and commitment, says Dr. Swencionis. Are you telling yourself you *can* change? Are you telling yourself that *maybe* you can change? Are you saying, "I can't" or "I probably won't stick with this"? Whatever you are telling yourself short of "I can" needs to be adjusted up at least one notch, says Dr. Swencionis. Correct that self-talk. If you're saying, "I can't," change it to "Maybe I can." If you're saying "maybe," change it to "I can." Because, says Dr. Swencionis, if you believe you can, you can. You're in control of this one.

Get it out. Don't hide your exercise equipment in the closet or in a crowded corner of the basement. Set it up in the open where it is convenient and easy to use—maybe in front of the TV. Seeing it can prompt you to use it.

Level Three Program

As you begin to enjoy the benefits of stretching and aerobic exercise, you may find yourself wanting to build muscle. That's a good time to turn to the Core Routine on page 121 and consider adding resistance training to your program.

"Resistance exercise increases stamina, strength, endurance and power," says exercise physiologist John Amberge, director of corporate programs for the Sports Training Institute in New York City.

You're on a roll when you hit Level Three. Exercise is becoming a habit. It actually becomes something you look forward to much of the time. It's a break, a stress-buster, a time to play.

At Level Three your big challenge is to keep rolling. Stay vigilant.

"It's important for health," says Jonathan Robison, Ph.D., an exercise physiologist, nutritionist and executive co-director of the Michigan Center for Preventive Medicine in Lansing, "that you accumulate about 30 minutes of moderate-intensity physical activity daily. I don't believe that working out on stair-climbers and bikes and treadmills is what most people are going to do. You can do other things and be healthy. You can garden. You can walk the dog. You can park the car two blocks away from your appointment and walk. It all counts. It's the total amount of activity in a week that matters, as far as health is concerned."

Keep that in mind should you find yourself resisting or falling away from a particular exercise routine. We all do fall away at times.

You can be a world-class exerciser and then get sick, or go on vacation, or get injured or pack up and move and, suddenly, you're not exercising anymore. You may not even be thinking about exercising any more. You may be telling yourself that you don't want to exercise, says Dr. Swencionis.

That's okay. Everybody falls off the treadmill at times, says Dr. Swencionis. The key is to realize that. Understand that getting back on is part of the process, and try to limit the downtime, he says.

Use every bit of motivation that got you to exercise in the first place and get going again at an easy pace so you don't injure yourself, he says. You can't enjoy the benefits without doing the work, and just because you stopped for a while doesn't mean you must stop forever.

Actively start thinking your way back into exercising; picture yourself exercising and enjoying it. And then, doggone it, do it. Force yourself. But restart gently. You'll be surprised that suddenly you find yourself enjoying it, wondering what the big deal was.

The Career Man

Who predicted the seemingly endless 60-hour work-weeks that so many of us battle through at the close of the twentieth century? That so many of us would be self-employed, searching for business seemingly round the clock? That company allegiance would become more a liability than an asset? That we would have to scramble so incessantly just to stay one step ahead of changing technology, corporate layoffs and downsizing. All the rules seem to have changed for the typical working man these days, and yet the old saying rings truer than ever: A man's work is never done.

The scramble to make a decent living in these modern times requires sacrifices—mostly of personal time. And one of the first things to get set aside is exercise. The quality of our lives, our health and even our work suffers as a result, says Charles Swencionis, Ph.D., head of the health psychology program at Yeshiva University in New York City and co-author of *The Lazy Person's Guide to Fitness*.

"The problem is that man was made to be physically active, not to sit at desks and stare at computers," says Jonathan Robison, Ph.D., an exercise physiologist, nutritionist and executive co-director of the Michigan Center for Preventive Medicine in Lansing.

Why We Must Exercise

We can't perform at our peak—at work or play—if we give up physical activity. So it's time we work smarter, not harder—to parrot the mantra managers chanted during the initial frenzy of corporate downsizing.

Working smarter means fitting regular workouts into our daily work routine. Rather than squeezing us for time, they help us do our work better and more effectively—and they blow away stress, say Dr. Swencionis and Dr. Robison.

Ever notice how much more clearly you think, how much easier the thoughts flow after a few minutes of vigorous walking? That's one of the immediate benefits of exercise.

It's simply part of our physiology, says Dr. Robison. Our brains, hearts, muscles, and joints all were designed to work more efficiently when regularly exercised.

"The challenge," says Dr. Swencionis, "is to find creative ways to squeeze exercise into our busy lives." Fortunately, once we understand what's needed, we can find many ways to provide it, says Dr. Robison.

The Busy Man's Needs

Being in peak condition means more than just looking good in your gym shorts, according to Dr. Robison. It means having a

Why Bother?

Why should we juggle impossible schedules to fit exercise into our already too complicated lives?

Here are a few reasons from Susan Lark, M.D., who has written a book on stress and exercise. Exercise, Dr. Lark says:

- Improves brain function
- Increases the output of feel-good brain chemicals, so we feel better physically and emotionally
- Dissipates pent-up frustration and aggression
- Loosens muscles, easing physical tension
- Improves digestion
- Stabilizes blood sugar
- Reduces blood pressure

balance in all aspects of our lives.

"Yes, physical activity is important," he says. "Yes, reasonably balanced nutrition is important. They're part of the bigger picture of physical, emotional and spiritual balance."

A well-designed peak conditioning program uses good nutrition as a base, says Dr. Robison. For the super-busy corporate man, the plan blends in efficient aerobic, resistance and flexibility workouts, along with mental and physical relaxation routines.

Let's look again at each of those elements more closely, as they pertain to the working man.

- Aerobic exercise is anything that gets your heart rate up higher than normal, but not at a rate so high that you can't carry on a conversation, and holds it there for 12 minutes or more. It could be vigorous walking, bicycling, rowing, dancing, racquetball, jogging, basketball, soccer and so on.
- Strength training, also known as isotonic or resistance training, builds muscle by resisting its natural movement with weight—even body weight.
- Stretching alternately tenses and relaxes muscles, increasing flexibility and blood flow.
- Relaxation can be as simple as breathing rhythmically and gently pruning the mind of all but one thought, phrase or image—and can even be done while working out.

An ideal prescriptive program might involve devoting an hour or more a day to a balanced combination of all those exercise components. But most people don't follow exercise prescriptions. "Doctors have almost given up telling people to exercise," says Dr. Swencionis.

Realize, says Dr. Robison, that while we need all these components in our daily life, we don't need to

do them by rote, all at once. That is, we don't have to spend 20 minutes on the treadmill, followed by 20 minutes lifting weights, and then 20 minutes stretching and relaxing. Rather, we can accumulate bits and pieces throughout the day, in a variety of ways, and achieve the basic benefits.

In fact, if we make the process enjoyable, helpful and re-energizing, we gain even more benefits.

Walking the dog counts. So does gardening and taking the stairs instead of the elevator. So does two minutes of peaceful daydreaming, visualizing lying on a beach in the South Pacific, while bumping around on the cross-town bus.

In a moment, we'll explore numerous ways of accumulating activity of all sorts throughout the business day. But some men do prefer to block off specific time on their schedules for regular workouts. Here are two super-efficient routines for time-managers.

The Busy Man's 30-Minute Workout

To gain the invigorating, life-preserving benefits of physical activity, research suggests we need to accumulate a minimum of 30 minutes a day of moderate-intensity physical activity, says Dr. Robison.

An easy way to do that, he says, is walking.

"You don't have to learn how to walk. You can do it almost anywhere. You can walk around the block. You can walk around a hotel. You can walk around the office," he says.

So walking is the first element in Dr. Robison's really-strapped-for-time busy executive's workout on the run. You should try to get at least 30 minutes, but for this quick, on-the-fly routine, you could get away with 15 minutes.

"Let's say a man is really strapped for time," says Dr. Robison. "In addition to walking, at the very least, he can do push-ups. They're pretty good all-around upper-body conditioners. You don't have to spend much time doing push-ups. They're certainly something you can do anywhere for a couple of minutes. Then do five minutes of stretching, or a few Yoga poses. And then five minutes of sitting doing nothing—trying to just get in touch with yourself at the present moment and not *doing*, because people are always so busy *doing* that we hardly ever end up just *being* in the moment. You can do that while stretching. So, 15 to 20 minutes walking, a couple minutes doing push-ups, five minutes stretching and meditating, and you've had a quick workout."

The 60-Minute Gym Workout

If you *can* hit the gym for an hour, three days a week, here's what exercise physiologist John Amberge, director of corporate programs for the Sports Training Institute in New York City, would suggest.

Start with 20 to 30 minutes of aerobic exercise

(start slowly to warm your body up). Then go through a full-body muscular strength routine for 20 to 25 minutes. Our Core Routine, with one set of each exercise, will work. Then cool down with abdominal exercises and whole-body stretching. "You'll be in and out in an hour, as long as you don't rest longer than one minute between each set," Amberge says. "You could even do this on a lunch break."

Specific Exercises

Obviously, calendaring an hour a day, three days a week, for total workouts in or out of the gym, plus accumulating at least 30 minutes of physical activity on each of the other days, is the ideal, says Dr. Robison. The point here is that most of us busy men feel we don't have time for that. We're too busy earning a living, remember?

Here are some surefire ways to easily fit working out into your work days. Many of these activities combine one or more of the exercise elements, such as cardiovascular work *and* strength training. As a bonus, we'll toss in a series of stretches you can do while sitting at your desk. As a double bonus, we'll offer a resistance workout you can do in your office with some high-tech gym equipment that will cost you less than $20 and fit in the corner of a desk drawer or in a compartment in your briefcase.

Cardiovascular Work

Unfortunately, there are no shortcuts for this one. The very nature of aerobic exercise—pumping up your heart rate and then sustaining that heightened level for a time—mandates that it eat into your day. Here are tips for getting the time or motivation to work aerobic exercise into your busy day.

Take a walk. This is the number one solution. No clothes changes, no equipment, and the clock starts running the second you get out of your chair. Switch to dressy walking shoes or carry sneakers with you for a quick change, recommends Amberge. Walk to appointments and to lunch. "Make it a point during the day to get out and walk around the block or around the building for 15 minutes," Amberge says. Use stairs instead of elevators. "You can use the flights of stairs in your building and do 15 minutes of stair-climbing for a cardiovascular workout," he says.

"Take the subway or train and get off a couple of blocks early and walk the rest of the way," suggests Dr. Robison.

Forget shortcuts, says Dr. Robison. Take the long way. "Park a couple of blocks away from your destination and walk the rest. If the weather is reasonable, walk to work if it's possible and safe, or find a garage or parking lot away from your office and park there most days and then walk."

Eating Right

Being in peak condition is more than hefting weights a carnival strongman might shy away from, notes Jonathan Robison, Ph.D., an exercise physiologist, nutritionist and executive co-director of the Michigan Center for Preventive Medicine in Lansing. It also involves putting a relatively healthy combination of fuels into our bodies, he says.

We need a proper balance of nutrients to maintain our body's ability to resist disease, repair damage, think clearly and quickly, and otherwise function optimally. That doesn't come from skipping breakfast, gobbling sugary and greasy snacks, guzzling soft drinks and grabbing burgers on the run, notes Margaret A. Caudill, M.D., Ph.D., associate professor of medicine at Harvard Medical School.

Instead, pack in three meals daily teeming with fresh vegetables and grains and other high-fiber foods, says Dr. Caudill. Add snacks of fresh fruits. Drink plenty of water. Learn to plan meals and snacks based on the government's food pyramid guidelines. And learn to listen to what your body is telling you it needs, she says, because nutritional needs vary from person to person.

Join a gym. Find one close to your office, one you must pass every morning and evening. Make it easy to drop in for a few minutes or to run over to it during lunch. Better yet, go before or after work: This saves the most time since you only have to change clothes once (that is, you can leave your house in your workout clothes in the morning and dress for work at the gym). Get in a quick game of racquetball or basketball, or swim or hit the workout machines or weights, says Dr. Swencionis.

Log your activity. So advises Dr. Swencionis. Studies show that people who keep track of their daily physical fitness efforts tend to place more importance on fitness and are more likely to find time for it.

Accumulate activity. Garden, walk the dog, carry trash, mow the lawn, trim the hedges, split logs. Discover ways to avoid labor-saving equipment and go ahead and use your muscles, says Dr. Robison.

Ride a bike. Ride to work some days if that is feasible. Ride your bike on errands. "Five or six miles on a bike is a great workout," says Dr. Robison. And, he notes, it's a lot more fun to do it outdoors than in a gym on a stationary cycle. And the very act of balancing on a real bicycle adds a fitness element that you miss on a stationary bike, points out Covert Bailey, a popular fitness writer and author of *Smart Exercise*.

Flexibility and Relaxation Exercises

First off, study ergonomics, suggests Amberge. Ergonomics is sort of the science of sitting at a desk without hurting yourself. It is serious business, since humans weren't created to sit at desks. Most personnel departments have brochures produced by workers' compensation insurance companies that demonstrate proper postures for various tasks, and libraries have books on the subject. An important ergonomic factor, Amberge says, is movement. "Get up from your desk and move around regularly," he says. This stretches muscles, helps blood move and works out kinks that can otherwise turn into problems.

In fact, tense, relax and stretch your muscles throughout the day, says Dr. Robison. The following stretching exercises can all be done while sitting at your desk. In the next section, we'll toss in some strength-builders you can do at your desk that are recommended by Dr. Robison.

Arm Muscle Toners

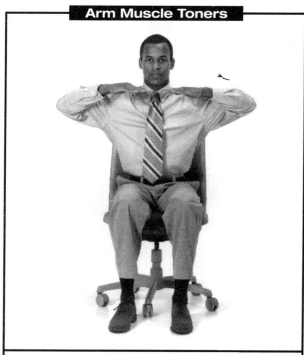

◄ Arm Muscle Toners

Raise your elbows to shoulder height and bend your arms so your fingers are in front of your chest. Your arms and fingers should be parallel to the floor.

Push your elbows out as far to the sides as possible. Hold for five to ten seconds, then relax. Repeat five times.

Mid-Back Stretch

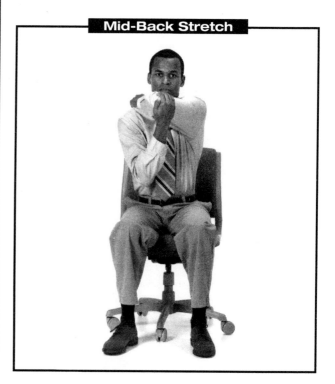

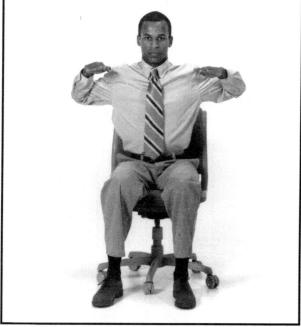

Mid-Back Stretch ▲

Draw your left arm across your chest in front of you. With your right hand, grasp your arm just above the elbow and pull it, gently, toward your right shoulder. Hold the stretch for five seconds. Do the other side. This stretches and increases flexibility in the upper and middle back.

Shoulder Hugs

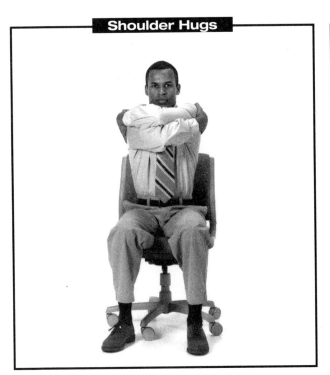

Side Stretch

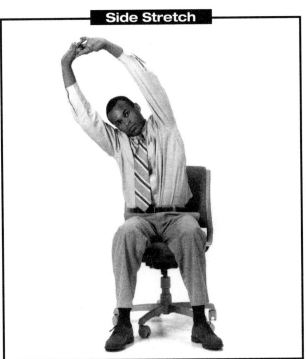

Shoulder Hugs ▲

Cross your arms around your chest, reaching your fingers around your shoulder blades. This relieves shoulder and upper-back tension.

Lower-Back Relaxers

Sit upright in your chair with your legs spread slightly. Droop forward, dropping your neck and shoulders and then your arms, bending down between your knees as far as possible. Then sit up and relax.

Windmills

Sitting upright on your chair's edge, reach down and touch your left foot with your right hand while reaching your left arm up into the air. Slowly alternate sides. This stretch is good for the hips and waist.

Arm Circles

Stretch your arms straight out to the sides with your elbows straight. Slowly whirl your arms, defining small circles with your pointed fingertips. First go forward, then backward. This improves shoulder mobility.

Shoulder Rolls

Sitting up, gently roll your shoulders forward five times, then backward five times. Great for dissipating tension buildup in the neck and shoulders.

Finger Relaxers

With your palms down, spread your fingers and thumbs as far apart as possible, hold for five seconds, relax, then repeat. Particularly good for relieving tension in fingers tired of dancing on a keyboard.

Side Stretch ▲

Clasp your fingers together in front of your chest. Turn your palms outward and lift your arms over your head, keeping your fingers interlaced. Push your arms back as far as they comfortably will go with your elbows straight, then lean to the right as far as comfortable and then to the left. This works and stretches your side muscles from your arms to your hips.

Upper-Back Relaxers

Sitting upright, place the tips of the fingers of your right hand on your right shoulder and the tips of your left fingers on your left shoulder, while pointing your elbows straight out to the sides. Then slowly draw your elbows together in front of you as close as is comfortable, stretching the muscles in your upper back and shoulder blades. Then return to the starting position. Drop your arms and relax with your hands in your lap. Then repeat.

Shoulder Stretcher

Reach over and behind your head with your right hand, resting it as low as possible on your left shoulder. Bring your left hand up behind your back and try to touch or interlock the fingers of both hands. Repeat on the other shoulder.

Neck Stretcher

Sitting upright, slowly drop your chin to your chest. Then slowly tilt your head backward as far as possible and stare at the ceiling. Return it to the normal upright position so that you're staring straight ahead. Now slowly tilt it as far as possible toward your right shoulder. Bring it back to the center upright position, then lower it to the left.

Strength-Building Exercises

You don't have to buy a lot of expensive gym equipment to get a good resistance workout. You don't even need to buy weights, says Amberge.

You already have the weight. Your body weight. Remember the mat exercises the P.E. coach led you through back in high school? The push-ups, the squats, the lunges, the crunches and so on? Add "step-ups, pull-ups, chin-ups, wall sits—these are all good resistance exercises that use your own body weight and can be done anywhere, without special equipment," says Amberge. There are many other exercises as well.

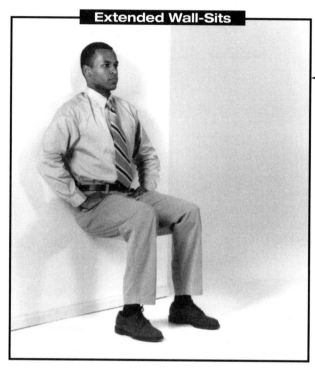

Extended Wall-Sits

◄ Extended Wall-Sits

This is great for building muscular strength and endurance in your quads, hamstrings and glutes, says Amberge. Start by standing with your back against a wall, feet about hip-width apart. Then slowly slide down and walk your feet out until it is almost as though you are sitting in a chair—but there is no chair. Your back is supported against the wall; your quads, hamstrings and glutes are contracting to support your body weight. Start slowly by holding for a count of five to ten seconds, then slide back up. Repeat five times. You may progress to the point where you can hold the wall-sit position for several minutes. Don't go below a 90-degree angle at the knee joint in the seated position, nor allow your knee to go in front of your foot, Amberge warns.

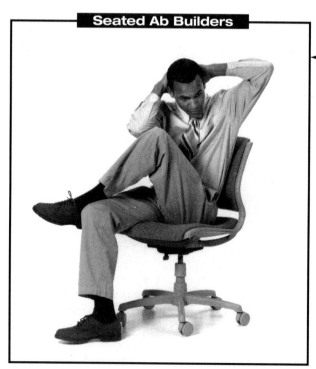

Seated Ab Builders

◄ Seated Ab Builders

While sitting upright, link your fingers behind your head. Lifting your left knee, bend and touch it with your right elbow. Then return your left foot to the floor and lift your right knee and touch it with your left elbow. Do at least five in a set.

Seated Quad Builders

This also builds abs. Sitting upright in your chair, lift your legs straight out in front of you, so your body is making an L-shape. Hold for five seconds, then repeat.

Back Strengtheners

Here's one you can do lying in bed, says Dr. Swencionis. Roll over on your stomach, put your hands at your side and lift your head and shoulders up off the bed—keep your head and neck straight. Hold the position for a few seconds. Do it in sets of five.

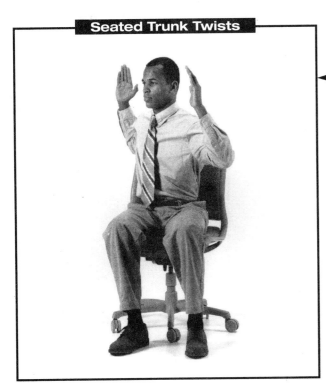

Seated Trunk Twists

◄ Seated Trunk Twists

Sit on the edge of your seat and hold your arms straight out to the sides, then bend them up at the elbows at right angles. Turn your entire upper body (turning your head with your trunk) to the right as far as comfortable, hold for a couple of seconds, then return to center. Repeat three times, then turn to the left. This is good for the abs and pecs and for relieving back tension.

Seated Pec Stretch

While sitting upright, link your fingers behind your head and push your elbows back as far as comfortable. Hold for a few seconds, then relax and return to the starting position. Drop your arms to your side and then repeat several times.

The Tube Workout

Tubing is an amazing fitness tool. Fashioned from surgical tubing, it is sold in varying lengths and thicknesses, sometimes with handles attached to the ends, in some fitness stores. It's inexpensive and takes up little space, yet can replace a full set of weights.

"With tubing, you can do a workout simulating all the muscle group isolations just as you would with free weights or gym equipment," enthuses Amberge. The various thicknesses of the tubing create various levels of resistance. "You can wrap one end around a door knob or the leg of a desk or some other immovable object and use the other end like a weighted pulley on gym equipment," he says.

Tubing easily fits in a briefcase, and so it travels anywhere. Most manufacturers include instructions showing a range of exercises that can be combined for a full-body workout. But to start, here are three great exercises to do with six-foot tubing.

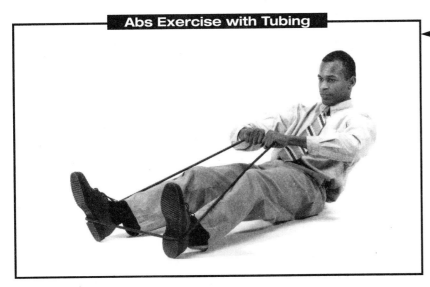

Abs Exercise with Tubing

◄ Abs Exercise with Tubing

Stretch the tubing across the bottom of your feet (cross in the arch area) while sitting on the floor. Both legs should be extended in front of you, knees bent slightly, feet pointed up and slightly out, about two feet apart. With a handle gripped in each hand, bring your hands together in front of your chest and, holding them there, slowly lower your upper body back toward the floor while tightening your abs. (You need not touch the floor.) Pause. Return slowly to the starting position. Do sets of five reps.

Seated Rows with Tubing

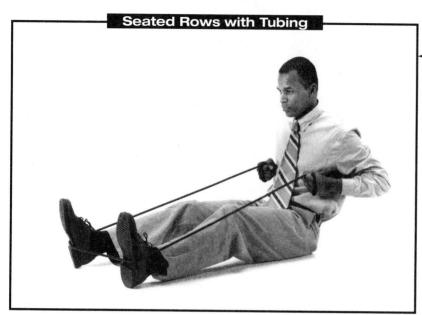

◄ Seated Rows with Tubing

Sit on the floor, legs extended in front of you, knees slightly bent, feet pointed up or slightly out. (For added resistance, you may spread your feet shoulder-width apart.) Stretch the tube around the bottom of the arches of your feet. Wrap the ends of the tubing around your hands to create resistance. Your palms should be facing inward. Pull your elbows back evenly until your hands are near the midline of your torso. Then pause and slowly return to the starting position. That is one complete rowing motion.

Triceps Press with Tubing

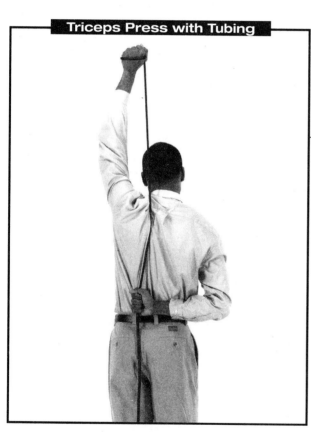

◄ Triceps Press with Tubing

Grasp one handle. Put that hand near the back of your neck and let the tubing fall down your back. With the other hand, reach behind your back and grasp the tubing at a place that feels comfortable and hold it there, taut between your hands. Slowly raise the hand at the back of the neck, extending the arm upward (but not locking the elbow), keeping the elbow close to your head. Slowly return to the starting position.

The Traveling Man

Sticking to your workout is hard enough when you're close to home. But when you throw in an out-of-town conference here, a weekend excursion there, a regular exercise routine becomes even tougher to sustain.

If travel is a regular part of your job, you have some inkling of what we're talking about. When you travel to another city, you're in unfamiliar territory and often an unfamiliar time zone. Fatigue takes its toll on your plans for an evening run; daylong meetings quash your opportunity for a morning workout.

"If you're trying to stay fit, travel's tough on you," says Sandra Fisher, exercise physiologist and owner of New York City's Fitness by Fisher, an exercise consulting firm. Fisher works closely with corporations whose employees travel a great deal and devotes much of her practice to helping busy executives exercise on the road. "It's not just the issue of making time for exercise while you're traveling. Just as big a question is: Where can I go to exercise?"

Taking Your Workout on the Road

Fisher calls them the twin demons of travel fitness—finding time to work out, and finding a place to work out once you do find the time. But you can exorcise these demons once and for all with a little ingenuity. And we're not just talking about calling ahead to make sure your hotel has an exercise facility (although that's a great idea). One of the factors that made man the dominant species on the planet was our ability to adapt to changing surroundings, improvise with the materials at hand and overcome the obstacles to our survival.

And so it is when you're on the road and there isn't a barbell around for miles. Now, the point isn't to try to duplicate your at-home workouts. The idea is to do enough substitute exercise so that when you can resume your regular exercise routine, you won't have lost any ground on your physical fitness. If you want to ensure the survival of your fitness in those situations, try these expert tips.

Pack for a workout. The easiest way to miss out on exercise is by conveniently forgetting to pack appropriate exercise clothes. "I'd make it a habit to always keep workout clothes in one of your suitcase pouches," says Fisher. "If they're always in that pouch, you'll never have the excuse that you forgot your clothes." Wrap the clothes in a plastic bag, though—you wouldn't want your suit smelling like sweat socks.

Ask at the front desk. If your hotel has a weight room and a couple of stair-climbers, or a pool where you can do a few laps before bedtime, then you're set. But even hotels that don't sport these healthful facilities do have at least one useful exercise resource—the concierge.

"It never hurts to ask at the front desk where you can go for a workout," says Fisher. At the very least, a concierge can

Packing for Fitness

Before you head out the door on that next road trip, go to the kitchen and grab yourself a garbage bag. We're going to make an exercise survival kit that you can take with you. We can't guarantee it'll keep you in shape until you get back home—only you can do that. But this kit will sure make it harder for you to blow off exercise while you're traveling. Sandra Fisher, exercise physiologist and owner of New York City's Fitness by Fisher, an exercise consulting firm, suggests that you fill that bag with:

The Essentials

- Athletic shoes. For versatility, cross-trainers are your best bet. If you're a runner, though, pack only running shoes; you'll need the support.
- T-shirt.
- Sweatshirt. Just in case it's cold.
- Shorts. You'll want them to double as a swimsuit, so pack shorts made of a synthetic material. Cotton will sag when it gets wet, which could be pretty embarrassing when you're poolside.
- Athletic socks. Two pairs.
- Fanny pack. Or anything that will securely hold your ID, hotel keys and a little bit of cash.

Recommended Options

- Reflectors. On the road, the only time you can work out might be at night. Carry these when you're running or walking, and you'll help ensure a safe workout.
- Personal stereo. Listen to music or an audio book while you're working out. It's a great way to de-stress after a long day of travel. For safety's sake, don't use them when you are running or biking outside.
- Light hand weights. Not dumbbells, just a couple little hand weights. Carry them when you walk or run, or use them as part of your in-room workout.
- Jump rope. Handy for a workout anywhere. Also useful for lashing your suitcase together if it bursts open in baggage claim.

direct you to the local YMCA or the nearest squash court. And if you are an outdoor exerciser, the front desk can certainly tell you the safest places to do your exercise—an important consideration in a strange and unfamiliar city.

Walk when you can. One problem with traveling is the fact that we become overly reliant on vehicles to move us from place to place—the company car, the red-eye flight, the express train or bus. "It's easy to forget you have your own two feet to help you move around," says Charles Kuntzleman, Ed.D., adjunct associate professor of kinesiology at the University of Michigan in Ann Arbor.

So walk when it's practical. Take the stairs instead of the hotel elevator. Walk around the terminal while you're waiting for your connecting flight. Stop the car every two hours and saunter around the rest area. If you're taking a cab back to the hotel after your meetings are finished, have the cabbie stop about five minutes before you get there, and just hoof it the rest of the way. "Slip in a few minutes of walking here and there. If you tally it up at the end of the day, you might be surprised to discover you got 20 or 30 minutes of exercise," says Dr. Kuntzleman.

Seek out a partner. It may help to remember there are others of your kind—traveling men who would like to stick to their workout. "At conventions, I encourage people to check out the message boards you always see in the lobby. Lots of times, I've seen

messages announcing a morning fitness walk, or that someone was looking for a running or exercise partner," says Fisher. And if you don't see any messages, post your own. If you've made arrangements to meet someone to work out with, you'll be more likely to exercise than if you tried to go by yourself, says Fisher. "Plus, it's a novel way to network and make new contacts," she adds.

Visit the local clubs. If you belong to a fitness club at home, remember that membership may have its privileges, even when you're out of town. "A lot of health clubs have business relationships with clubs in other cities," says Fisher. Ask your club for more details; usually they can give you a list of affiliates where you can work out for a nominal "drop-in" fee or even at no extra cost. "Ask at your hotel, too," says Fisher. "Many of them have deals with local fitness clubs so that guests can exercise."

Make an appointment. At home, exercise is simply part of your routine—something you do at a set time everyday. When you're on the road, you don't have a routine, you have an itinerary. "You're on a travel schedule, so the routine goes out the window. It's easy to forget exercise. That's why I'd suggest actually scheduling exercise time. Put it in your daybook like any other meeting," recommends Dr. Kuntzleman. By actually building exercise time into your schedule, you're more likely to find time for it.

Exercising in Exile

Even when there's no weight room at the inn, and no fitness club where you can drop in, you can still get together a halfway-decent weight-training regimen. "Of course, you can always do exercises where you're using your own body weight as resistance," says Dr. Kuntzleman. "But over and above that, you can use items in your hotel room to help you do a makeshift workout."

But before you begin, a note of caution. Some of the exercises suggested here call for using furniture or hotel-room accessories that weren't designed for exercise. If we suggest using a bed, make certain the mattress is firm. If you're using a chair or luggage rack to do an exercise, test them, shake them, do what you need to do to ensure that they're stable and sturdy enough to support your weight. If they're not—or you're not comfortable using them—then skip the exercise.

"There's nothing wrong with being inventive and trying to develop a workout using materials close at hand. But it's important that you use common sense and be safe about it," says Dr. Kuntzleman. With that in mind, try these.

Hotel-Room Push-Ups

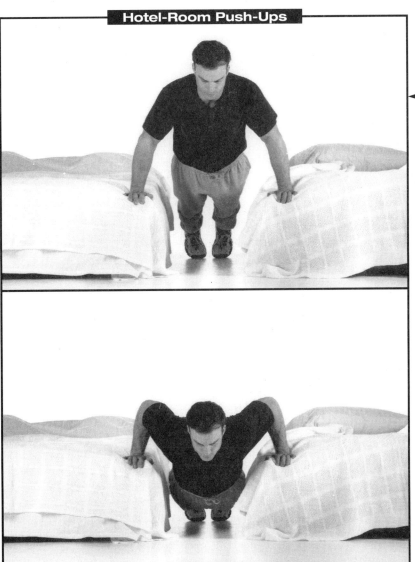

◀ Hotel-Room Push-Ups

Like the standard push-up, this exercise works your upper and outer pectorals. For this exercise, you'll need two beds side by side. If the beds are so far apart that you can't position your hands properly, then use two sturdy chairs.

Stand between the beds and get yourself in standard push-up mode—legs extended behind you, toes touching the floor. Place a hand flat on either bed, fingers pointing straight ahead—your hands should be about shoulder-width or slightly wider apart. Your arms should be extended so your upper body is elevated slightly above the level of the bed.

Now slowly lower yourself down toward the floor. Keep your back and legs straight and bend your arms; your elbows should be close to your sides. Lower yourself so your chest is in line with the beds. Pause, then raise back up.

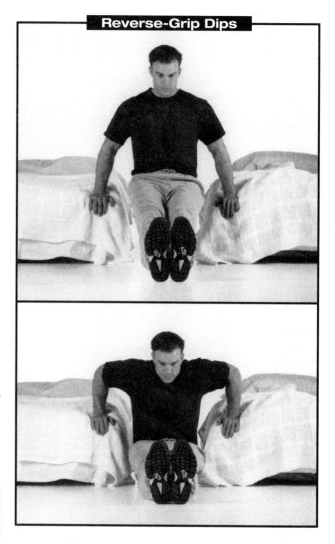

Reverse-Grip Dips ➤

This dip works your lower pecs and triceps. Start by standing between the beds or two chairs.

This time, your legs will be straight out in front of you, toes pointing up, heels touching the floor. Place a hand on each mattress and extend your arms so you're holding your butt off the ground. Your fingers point straight ahead, parallel to the sides of the bed.

Now slowly bend at your elbows and lower your butt toward the floor—but don't let it touch. Pause just above the floor, then raise yourself back up to the starting position.

Note: If the mattresses aren't firm enough, slide your hands under the mattresses and support yourself on the box springs.

Luggage Rack Shoulder Raises

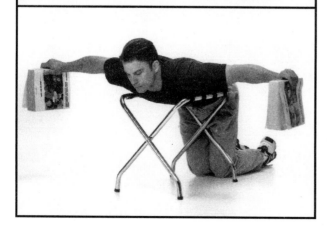

◄ Luggage Rack Shoulder Raises

For this exercise, which works the top and back shoulder muscles, you'll need one of those fold-out luggage stands (check the closet), which will act in place of a weight bench.

Note: Test the rack to make sure it doesn't wobble and that it will support your weight. If you don't think the luggage rack is sturdy or large enough to support you, do these luggage rack exercises on the bed, working one arm at a time. If you haven't brought a set of light weights with you, use a couple of heavy books, like the telephone directory or the Bible in the nightstand.

Kneel facing the luggage rack, using it to support your upper body. Let your arms dangle off either side of the stand. Hold a weight in each hand, palms facing inward. Your arms should be fully extended. If your arms are long enough to touch the floor, raise them slightly so they're no longer touching the floor.

Now raise the weights in a semicircular motion, keeping your arms as straight as possible without locking your elbows. Raise your arms to shoulder height, then lower and repeat.

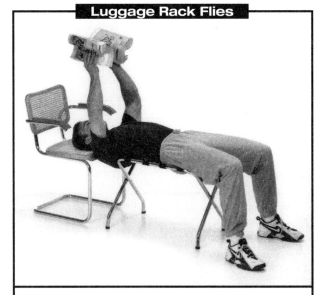

Luggage Rack Flies

Luggage Rack Flies ➤

You'll need the luggage stand and a chair for this pectoral exercise. If the stand is not sturdy enough, do this on the bed, working one arm at a time.

Push a chair up to one end of the luggage rack. This time lie on your back on the luggage rack, with your knees bent so your feet are touching the floor. Support your head on the chair. Extend your arms up so you're holding the weights above your chest. You should be holding the weights so your palms are facing each other.

Keeping your arms as straight as possible (it's okay if they bend a little), lower the weights in a semicircular motion out to either side of your chest. Lower until the weights are even with your chest, but back slightly so they're in line with your ears. Pause, then raise the weights back up. Repeat.

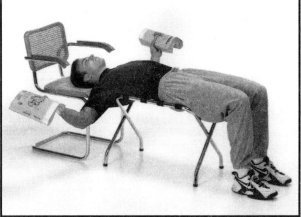

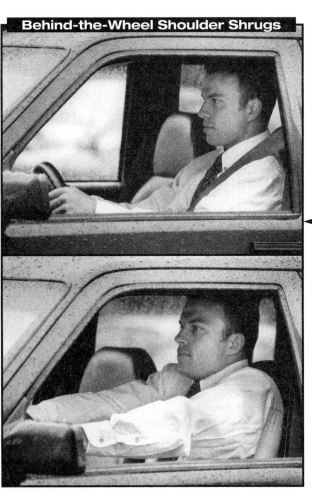

Behind-the-Wheel Shoulder Shrugs

◄ Behind-the-Wheel Shoulder Shrugs

Try this exercise the next time you're caught in traffic—it not only reduces stress but it also works the trapezius muscles of your shoulders.

Hold the steering wheel with your left hand on the nine o'clock position, right hand on the three o'clock. Try to keep your arms as straight as possible.

Now raise your shoulders. When they've reached the highest point, rotate them forward, then roll them back to the top and toward your back. Lower and repeat.

Push-Ups

There are darn few hotel rooms too small for you to stretch out on the floor and do some push-ups. "That's the great thing about push-ups—you can do them anywhere. And you can modify them to work different parts of your arms and upper body," says Dr. Kuntzleman. Just squeak in a quick 10 or 20 before you jump in the shower every morning. You'll get your engine revving, you'll be ready to start the day and you'll have had a little exercise to boot. If you can't do regular push-ups, Dr. Kuntzleman suggests doing bent-knee push-ups or inclined push-ups.

Crunches

Same deal. You have the time, so do them slowly and carefully. Mix up your abs exercises to get a complete workout. That means reverse crunches, oblique crunches, cross-over crunches, raised leg crunches, frog crunches and so on.

Jump Rope

When you're packing your workout clothes, make sure you slip a jump rope into that plastic bag.

"It's the perfect exercise equipment for traveling," enthuses Dr. Kuntzleman. "You can slip it in your briefcase, and you don't need a lot of space to get a great workout, just jump rope for 20 or so minutes." Hint: Do be mindful of your fellow travelers, especially the ones trying to sleep in the room below you—they might not appreciate the rhythmic pounding overhead.

Stretches

Stuck in a hotel room for an hour with nothing to do and no one to do it with? Do a slow, relaxed, whole-body stretching routine. We assume that since you work out, you know the basic stretches. But this time, instead of hurrying through them to get to the rest of the workout, make the stretches the entire workout. Take a few minutes to give each muscle group a slow, careful stretch. Just don't overextend— your body may not be used to the pressure. A well-done 30-minute stretching program can give you a far better workout and relaxation response than you might realize.

The Family Man

Are you in good enough shape to be a father?

Do you have enough strength to carry a baby in one arm, a bag of groceries in the other, and walk with both for a half-mile?

Can you, after a full day of work, come home and still wrestle with the kids, pick up toys, carry out the trash, mow the lawn, play a little basketball with the teens and have enough energy left over to enjoy the activity that got you into the daddy business in the first place?

These are not trivial questions. The years in which you are raising young children—your twenties and thirties—are often the years you are working hardest to get your career on track, and these are not easy times for worker bees. Throw in a family, and chances are you are struggling to find the time, the energy, the motivation to meet all the demands on you. And yet, you're not willing to sacrifice any of it.

So if the idea of working out to be a better father seems odd, think again. Exercise will give you the stamina, strength and flexibility you need to be the best dad—and husband—you can be. And what's more important than that?

What a Family Man Needs

The best program for dads would be well-rounded, says Bob Glover, who runs a New York City fitness consulting firm and who co-authored *The Family Fitness Handbook*. You need cardiovascular strength to have the energy to last through those days in which you are going nonstop from 6 A.M. to midnight. You need flexibility for all that wrestling and carrying and fixing and cuddling. And you need powerful muscles so that an hour

with a push mower doesn't sap you for the rest of the day. Just as important, you need your family's help and understanding.

"They need to see this as a regular part of your daily routine and respect that," says exercise physiologist John Amberge, director of corporate programs for the Sports Training Institute in New York City. "Then not only will you stay in shape but you'll also set an example that may get your whole family into the idea of exercise." Here are a few suggestions for accomplishing all these goals in a few simple steps.

Get into the home stretch. Devote a few minutes every day to stretching, either first thing in the morning or right when you get home. First do a couple minutes of warm-up by running in place or playing tag with the kids—you never want to stretch a cold muscle. Then get down to business.

"Stretching does more than aid flexibility. Since it increases blood flow and reduces stress, a regular stretching program is going to revitalize you and give you more energy, which you can use with your family," says Amberge. Plus, a few good stretches will loosen up the muscles that always cramp up from ceaseless baby-carrying, swing-pushing and general roughhousing.

Don't slink off and do your stretches in the bedroom or basement, though. Do them in the living room, in front of your kids. "They'll probably want to do them along with you, and that way they'll pick up a good habit," says Amberge. If nothing else, they'll be vastly amused by the faces and strange noises you'll be making.

Find family-friendly aerobic exercise. As Glover observes, dads need aerobic activity. Good cardiovascular strength ensures you'll have the energy to keep up with your family. It will also help you to stay around long enough to keep up with your grandchildren.

Whatever cardiovascular activity you choose, make it one your family can do with you. Brisk walking, running, cycling, rowing, skating, skiing, swimming or vigorous walking all qualify for cardiovascular fitness points—and they're all activities you can do with your wife and kids, points out Jonathan Robison, Ph.D., an exercise physiologist, nutritionist and executive co-director of the Michigan Center for Preventive Medicine in Lansing.

Set your pace according to the slowest family member, says Glover. It may not be a very satisfying or effective workout for the more-conditioned family members, but that's okay, he says. "Enjoy the time together. Use it as your warm-up. Then, after family time, go on out and get in your real workout," he says.

Build a home gym. Families are a fitness catch-22. As your family grows, your need for physical strength and fitness grows with it, but the time you have to build that fitness only dwindles. Between recitals and varsity football and building stage props for the school play, you'll have less and less time to get to the gym.

If you haven't done it before now, think about investing in a home gym, suggests Amberge. Nothing fancy—a standard Olympic weight set, a few dumbbells and a good weight bench are all you need. Set it up in your basement or den. Now you can do a workout whenever it's convenient for you—first thing

in the morning or after the kids have gone to bed. Make sure to include equipment for a cardiovascular workout, such as a stationary bike or rowing machine, he suggests. It can be as simple as a video and a step for step aerobics.

"If the equipment is available, you'll be more likely to use it," says Amberge. Plus, you've eliminated the hassle of driving to and from the club, changing, showering and waiting in line to use the equipment. As your kids get older, you can teach them how to use it, thus reinforcing their interest in fitness while giving yourself one more thing you can do with your family.

A special caution: If you still have small children, keep your equipment in a locked room or inaccessible place. According to the U.S. Consumer Product Safety Commission, home exercise equipment accounts for as many as 30,000 emergency room visits a year—roughly half of those visits involve children under 15. At the very least, teach your kids that Dad's exercise equipment isn't a toy.

Don't forget Mom. As soon as you've developed a fitness routine that works for you, teach it to your wife. Chances are, as mommy, she needs it even more than you, says Glover. Better yet, seek out exercises that you can do as a couple. We've outlined some suggestions in the Partners chapter on page 163.

The Family Man's Fitness Plan

Our specific prescription for paternal power has special emphasis on two key areas. First, we've doubled up on stretches, which increase energy while reducing pain, according to Charles Swencionis, Ph.D., head of the health psychology program at Yeshiva University in New York City. Second, whether it's a stretch or a weight-lift, we've thrown in plenty of exercises for the back so you won't be throwing yours out. Whether you're pressed into service as a makeshift stallion or stooping down so you and Junior can see eye to eye, there isn't a dad out there who couldn't use a stronger back.

Or a stronger body, for that matter. So in conjunction with our Core Routine for strength building, find a way to work these exercises recommended by Amberge into your schedule. Do them three days a week and your kids will be bragging, "Our dad can beat your dad."

Side Stretch (Holding Wrist)

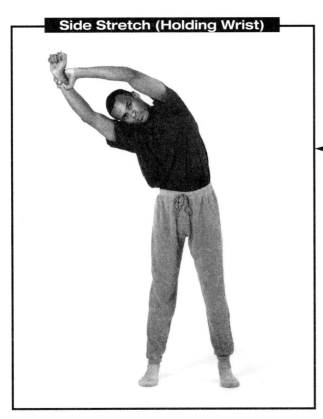

◄ **Side Stretch (Holding Wrist)**
Stand with your arms stretched over your head. Holding your right wrist with your left hand, bend over to the right as far as is comfortable and hold for 20 seconds. Return to center position. Grasp your left wrist with your right hand, lean to your left side and hold for 20 seconds.

Forward Stretch

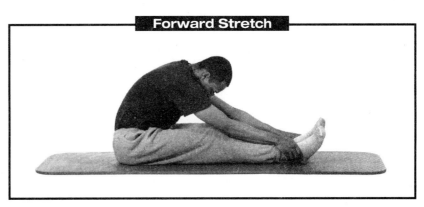

Forward Stretch ►
Sit with your legs together, stretched out in front of you. Bend forward at your waist and grasp your ankles or feet. Hold for 20 seconds.

Extension Stretch

◄ **Extension Stretch**
Sit on the floor with your legs spread as far as possible, heels on the floor, feet pointed upwards. Lean forward and grasp your ankles. Hold for 20 seconds.

Knee Pulls ➤

This one is part of our total flexibility routine (page 33). Lie flat on your back with your legs straight. Bring one knee toward your chest. Interlace your fingers behind your thigh and draw your knee as close to your chest as possible for 20 seconds. Relax and repeat with the other knee.

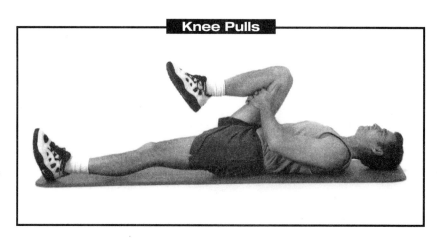

Knee Pulls

Lying Side Stretch ➤

Start flat on your back. Bend your right leg across your body to your left side. With your left hand, hold your right knee down and roll your head and shoulders back to the right. Hold this position for 20 seconds, then relax and stretch the other side.

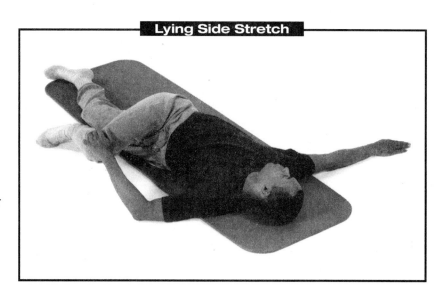

Lying Side Stretch

Lying Back Stretch ➤

This is a great lower-back pain reliever and stretcher. Start by lying flat on your back. Bring both knees toward your chest and pull them closer by wrapping your arms or hands around the backs of your upper thighs. Your hips should curl slightly off the floor. Hold for 20 seconds, feeling the stretch, then relax. Repeat several times.

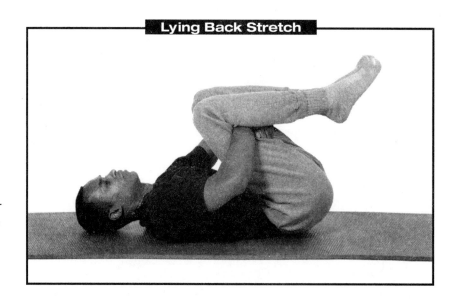

Lying Back Stretch

Shoulder Exercises

Your shoulders know all about the stress of raising children—literally. Between lifting, holding and carrying your kids on marathon piggyback rides, your shoulders go through pure hell. You can keep them strong, and relax the tension you'll inevitably feel in them, by doing several shoulder exercises, especially shoulder shrugs and the alternating dumbbell press.

Crunches

Good abdominals are important for fighting off lower-back strain. Plus, you'd be surprised how much you need your abs when you're hauling one of your chubby cherubs around. For the busy family man, Amberge says crunches are the easiest way to go. They require no special equipment, and you can do them in the backyard, on the living room floor—anywhere you want.

Back Extensions

Again, the stronger you can make your back, the better and more pain-free you'll be. Back extensions, both with and without weights, move your back through a broad range of motion, which also helps keep you limber and flexible.

Rows

Although the pangs of fatherhood seem to concentrate themselves in your lower back, your upper back does more than its share of muscle work. Upper-back muscles not only help you bend over and lift but they also support your shoulders and chest. Bent-over rows and one-arm dumbbell rows will target those hardworking upper-back muscles.

Fun and Fitness for the Family

When we interviewed Edmund Connors for this book, he had just come from an all-out hockey match against his grandchildren.

"They're five and seven years old, decked out in full hockey equipment, playing against me and my son-in-law," he says. "We didn't stand a chance."

Connors's grandkids get their love of hockey from Connors himself, a certified strength and conditioning specialist in Hingham, Massachusetts, who has trained hockey players currently playing for the Boston Bruins, the New York Islanders and the Chicago Blackhawks. Connors also teaches physical education from kindergarten to the sixth-grade level, a key time when dads should be exercising with their children, he says.

"Children need to be exposed to a lot of different kinds of physical activity. It's when they're growing up that your children are going to benefit the most from the example you set in physical fitness," he says.

If your kids are already adolescents, they can do many of your favorite fitness activities with you. "Running, cycling, skiing, whatever. At that age, they'll probably leave you in the dust," says Connors. If they're younger, though, you need to modify your personal fitness program to fit your children's level of physical development. Remember that when your children run with you, because of their shorter legs, they are taking twice as many steps as you.

"Younger children aren't mature enough to grasp the idea of fitness as something that's good for them. They just want to do something that's fun," Connors says. "If you set up certain rules or routines that get them interested in fitness early on, when they're older, they'll be predisposed to exercise because it's something they've always done and always enjoyed." We've mixed together some sensible fitness rules, a few creative calisthenics and some favorite childhood activities to get you going.

Ration TV time. If a family fitness routine is going to work, it will need some ground rules as well as a minimum of distractions. "In other words, you need to get them away from the TV," says Connors.

The best way to do this, Glover recommends, is to ration television-watching time to, say, three hours per week and stick to it. Not only does this free up more time for exercise but it also helps your kids to be more discriminating about what they watch.

Make indoors out-of-bounds. As a corollary to the TV Law, you could add another house law: that certain times will be decreed "outdoor time."

"Maybe it's an hour every afternoon or a few hours on the weekends. The idea is, unless it's really awful weather or the child is sick, they're not allowed indoors," says Connors. "When children are outside, odds are they're going to do some physical activity—riding a bike, playing in the park. There's no couch, no TV, no Nintendo outside, so they're much less apt to sit around and do nothing." Just make sure you adhere to the outdoor rule too, Dad.

Play tag. Now that you're outdoors, you'll need some activities to keep you busy and fit. Remember how out-of-breath you felt when you played tag as a kid? Glover recommends it as a solid exercise. Between the running and diving and stretching to make the tag or latch onto the tree you've designated as your safe zone, you have a terrific aerobic workout. It's one you can do year-round, too. For example, in the winter, play snowball tag—whoever gets hit is it. Just make sure the rules call for soft snowballs, not ice balls. And no hitting in the face.

Play ball! With a soft kickball or beachball, you can get your family involved in any number of fun exercises. Don't just play obvious games like kickball, soccer or catch. Play dodgeball or keepaway, too.

Do animal aerobics. Both Glover and Sara Black, fitness expert and co-author of *The Supple*

Sport Smarts

Sports and exercise do more than keep your family healthy. They also broaden your kids' horizons and teach them valuable skills they'll need throughout life.

"As a rule, you should be helping your kids to sample a broad variety of physical pursuits—that way they can find out what their gifts are, what they're good at," says Edmund Connors, a certified strength and conditioning specialist in Hingham, Massachusetts, who has trained hockey players currently playing for the Boston Bruins, the New York Islanders and the Chicago Blackhawks. Here are some of the most valuable activities your children can enjoy. You can—and should—share these pursuits with your children as much as possible.

- Swimming. Besides building balance, coordination and good cardiovascular health, swimming is a vital life skill that every child should learn. "There aren't many sports you can play that might one day save your life or someone else's," says John McVan, aquatic specialist at Iowa State University in Ames. "But swimming is one of them. Probably the most important one." Your local parks department and most YMCAs offer a full range of swimming courses. Call the one near you for more information.

- Bicycling. It's a rite of passage, teaching your kid to ride a bike. Don't just teach them how to keep their balance, though. Buy them proper helmets. Make sure their bikes have proper reflectors. Sign them up for a bicycle safety program. "This is how kids start to learn the rules of the road," says Connors. "It will make them more aware of their surroundings. It might even make them better drivers one day."

- Martial arts. Whether it's karate or tae kwon do, sign your kids and yourself up for at least one session of martial arts instruction. "This isn't to teach your kids how to fight," says Connors. "Martial arts are really very physical philosophy courses—you're learning how *not* to fight." At the same time, your child learns the basics of discipline and improves his self-confidence, flexibility and physical coordination.

- Team sports. You probably had this one figured out for yourself. "Team sports can be great," says Connors. "Your child learns how to work with others, how to make more friends. He learns how to function as part of a team, to work toward a greater good." Not bad for a few afternoons of Little League.

However, just because you won the soccer championship when you were a kid, don't force your child to follow in your footsteps. "Give your children the freedom to pursue whatever sports they like. If you force them to play baseball or soccer when you know they hate it, you're doing them a disservice," says Connors. If your child doesn't like it, let him choose something he *does* like. "There are too many sports out there for you to force him to play just one. Let him shop around, find what he likes. He'll thank you for it," says Connors.

Body, recommend "animal" exercises as a fun way to exercise with your family. The idea is that each of the exercises mimics a certain animal. While you and your kids are playing, you're doing dynamic stretches and aerobics at the same time. Here are some examples.

- Elephant walk. Stand with your feet about hip-width apart. Bend over at your waist and place your palms flat on the floor. You may have to bend your knees, but try to hold your legs as straight as possible. Now move your right hand and foot forward at the same time. You've just taken your first elephant step. Now do the same on your left side and repeat.

- Rhino hip roll. Stand and rotate your hips in a big circle, first one way, then the other.

- Cat back. Get on your hands and knees, arch your back up, tuck your chin toward your chest. Then reverse direction and hiss like a cat.

- Chicken wings. This is a great shoulder exercise. Make fists with both hands and place them in your armpits. Now walk around, flapping your "wings" and clucking at each other.

- Safari aerobics. Glover recommends a faster drill of several animal activities, one after the other. First, run like a lion, then bend over and wiggle like a snake, then hop like a bunny, then lope along like a gorilla, then flap your wings like an eagle. Do each of them for about 10 to 20 seconds in quick succession, and you'll have a fast-paced, high-energy workout that will leave you and your kids in a heap, gasping and giggling.

Give a no-pressure guarantee. Somedays, a child just won't feel like doing what Dad or his brothers and sisters are doing. If you have a dissenter in the ranks, that's okay once in a while.

"You don't want to put too much pressure on a child to do some fitness activity all the time. If he feels pushed into it, he won't want to do it," says Connors. As an alternative, ask your child if there's anything he wants to do. "He may just want to play cops and robbers. So play cops and robbers. Just make sure there's a chase scene. Chances are, whatever your kids want to do, you can find some ways to sneak in exercise," says Connors.

Partners

You're by yourself on the running track, and you can't find the energy to go one more lap. You're huffing and puffing all alone at the gym or in the basement, and you decide to skip the next set of weights. Your heart's just not in it. You can't motivate yourself. Something's missing, you decide.

Maybe that something is actually some*one*. As in your partner.

Now, we're not talking about a guy to spot you while you bench press. We're talking about your girlfriend, your wife, your significant other. If you've never before thought of your helpmate as an exercise mate, fitness experts say there's plenty of reason to start.

"Working out together can be a bonding experience. It can be good for the relationship, and you can actually exercise very effectively with someone else," says Sandra Fisher, exercise physiologist and owner of New York City's Fitness by Fisher, an exercise consulting firm.

Here's why: When you exercise with a partner, you're less likely to quit. "When men work out together, there's kind of a competitive edge that keeps them both going," says Al Paolone, Ed.D., professor of exercise physiology in the physical education department at Temple University in Philadelphia. With your wife or girlfriend, you probably won't feel as great a need to

bench-press more than she, but you'll still benefit from working out with her. "Your partner can offer you a lot of positive encouragement just by being there, and vice versa," says Charles Kuntzleman, Ed.D., adjunct associate professor of kinesiology at the University of Michigan in Ann Arbor.

Pairing for Performance

Now, it's true that men and women have different aptitudes when it comes to exercise. Women tend to be more inclined toward individual, aerobic exercise; men lean toward rough-and-tumble sports or weight-bearing activities. In other words, you'll probably make about as good an aerobic dance partner as she would a barbell spotter. The trick to being a dynamic duo, then, is to find activities you can do together, or to find ways to modify your favorite exercise activities so that you can do them as a twosome.

"If you're at different levels of proficiency at certain exercises, it can lead to frustration. For example, if you're running and trying to keep a good pace, but she's slower, you'll feel like you're not getting a good workout. She feels like she's slowing you down," says Dr. Kuntzleman. Either way, the workout starts to become just a lot of work, and absolutely zero fun.

In situations like this, look for ways to level the playing field. To give you an idea, we've listed some popular sports and ways

The Power of Two

Doubles tennis the best you could come up with in the way of a couple-friendly sport? You can do better. Here are a few more exercises-built-for-two, guaranteed to keep both your pulse-rates up.

• Kissing. Yes, mere necking burns calories, roughly 6 to 12 calories per smack. For a varied workout, mix long, slow deep kisses, with bursts of multiple, short pecks. Consider it a warm-up to heavier exercise (see the bottom of the list).

• Tandem bicycling. Rent a bicycle-built-for-two for a few hours; call and reserve yours today. When you use it, sit in the back. That way, she won't see when you're slacking off on the hills.

• Wrestling. We're not talking Hulk Hogan–style head slams and knee drops—just plain ol' wrasslin' 'round on the living room rug, with plenty of pillows lying around in case one of you needs to take a swing. Winner gets control of the remote. To make it more interesting, move it into the bathroom or backyard; add Jell-O or mud. Or subtract clothes. Which brings us to . . .

• Sex. The greatest aerobic exercise ever devised truly requires a partner's help to be done effectively. Sexual intercourse burns about 315 calories per hour. That's the same as doubles tennis—but your partner is less likely to fault you for your service.

---

to increase your workout by the power of two.

• Aerobics. No, we're not suggesting you go to her aerobics class (although one session won't kill you). But if you both go to the gym, Fisher suggests doing some of your warm-up and aerobic work together. Get machines side by side, be they stair-climbers, stationary cycles or treadmills. You can set the machines to your individual skill levels, so you don't rob yourself of a workout—and you get to be together.

• Cycling. The better cyclist can ride in a lower gear. This slows him down considerably, but still gives him a terrific leg-burner and aerobic workout.

• Hiking. As men, evolution has pegged us for packhorses. Make the most of that by carrying most of the heavy gear. Then, the numerous stops you'll make won't be because you're waiting for her to catch up, but because you're trying to catch your breath.

• Running. The faster runner can run with light hand weights. If only one of you runs, the non-runner could ride a bike. "Then that person still exercises with you, and they can be kind of a running coach, offering encouragement along the way," says Dr. Kuntzleman.

• Weight training. In the gym, plan one day a week that you'll work out together. Odds are she won't be able to lift as much as you, but that's okay. It only takes a few extra seconds to unload weight plates so she can take her turn. Take your time during this workout. "If you work out three days a week, you have two other days to really go all out. Make this a relaxed, slow-tempo day in which you keep pace with her," says Dr. Kuntzleman.

Note: If she's not strong enough to spot you during your heavier lifts, ask someone nearby to spot you for those few lifts. Otherwise, skip those exercises for that day.

• And other favorites. To be better partners—and possibly better workout partners—share a little in what each of you enjoys, suggests Fisher. If she swims laps, head to the pool with her one day a week. If you're into circuit training on the weight machines at the gym, take her in and show her your routine. She may want to start circuit training herself.

• New sports. One of the best ways to exercise together is for both of you to adopt a brand-new sport at the same time. "It could be tennis, racquetball, mountain biking—doesn't matter. If neither of you has done it before, you're both starting from the same skill level, which is good. Plus, you'll have a partner to motivate you and to practice with," says Joel Rappelfeld, in-line skating instructor and author of *The Complete Blader.* Rappelfeld says many couples sign up together for his skating courses in New York City. "They do a lot better than those who don't have someone along to encourage them," he says. But always keep it fun, not competitive, Rappelfeld adds. Otherwise, you could end up rolling away from each other.

Couples Calisthenics

With a little extra effort and improvisation, working out as a twosome need not be restricted to doubles sports or exercises you can do individually in the same room.

"There are many ways a couple can truly work out together—physically rely on one another for their workout," says Dr. Kuntzleman. The principle is called isotonics, where you work muscles using resistance that your partner applies. Granted, it's not as effective as working with weights, but you can get a decent workout. And it's a heck of a lot of fun. We've provided a few examples from Dr. Kuntzleman to get you started.

Kneeling Curls

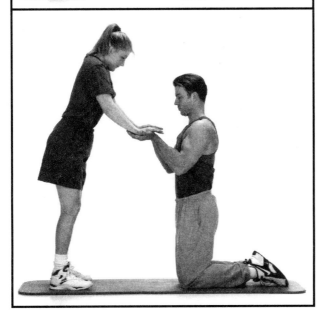

◄ **Kneeling Curls**

Start by facing each other, standing only a couple of feet apart. Get down on your knees. Bend your arms, keeping your elbows close to your sides, and hold out your hands toward her. Your hands should be palms up, fingers pointing toward her. Have her place her palms on yours and bear down slightly.

Now slowly curl your arms up, bringing your palms toward your shoulders. As you curl, she should press against your palms, bringing more of her weight to bear on you. Keep trying to curl your arms for a count of 12, then relax and repeat. When you've done 8 to 12 reps, switch places.

Kneeling Overhead Press

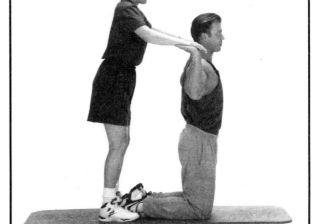

Kneeling Overhead Press ►

This time kneel and place your hands over your head. Bend your elbows so your hands are behind your ears, shoulder-width apart, palms up. Have your partner stand behind you, facing the same direction you are. Have her place her palms flat against yours.

Now push upward as she presses down, bringing her weight to bear on your hands. Lift against her pressure for a count of 12, then relax and repeat. When you've done 8 to 12 reps, switch places.

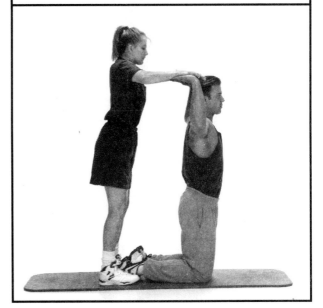

Abductor/Adductor Lifts

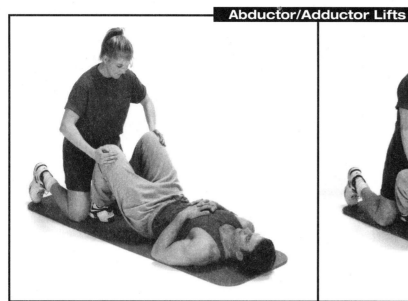
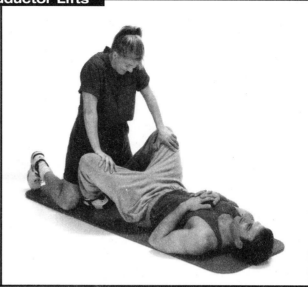

Abductor/Adductor Lifts ▲

To work the outer-thigh muscles, lie on your back on the floor. Bend your legs and place your feet flat on the floor, knees together. Have your partner kneel opposite you, with her hands on the outside of your knees. Now try to spread your legs, bringing your knees apart. While you do this, your partner should be applying inward pressure.

For your inner-thigh muscles, assume the same posi-

tion. Only this time, put the soles of your feet together, knees pointing outward. Your partner should apply pressure to the inside of your knees while you try to bring your legs together.

Do each exercise for a count of 12, then relax briefly and repeat. When you've done 8 to 12 reps of each exercise, switch positions with your partner.

Crunches

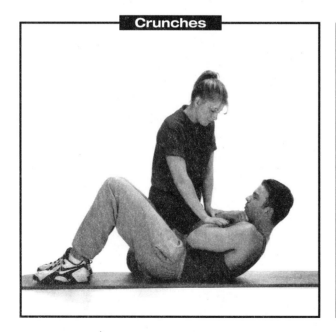

Push-Ups

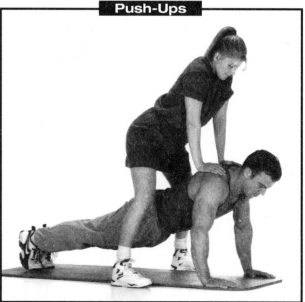

Crunches ▲

Lie on your back, with your knees bent and feet flat on the floor. Fold your arms across your chest. Your partner should be kneeling at your side, with her arms outstretched, hands lightly placed on your arms. As you lift your shoulders to do your crunch, she should press against your arms. Try to push against her for a couple of seconds, then relax and repeat. Do as many as you can.

Push-Ups ▲

Assume push-up position—feet together, legs extended behind you, hands slightly wider than shoulder-width apart, palms flat on the floor. Have your partner stand, straddling you. Then have her bend down and place her hands on your shoulder blades. Her legs should be bent to avoid undue strain on her back. She can apply pressure as you push up. Do as many as you can.

Flexibility Exercises

Once you're done with your workout and it's time for cooldown and stretching, you and your partner can work together on your flexibility, too. In their excellent book, *The Supple Body*, fitness experts Sara Black, Sarah Clark and Liliana Djurovic outline several fun and effective stretches couples can do together. Remember, don't stretch farther than you and your partner can comfortably go. Try these.

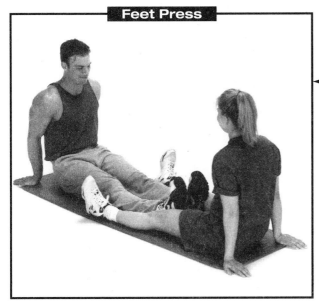

Feet Press

◄ Feet Press

This exercise limbers up inner- and outer-thigh muscles as well as the hips. Sit on the floor, facing each other.

Place your legs together and extend them so they're between your partner's legs—you should be sitting far enough apart so that your feet are about even with her knees. Now try to push your partner's legs farther apart. Hold for 30 seconds. Then for another 30 seconds, she should try to push your legs together. Then switch places, with her legs between yours, and reverse roles.

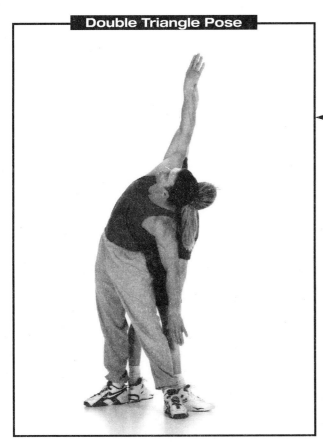

Double Triangle Pose

◄ Double Triangle Pose

This is a good stretch for the arms and upper body. This works best with partners of similar size. Stand back to back with your feet wider than shoulder-width apart. Extend your arms and raise them to shoulder-level. Turn your hands so your palms and your partner's are facing each other. With your hips and chest facing front, turn your right foot so it's at a 90-degree angle to your left.

Now with your palms and backs together, you should reach down to the left; your head should be turned right. Your partner mirrors your movement. At the bottom of the stretch, your fingers should be as close as you can get them to your left ankles; your right hands should be straight up in the air. Hold as long as possible; then return to the starting position. Repeat on the right side.

Shoulder Lifts ➤

This exercise is part stretch, part weight-lift. For the one standing, you'll be working your side and leg muscles. For the one sitting, it's a great arm, shoulder and back stretch.

Have your partner sit cross-legged on the floor, hands clasped above her head, arms extended (elbows should not be locked).

Now stand behind her, perpendicular to the direction she's facing. The side of your right leg and knee should be resting along her back. Bend down and get your shoulder under her clasped hands; grab her left forearm with your right hand. Slowly shift your weight to your left leg, pulling and lifting up and back. Lift as much as is comfortable for your partner; hold for 20 seconds at the top of the lift, then relax. Now switch sides and repeat with your left arm and leg resting along her back. When you've finished, switch places so you can both take turns being stretcher and stretchee.

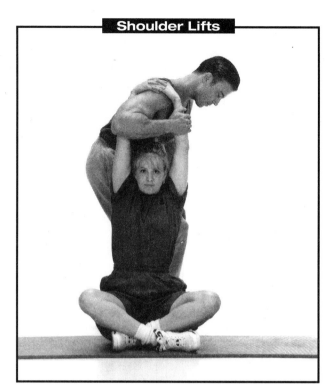

Shoulder Lifts

Better Sex

What does it mean to have "great sex"? Ask a thousand people, and you'll get a thousand answers. Sex is a complex mix of the physical, the mental and the spiritual, and for each man and woman, the optimal balance is different. For some, brain stimulation—romance, mystery, love, even danger—dominates the sexual encounter; for others, the greatness is all in the technique, the sensations.

Sorry, but we're not going to focus deeply on those things. Instead, we're going to take one step back. Our perspective is that no matter how you define great sex, you won't be able to achieve it without plenty of stamina, energy and ejaculatory control. These we can teach you.

It's no small point. Few men past the age of 40 can claim the jackrabbit sexual energy or capacity they had in their teens. Likewise, how many men can say they have consistently good control over their private part's performance? And yet, with the right exercises, men can achieve a whole lot more sexual vigor than they likely would imagine. And who doesn't want more sexual vigor?

Improving Ejaculatory Control

First and foremost, the typical guy wants control over when he ejaculates. Problem is, the heat of the moment always interferes. We're chugging along, enjoying the ride, when suddenly things pick up speed. Too late, we realize we're on the express train to Orgasm Junction, when what we really wanted was the slow route so we could take in the scenery along the way.

Although the delicious sensations of sexual contact are the main triggers of an ejaculation, there are a number of bodily processes that control the physical act of ejaculating. Many of these processes are completely involuntary, but there are some key functions that you can learn to control.

"You need a lot of different events to occur in the body for ejaculation to happen," says William Hartman, Ph.D., co-director of the Center for Marital and Sexual Studies in Long Beach, California. "There's muscle contraction, there's breathing, there's pressure you bring to bear on the penis. To a large degree, there are techniques any man can learn so that he can delay his orgasm and enjoy sex for longer periods of time." Here are some tried-and-true methods.

Learn to block. Okay, these tips don't fall in the category of training your body for long-term control. But if you want to slow things right away, as in tonight, here are three ways to do that, according to Dr. Hartman.

1. When you feel like you are about to ejaculate, firmly press and hold the underside of your penis. The idea is to block the ejaculate from passing through your urethra.

Hold still for 12 seconds. You could involve your partner and ask her to hold you tight "down there." Once the sensations pass, you can resume your business.

2. Again, just prior to ejaculating, place your fingers against your perineum (that's the space between your penis and anus) to block your testicles from retracting into your body. Do that correctly and it will keep you from ejaculating.

3. A third method is the start-and-stop. Essentially, when you begin to feel an orgasm coming on, slow down your motion, even coming to a halt if need be. Let the sensation pass before starting up again. Let your partner know what you are doing, though—she might get frustrated otherwise.

Clinch it with Kegels. Your lower pelvis is home to some pretty powerful muscles. Take the pubococcygeal (PC) muscles. They're the muscles you use to stop urinating midstream. They're also the muscles you feel contracting when you ejaculate. If you do an exercise known as a Kegel, where you clench and unclench your PC muscles, you can build control over them and prolong ejaculation. "The idea is that, at the point where you're about to ejaculate, you clench the PCs hard, and that prevents the ejaculation," says E. Douglas Whitehead, M.D., director of the Association for Male Sexual Dysfunction in New York City. "But first, you'll have to do a lot of Kegels."

Luckily, you can do them anywhere, and you should, several times a day. Do a short clench, relax for a moment, then try to do a longer clench for about 10 to 15 seconds. Do about ten of these exercises at least three times a day. Gradually increase the number over time. The more you do them, the better your control will be, according to Dr. Whitehead.

Take a deep breath. A common route to quick ejaculation lies in the way we breathe. "In the heat of the moment, you start breathing heavy, your heart starts racing and everything moves faster, including the time it'll take you to ejaculate," observes Dr. Hart-

Remember Your Kegels

By now, you've probably heard about Kegels—the exercise where you clench the same muscles you use to control urine flow. The idea is that Kegels will make those muscles stronger, and you'll therefore be able to improve your ejaculatory control. The goal is about 100 flicks of those pubococcygeal (PC) muscles a day, according to William Hartman, Ph.D., co-director of the Center for Marital and Sexual Studies in Long Beach, California.

The problem is remembering to do them. After all, it's not like there's a Kegelcisor exercise machine sitting in your living room or basement, reminding you to do your sexercises. So here's a short list of tips to remind you of the simplicity and beauty of Kegels, which you can do anytime, anywhere.

• Kegels and bagels: Ah, breakfast, the most important meal of the day. And no better time to start your daylong Kegel routine. Clench your PC muscles with every bite you take of breakfast. Try to hold the clench for as long as it takes you to sip and swallow a mouthful of coffee.

• Kegel and Hegel: The German philosopher claimed that reality was based in ideas, not in things. Remember that as you're explaining your ideas at the next meeting. And take a minute to ground yourself in your own reality. Do a few quick PC clenches while your boss is mulling your ideas over. Heck, he might be doing the same thing.

• Kegel and finagle: Buying a new car, but don't feel like paying new car prices? Or maybe you're at the local flea market, trying to get that antique dresser for a steal. It doesn't matter; just remember to clench while you're trying to clinch that deal. Even if your finagling doesn't get you the price you want, your ejaculatory muscles—and your partner—will consider it time well-spent.

• Kegels and Eagles: Or Jets. Or Cowboys. Or Raiders. Yes, even when you appear to all the world to be a couch potato, absorbed in the afternoon game, you know that you're working to gain yardage in the great gridiron of your bedroom. Do a Kegel every time the teams come to the line of scrimmage. Hold the clench for the duration of every pass or kick. And every time someone makes a touchdown, do as many as you can in the space of a couple seconds. In the game of sex, there are players and there are punters. Be a player.

• Kegel and Nagel: You're wandering around the local art museum, trying to make sense of paintings that appear to defy all reason for existence. When the gallery before your eyes doesn't meet your high artistic standards, summon up a vision of the Birth of Venus, or a nice marble statue of an ample Italian beauty or the smooth, electric lines of a Nagel nude. Kegel your way past the modern art. If you see something that catches your eye, hold the clench for as long as you can. Think of the strokes you'll be adding later to the great masterpiece that is your sex life. Now, that's art.

man. "Instead, I counsel patients to concentrate on taking long, slow, deep breaths." This gives you better oxygen flow and helps equalize everything even when you're stroking your way vigorously through some scorching sex.

Don't desensitize. Most guys try to hold off as long as they can by focusing on something other than sex—usually something mundane such as baseball stats or going down the list of chores you have to do around the house. This is the wrong way to go about it, according to Dr. Hartman. "You might think you're avoiding ejaculating, but what you're really doing is cheating yourself out of the pleasure of sex," he says.

Dr. Hartman has male clients practice something called sensate focusing. "Don't concentrate on the genitals; focus on the whole body. When you touch your partner, focus on what your hand is feeling. When you kiss her, concentrate on the signals you're getting from the lips. Don't think about baseball averages; don't distract yourself. Concentrate on the feeling of your partner's body against your body," he says. At first, this may make ejaculatory control a bit iffy. "But ultimately, you'll find it makes your control stronger. You'll get better with practice," Dr. Hartman insists.

Master your feelings. One of the best ways to practice ejaculatory control is by yourself.

"Masturbation can help you to learn what your limits are. You can determine what feels good and what feels *too* good, to the point of losing control," says Dr. Whitehead. Masturbation also helps you control ejaculation another way. If you masturbate within a few hours of when you think you're going to have sex, you'll take the edge off your anticipation and be able to go longer, points out Dr. Hartman.

Be a lord of the rings. If you and your partner are not opposed to the idea of sex toys and other equipment, consider investing eight or ten dollars in a penis ring, a constrictive device that you slide or snap over the base of the penis. Similar devices are available from medical supply houses but should only be used under the direction of your physician, according to Dr. Whitehead. The ring traps blood in the penis and helps you maintain hard erections for longer periods of time. They also have the side benefit of blocking ejaculation, he adds.

Two caveats: Don't wear it for longer than 20 to 30 minutes at a time—cutting off blood flow to the penis for too long can cause tissue damage, says Dr. Whitehead. Also, you may find that ejaculating while wearing the ring may cause a retrograde ejaculation: Semen can't travel via its normal route, so it backwashes into the bladder. It's not harmful, but you might find it uncomfortable, according to Dr. Whitehead.

Fitness for Better Sex

Sex experts are forever saying the key to great sex is all in your head. But for our purposes, let's look at the other love machine—your body. Mental sex isn't much good without a body that can deliver the goods the mind has promised itself.

"There's no doubt that there's a link between libido and fitness," says Eric Gronbech, Ph.D., a professor at Chicago State University who researches the link between fitness and libido. Actually, there are two links: First, when you exercise, you prepare your body for better sexual performance. "There's been evidence to suggest exercise increases your testosterone levels," says James White, Ph.D., professor emeritus at the University of California, San Diego, and author of *The Best Sex of Your Life*. Not only will exercise help increase your sexual activity but it also lets you build the cardiovascular and physical fitness that's going to help you perform for as long as you want.

The second link is more psychological. "As you exercise, you tend to feel better about yourself," says Dr. Gronbech. You feel more confident, and your appearance improves, as does your overall ability to draw a few delicate moths to the glorious flame that is your golden self. So in addition to your core workout of lifts that work all your muscle groups (see the Core Routine on page 121), here are some specific suggestions, stretches and routines to turn your body into a total sex machine. You can even do some of these on your bed while you're waiting for your partner to join you. Just make sure you have a firm mattress. If you have an old mattress or a waterbed, use the floor or a weight bench instead.

Do aerobic exercise for amore. Sex is not a sport of power; it's one of endurance. The best way to build endurance is by improving your cardiovascular fitness with aerobic exercise like jogging, swimming, cycling or stair-climbing. In one of Dr. White's studies, men who performed aerobic exercise reported increases in libido. But more important, they reported having 30 percent more sex and 26 percent more orgasms. "Overwhelmingly, they reported more sexual satisfaction than those who didn't exercise," says Dr. White. Try to keep your aerobic exercise to at least three sessions a week, 30 to 45 minutes at a time.

Pump up a pleasure chest. Cosmetically, it's obvious why you'd want a well-muscled chest—to attract more mates for sex. Seriously, though, your chest muscles help support your arms and shoulder muscles, which you need any time you're on top, especially in the missionary position. Keep doing those bench presses.

Work your gut. Your abdominals do more than give you thrusting power; they also help you make subtle changes in the angle of thrust and your position relative to your partner. To keep your abs sexually potent, do a variety of crunches, such as crossover and oblique. Dr. Gronbech suggests starting out with three sets of 10 reps, and working up to 20 reps.

Push-up for passion. Shoulders play a key role in the missionary position as well as many other sexual anglings, Dr. White notes. Push-ups work the muscles essential to good sex. Other shoulder-builders include shrugs and upright rows.

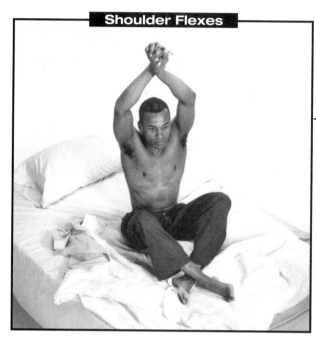

◄ Shoulder Flexes

Sit up in bed, hold your arms above your head and cross your wrists, grasping your fingers.

Straighten your arms and extend them back behind your head as far as you can, while still keeping your wrists crossed. Hold at the furthest point for a count of 30, then relax.

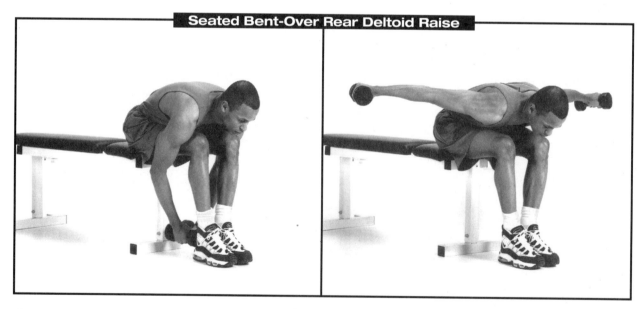

Seated Bent-Over Rear Deltoid Raise ▲

Hold a dumbbell in each hand, palms facing in. Sit toward the end of a bench, keeping your feet together and planted firmly on the floor. Bend forward so that your chest almost touches your upper thighs. Let the dumbbells hang behind your lower legs. Keep your arms slightly bent.

Lift your arms straight out in a semicircle. Raise the weights to shoulder height and hold for a moment. Slowly lower to starting position and repeat for 8 to 12 reps.

Butterfly Stretch

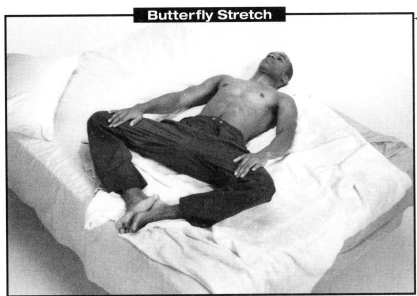

◀ Butterfly Stretch

To keep your groin muscles limber and flexible for an all-night lovemaking session, lie on your back, knees bent, feet flat on the bed. Pull your heels towards your butt; turn your ankles so the soles and heels of your feet are touching. By now, your knees should be pointing out to the sides.

Let your knees slowly drop toward the bed. Gravity should naturally pull them in that direction, but you may want to put your hands on your inner thighs and apply slight downward pressure. When your knees are as far apart as possible, count to 30, then relax.

Hip Stretches

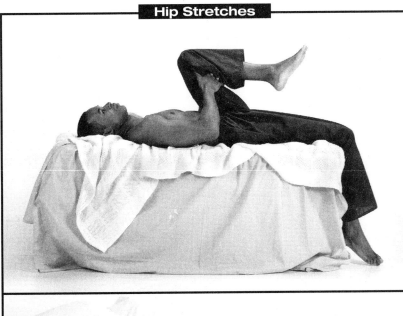

◀ Hip Stretches

To keep your thrusting muscles loose, lie on your back, with your knees dangling off the bed. Put your hands behind one thigh and pull your knee toward your chest. Hold for 30 seconds. Switch legs and repeat.

Next, sit on the bed or ground and spread your legs out. Put your hands in front of you and lean forward from the hips. Keep your legs relaxed, back straight and feet upright.

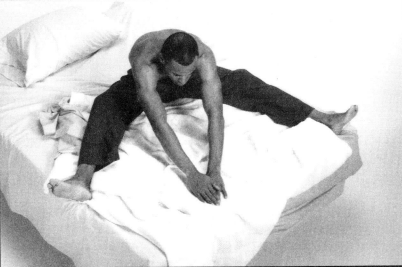

Pelvic Lifts ➤

To strengthen your pelvic and butt muscles at the same time, lie on your back, with your knees bent and feet slightly apart, flat on the floor. Keep your arms at your sides, hands also flat on the floor.

Clench your buttocks and raise your pelvis off the floor. Keep your butt clenched through the lift. Raise your pelvis until your back is straight, but not arched. Lower, then repeat.

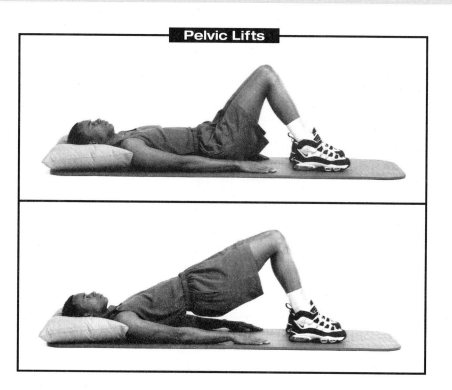

Pelvic Lifts

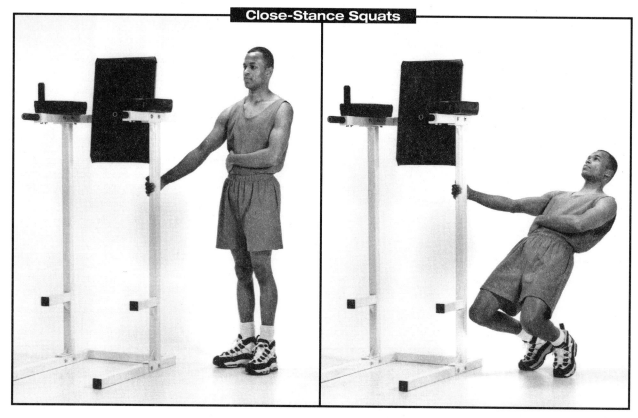

Close-Stance Squats

Close-Stance Squats ⋀

Lamentably, this squat is also known as the sissy squat, but don't let that mislead you—this is a man's exercise, a true thigh- and butt-burner. Start by standing with your feet a few inches apart, toes pointed slightly outward. Hold onto a bedpost, weight machine or other tall, stable object.

Lean back and lower your body by bending your knees. Shift your weight up onto your toes. Lean back until your thighs are as close to parallel to the floor as you can get them. Hold the position for a moment and clench your butt muscles as you go. Keep your back straight. Return to the upright position. Do five reps.

How to Become a Sex Master

As you've probably learned by now, sex is a lot more than just ejaculating. "It's unfortunate that men are as tight-lipped as they are about sex," says Dr. Hartman. "If they weren't afraid to ask their doctors or talk with their partners or other men, they could open themselves up to a wealth of information that could help them improve their sex lives."

To save you a little trouble, we went out and asked some experts for you. Here's a roundup of their best all-around suggestions for greater and greater sex. Be warned: Some of these tips may be more fun to follow than you were expecting.

Have more erections. What did we tell you? For men, sex is a use-it-or-lose-it proposition. The more frequently you have erections, the more you'll have and the firmer they'll be over time. "More erections means the various tissues and chambers in the penis will stay strong and expandable," says Irwin Goldstein, M.D., professor of urology at Boston University Medical Center. "Less erections means that over time, the tissue inside the penis will become more scarred. That translates into softer erections or even impotence as you get older." So have more erections—of course, how and when you choose to generate those erections is entirely your business.

Don't mix sex and drugs. If your sexual prowess has been declining, you may find the explanation in your medicine cabinet. "A lot of prescription and over-the-counter drugs can decrease libido, limit the amount of blood that's going to the penis, or both," says Dr. Gronbech. Some of these drugs include blood-pressure medications like Procardia, tranquilizers and antidepressants, anti-epilepsy drugs like Dilantin and anti-ulcer drugs like Tagamet. If you suspect a medication is hurting or inhibiting your sexual performance, see your doctor, who might be able to prescribe a substitute medication.

Warning: If you're on a prescription for these drugs, do not limit or discontinue using them without consulting the doctor who prescribed them. Going off heart medication could kill you—and that would really put a damper on your sex life.

Ask and ye shall receive. We're assuming the sex you're having involves another person. You should, too. "A lot of men don't take the simple step of asking their lover what they want, what feels good to them," says Arlene Goldman, Ph.D., coordinator for the Jefferson Sexual Function Center in Philadelphia. "Instead of expending all your energies running through the whole repertoire, you could save yourself some time and energy simply by asking what feels good." They may not like all your flashy moves, compared to one or two particular techniques. If you focus on those, you cut your work considerably and raise yourself up in her eyes as a sensitive guy who knows what makes her tick. "And don't be afraid to tell her what you want, too," says Dr. Goldman.

Don't do all the work. Sometimes we can overdo it in our vigorous sexual antics. We get to thrusting, and we start going too fast for our heart to keep up. When this happens, we wear out too soon, and a systems failure results. Pace yourself. "Let her do some of the work. It's like any exercise—when you start to feel winded, take a break," says Dr. Hartman. Or let her take over. Great lovers are unselfish lovers, he says.

Bicycling

Anyone who has bought a bicycle in the past eight years knows that the market has split into two camps: road cycling and mountain biking. Different mentalities, different bike styles, different pleasures, different goals. The road cyclist covers the miles, gets into a rhythm, a zone, and stays locked in, often for hours. He's more like a runner. The mountain biker is into the thrill, the flight, the risk, the bursts of power. He's more like a white-water rafter.

You can love one or the other or both. We take no stand over which is more fun. But what's certain is that the fitness needs of the two differ. If you want to ride a bicycle to your peak level, you first must determine how exactly you want to ride your bike (or bikes).

"Figuring out the right program for you depends first on the type of cycling you like to do. If you're strictly a road cyclist, you have issues of endurance and form to contend with," says Bill Strickland, contributing writer for *Bicycling* and *Mountain Bike* magazines, and co-author of several of the magazine's books of cycling hints and tips. You'll need a training program that emphasizes proper form while building up cardiovascular and lower-body power at the same time.

These are also important issues for mountain bikers. But because of the rough-and-tumble nature of off-road cycling, you'll need to work extra-hard to develop the skills and reflexes necessary to surmount countless obstacles and trail hazards. You'll also need to use equipment and conditioning techniques that will help minimize the pounding your body is bound to take on a mountain-bike trail.

"Cyclists used to think all they had to do for training was just ride their bicycle—a lot. But nowadays, no matter what type of bicycling they do, cyclists are seeing the value of strength training and conditioning off the bike. That's what will help them ride better and avoid injury when they're on the bike," says John Graham, director of the Human Performance Center at the Allentown Sports Medicine and Human Performance Center in Pennsylvania, and strength trainer of champion cyclist Marty Nothstein.

Taking It on the Road

For road cyclists, most of the pleasure of the sport comes from the exhilaration of getting into a good pedaling rhythm and just cranking down the road. Whether you're joyriding or competing, the only way to find that rhythm, maintain a good speed and keep your body in cycling trim is to get out there at least two or three times per week.

The more you bike, the more natural you feel doing it. That said, it's always wise to pay attention to form. Improper body

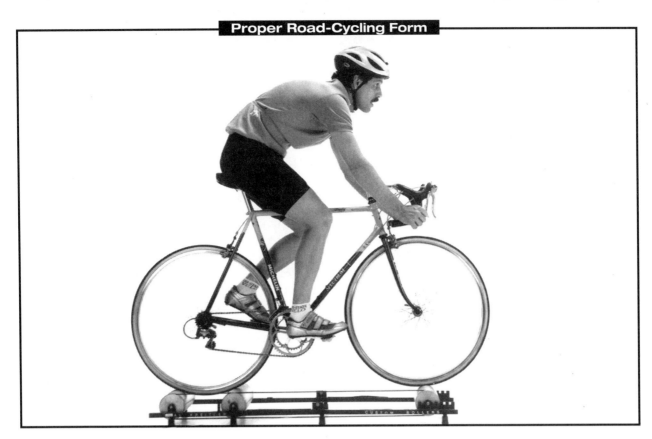

Proper Road-Cycling Form

alignment—and improper bike settings, for that matter—hurt performance. If you have any doubts about your form, check it against these specifications. With a few basic tools, you can make these adjustments yourself.

1. Handlebars: The top of your handlebar stem should be about one inch below the top of your bike saddle. As you get more experienced, you can lower the handlebars a little bit more—the lower you can go, the more aerodynamic your cycling form.

Make sure your handlebars are shoulder-width apart. Also, the bottom part of the handlebars should be level or pointed slightly down toward the rear-wheel hub.

2. Brakes: Brake levers should be positioned so your wrists are straight when you grasp the levers.

3. Top tube/stem length: To make sure your tube and stem length are correct, sit on the saddle and put your hands on the brake hoods (the tops of the brake levers). Look down. Can you see the hub of the front wheel? If yes, move slightly forward or backward until the handlebar blocks your view of the hub.

4. Saddle: Your saddle should be level or pointed slightly up at the tip. To determine proper saddle height, pedal a few strokes. If your knees are slightly bent at the very bottom of the stroke, your height is good. Never put the saddle so high that your knees lock.

5. Knee-over-pedal: When your pedals are level, check your forward leg. The bony part just below

your knee should be directly over the middle or axle of the forward pedal. If it's not, adjust the saddle forward or backward slightly until you get it right.

6. Frame: To make sure you have the right size frame, straddle the bicycle. There should be two to three inches clearance between the top tube and your crotch. Another guide is to check your seat post. Assuming your saddle height is correct, roughly four to five inches of the post should be visible. If you can see more than five inches of post, chances are your bike's frame is too small.

7. Feet: The widest part of your feet should be directly over the axles of the pedal. When pedaling, the angle of your feet should be natural—if it isn't, adjust the cleats.

8. Crankarm: To know the proper size crankarm for you, you'll need to know your inseam. As a rule of thumb, if your inseam is less than 29 inches, use 165mm crankarms; from 29 to 32 inches, use 170mm; 32 to 34, 172.5mm; anything more than 34 inches, 175mm.

Here are other tips for peak road-cycling performance.

Find your cadence. Pedaling fast and well is the absolute basis of powerful cycling. The trick is maintaining a consistent, even, speedy cadence—or leg speed—throughout a ride. Elite cyclists try to maintain a cadence where they are "spinning," a cadence that falls between 80 and 110 revolutions per minute (rpm). If you're training to be a fast road cyclist, you

Cycling Essentials

Hey, you on the bike! Don't you dare pedal another inch without making sure you have these velo vitals, says Don Cuerdon, senior writer of *Mountain Bike* magazine, and better known in the mountain bike community as "Captain Dondo."

- **Helmet.** Most fatal or crippling cycling injuries are the result of not wearing a bicycle helmet. Need we say more? "There's no excuse for not wearing a helmet, especially if you're going mountain biking," says Cuerdon. For around $25, you can buy a basic helmet and look smart. For around $100, you can buy the latest, aerodynamic, shock-resistant helmet and look smart *and* cool. "Did I mention there's no excuse for not wearing a helmet?" asks Cuerdon.

- **First-aid kit.** Skid on pavement or down a rocky slope even one time, and thereafter you'll be convinced of the need for a few medical necessities. Carry a few large adhesive strips, or a small roll of gauze and some waterproof adhesive tape. Also carry some antiseptic wipes, which are especially handy for cleaning out dirt and crud in cases of "road rash," if you're luckless enough to take a spill.

- **Patch kit.** Put enough miles on your bike and you're bound to suffer a flat. "Murphy's Law of Cycling absolutely dictates that will happen at the moment you are absolutely the farthest away from civilization," says Cuerdon. A patch kit will at least help you cope with the most obvious punctures. If you do mountain biking with any regularity, consider carrying a spare tube—insurance against the kind of off-road rips no patch kit can cure.

- **Bicycle pump.** The patch kit is useless without it.

- **Water bottle.** Feeling the coolness of the breeze against your skin may make you forget that you're sweating up a storm with all that pedaling. Be sure to carry at least one filled water bottle with you. Drink from it often—at least every 10 to 15 minutes.

- **Snack.** When you're cycling, you are your own engine—don't be caught in the middle of nowhere when you run out of fuel. Instead, bring your own, in the form of a sports bar, fig bars or even fruit.

- **Cash.** In case you forgot to bring a snack, a few bills tucked into a sock or sleeve could come in mighty handy. At the very least, carry a couple of quarters so if you or your bike gets hurt, you can call for a ride home. Assuming you can find a pay phone five miles from the trailhead, of course.

should work to get your cadence up to those levels, too.

Casual riders only need to keep their cadence to around 50 rpm—keep that number firmly in mind as your training minimum. To determine your cadence, you can either hop on a stationary cycle with an rpm register, or simply count the number of times your right foot comes to the top of your pedal stroke. Do this for 30 seconds, then multiply the number you get by two. That's your cadence.

Each week, work to increase your cadence by at least 10 rpm, until you find a rhythm that works for you. "Optimal cadence is a matter of personal preference and varies with terrain. Cadence decreases going up hills, for instance. Most accomplished cyclists keep their cadence in the 60 to 90 rpm range," says Don Cuerdon, senior writer of *Mountain Bike* magazine, and better known in the mountain-bike community as "Captain Dondo."

Stay narrow. The more your elbows and knees wing out away from your body, the more drag you'll create, and the slower you'll go. Instead, make a point of keeping your elbows tucked in as you ride, says Strickland. And if your knees are bowing out every time you pedal, take a look at your seat height—chances are it's too low for you.

Get flat. Even amateur cyclists know they should try to ride as low in the saddle as possible. Even though you feel like you're riding low, chances are you have an arch in your back, and that hump will make you less aerodynamic.

Practice flattening out your back and making adjustments in your form to make you even flatter, says Strickland. For example, rotating your hips forward in the saddle can help you straighten out and fly right. If you have an indoor wind-trainer or stationary cycle, set it up in front of a mirror. Or get someone to watch you on your bike. The point is to examine your form—are you doing all you can to keep your back flat and straight?

Don't stand for it. When you come upon a steep hill, the natural temptation is to immediately stand up in the saddle and crank furiously until you're over the top. The problem is that this position causes your heart rate to go way up, and you end up burning energy you might need later in the ride.

Instead, make a conscious effort to stay seated as long as possible. Switch to a lower gear if you have to, but keep your butt planted in the seat. Eventually, you may have to stand. "The point is not to make it an instinctive response—'Here's a hill; I have to stand up now.' The longer you wait, the more power you conserve," says Cuerdon. Practice this often enough and you may find you won't need to stand up at all to take most hills.

Use the big gears. One tip cycling coaches rec-

Proper Descent Techniques

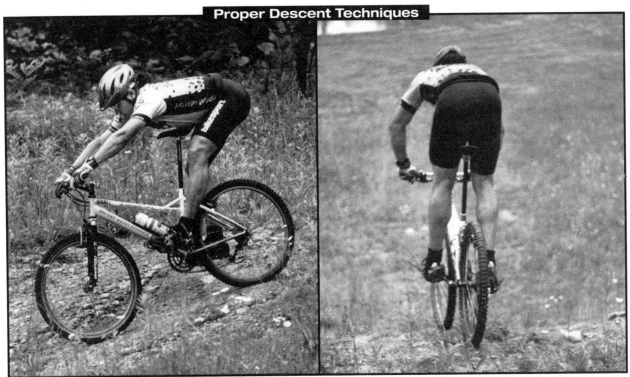

For maximum balance, extend your arms and slide your butt off the back end of the saddle.

For better control, squeeze the saddle with your thighs, and pump the brakes—don't jam on them.

ommend is deliberately cycling in the lower or bigger gears. This increases the resistance when you're pedaling and gives your legs a great workout. If you're going down a hill, don't shift to a higher gear. Stay in the big gear and pedal as fast as possible—it's a good speed-training technique, says Strickland.

Success on the Mountain

You don't need to be very streamlined on a mountain bike, but you sure need good form. "In mountain biking, good form means getting to the bottom of the hill in one piece," says Cuerdon.

That means building sharp reflexes and plenty of upper-body strength to help you steer the bike over outrageous obstacles. Good lower-body and cardiovascular power, meanwhile, will enable you to enjoy many hours of churning up and down hills and up and over logs, stumps and rocks. Here are a few wise words to help you accomplish all these goals.

Be a part-time roadie. Although some die-hard mountain bikers look down their nose at road cycling, doing so robs them of a great cardiovascular workout. "There's nothing wrong with taking your mountain bike out on pavement. Road cycling helps train your heart and lungs better. Believe me, that will come in handy when you're out in the woods trying to make it up a good, steep, crumbling hill," says Cuerdon.

Develop foresight. A mountain-bike trail is ab-

solutely studded with obstacles. "It wouldn't be a mountain-bike trail—and it wouldn't be fun—if it wasn't," says Cuerdon. What's not fun is hitting a rock or root and doing an endo—short for "end over end"—because you weren't prepared for it.

This most often happens because you overfocus on one object—the one right in front of you—and not enough on the rest of the trail. So work to widen your vision. Train yourself to see all the potential pitfalls on the next several feet of the trail—not just what's about to go under your wheel. "The trick is to see the log just ahead as well as the rocks two feet beyond that and the roots five feet beyond that," says Cuerdon.

Use the granny gear. When you're trying to crank up a hill, don't be afraid to shift up to the smallest front gear, also known as the granny.

"I think the name makes guys shy away from it. But it's there for a reason—to make your life easier. Go ahead and use it," says Cuerdon. As you climb, lean forward, almost putting your chest to the handlebars. This will make your climb easier.

Stay padded. In mountain biking, you might take harder knocks than you did in high school football—and you wore a lot more padding in football. To protect against some of the most common mountain-bike traumas, wear padded gloves and some sort of padding for your nether regions. "You don't have to be one of the shiny blue people, wearing those skin-tight, padded cycling shorts," says Cuerdon. If you want to be more discrete, you can buy padded underwearlike liners for your usual shorts. "Your butt will thank you," says Cuerdon.

Descend smartly. You're going down a steep hill, your speed's picking up, the bike's bouncing on rocks and sticks. Unless you learn how to control your descent, you might end up paying a steep price. Here's what to do, according to our experts.

Make sure your bike is in a high gear and pointed in the general direction of where you want to go. As you start downhill, don't let your weight slide forward—if you hit a big rut, you'll go flying. Instead, extend your arms and slide your butt back off the back end of the saddle. Keep your pedals parallel to the ground to avoid catching them on low obstacles.

For better control, squeeze the saddle with your thighs and pump the brakes—relying mostly on your front brake. Don't jam on them. When you get to the bottom of the hill, resume your normal position and start cranking.

Strength Training for Cyclists

Whether you're a road cyclist or a mountain biker, your workout is going to be pretty much the same.

"Cycling is universally hard on the legs and lower back. But because you're using your upper body to steer and help control the bike, you'll also want to pay attention to muscles there—that's something a lot of cyclists forget," says Graham.

The Core Routine on page 121 should help you keep a proper fitness balance between your upper and lower body. Meanwhile, to target your cycling muscles exclusively, include the following exercises in your workout, says Graham.

Arm Exercises

Whether you're bumping down a long, rough mountain or tugging on those handlebars as you climb a steep hill in the road, you're going to need strong arms to handle the job. "Barbell and dumbbell curls will strengthen the biceps, but don't forget the triceps for muscle balance and stabilization," Graham says. He recommends overhead triceps extensions. Also do wrist and forearm exercises, such as wrist curls and reverse wrist curls, to give you plenty of strength and endurance to keep the bike stable.

Rows

Along with your arms, your upper back is going to help you pull up on the handlebars when you're climbing; it also absorbs plenty of shock during a ride. One-arm dumbbell rows and bent-over rows will enhance muscle strength and endurance for the upper back.

Leg Exercises

Yeah, you'd think pedaling over hill and dale would be exercise enough for the legs. Don't believe it, says Graham. "Cycling really works the quads and the muscles on the outside of the thighs. The rest of the leg muscles don't get as much benefit." That's bad—it can lead to a strength imbalance in the leg muscles, which could in turn lead to a serious muscle injury that could take you out of the saddle for several weeks.

Focus on building well-rounded leg strength. Perform squats, leg presses and leg curls to ensure proper balance between the quadriceps and opposing hamstring muscles. Also, to strengthen your inner- and outer-thigh muscles, do some abductor and adductor lifts, either lying on the floor or using a cable machine.

When to Exercise

If you're the least bit competitive in your cycling—or you want to be—you need to partition your workouts according to the cycling season, off-season and pre-season.

Traditionally, the off-season, which runs October to January, is your time to focus on weight training. Do it three to four days a week. Keep your cycling muscles limber on a stationary bike or wind-trainer—use that as a warm-up or aerobic workout.

Long about February, you'll start to move into the pre-season phase. Here, Graham suggests riding more and cutting back weight training to two to three times a week. "Don't go easy on those days. Keep up the intensity of your weight training," he admonishes.

By April, you'll be getting into prime cycling season, and most of your exercise time will probably be devoted to riding. Don't abandon weight training, though. Graham recommends continuing to lift two days a week throughout the season. That should be enough to maintain your muscle until you get back into the off-season again.

Running

There's a simplicity, an almost zen purity to the sport of running. You, shoes, the open road. Nothing more, nothing less. Doing what man and animal has done for thousands of years. The most natural exercise of all.

And yet. Go to a bookstore and look at all the running books. There's more to this passion than meets the eye. There's a science to it all: how to train, how to prevent injury, how to breathe, how to condition your body for maximum results. Sure, you can go outside and just run. Children do it every day. But if you want to run well, you must do more.

Developing the skill, strength and endurance of a good runner—and keeping your knees, ankles, hips and hamstrings as injury-free as possible—requires a well-conceived training program, says Budd Coates, marathon runner, trainer, exercise physiologist and special consultant to *Runner's World* magazine.

The precise nature of the program depends upon what level of runner you are, of course. But, in general, "What you need to do over a seven-day period is introduce the body to endurance training, quality training and rest," Coates says. "When done in the right manner, at the right level of stress for the individual, you'll improve."

How Much Should You Run?

We'll get to stretching, strength training and other training tricks in a bit. But if you are a runner, your passion is the road, not the gym. So we'll start with what you love best: how much roadtime you need.

Coates notes that the majority of runners average 16 to 20 miles per week. If this is you, Coates recommends the following runs per week.

- One long run of about eight miles.
- One medium run of five to six miles that includes what Coates calls quality. "Quality is basically a run that involves more effort than the others," he says. "You could include cruise intervals, tempo runs, track intervals, some hill work."
- Two or three shorter runs of two to four miles, done at a comfortable pace.
- Two or three days of rest alternated into the schedule.

In all, it should add up to about 20 miles, says Coates.

Coates notes that each runner needs to adapt the basic seven-day-per-week running program to their level of strength and endurance. "The fact is everybody needs to do endurance work; everybody needs to rest; and everybody needs to do quality work," he says. "The exact ratio or recipe is really dependent upon where you're at and what you've done before."

The recommended program "could bury

someone who has just started running, and could be totally tedious for an experienced runner," he says.

For the more advanced runner, Coates says he "wouldn't make many changes—just the quantity. The long runs become longer. Rest days can be an hour easy run, and moderate days can be 12 to 15 miles. A hard day can be 15 to 20 miles with a variety of quality inside that mileage."

A beginning runner, on the other hand, should start off with walking and, after a couple of weeks, alternate between walking and jogging. After a couple more weeks, he should alternate between walking and running and, eventually, over a two-month period, work up to a steady run, says Coates.

Stretching

As with all workouts, it's important to get your blood flowing and your muscles primed with a short warm-up before diving into the main event. The same holds for running.

Through much of this book, we advise you to stretch both before and after a workout. Coates sees it differently for running: He suggests that you save the stretches for the end of the workout, which is what he does. "The key," he explains, "is that if you stretch after you work out, you will be ready for the next day's run."

Occasionally, he says, you may need to stretch early in your run "if you feel a muscle that's being kind of a squeaky wheel.

"But if everything is fine, after 10 to 15 minutes of comfortable running, just progress into the hard run and then stretch everything in general after the workout," Coates says.

Here are six stretches recommended by Coates that make up a good routine.

Total-Body Stretch

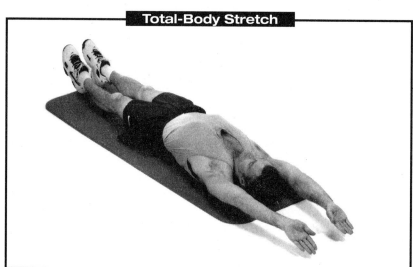

◄ Total-Body Stretch

Lie on your back. Fully extend your arms and legs and point your fingers and toes. Tense and stretch as far as possible for five seconds, then relax. Repeat three to five times. Do this to both begin and end your stretching routine.

Toe Touches

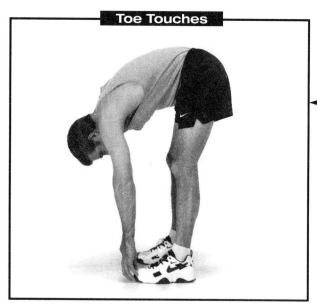

◄ Toe Touches

Stand with your feet about shoulder-width apart. Slowly bend over at your waist until you feel a pull at the back of your legs. Make sure your knees are not locked. Hold the position for up to 20 seconds. If you cannot actually touch your toes, that's okay. This stretch is good for the lower back, hips, groin and hamstrings and guards against pulls and injuries in those areas.

Runner's Terminology

Do-it-yourselfers and those relatively new to running may be unfamiliar with the following training techniques. Give them a try, suggests Budd Coates, marathon runner, trainer, exercise physiologist and special consultant to *Runner's World* magazine.

• Intervals. These are periods of hard running alternated with easier "rest" periods of jogging. They're great for increasing speed, says Coates. Hard running periods can be from 30 seconds to five minutes, and rest periods should be about the same time. Or you may be able to cut rest intervals down to half the time of the hard-run intervals.

• Cruise intervals. You'll need to have a good grasp on your speed and endurance capacities for this. Run for a period at a pace that is 15 to 20 seconds per mile slower than your ten-kilometer race pace; then jog for a period 20 to 30 percent as long (for example, ten minutes of running, two minutes of jogging). Do three or four, consecutively. The purpose is to raise the point at which muscle-tiring lactic acid begins to build up in your blood, thus increasing endurance. Increase distance, but not speed, as the training gets comfortable, advises Coates.

• Tempo runs. After warming up, run for 15 to 30 minutes at a pace 20 to 30 seconds slower per mile than your ten-kilometer pace. The object is the same as with cruise intervals, says Coates.

• Hill work. Run up hills at 85 to 90 percent effort, then jog down as a rest; repeat several times. The uphill part should take from 30 seconds to five minutes, and the recovery (downhill) portion 1½ to 2 times longer. You may want to add a 30- to 60-second surge in the middle of the downhill portion. The object is to increase your efficiency at running hills.

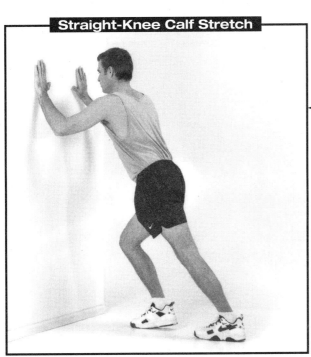

Straight-Knee Calf Stretch

◄ **Straight-Knee Calf Stretch**

Stand with your feet planted firmly on the ground, pointed straight toward a wall two to three feet away. Lean forward and put your palms on the wall. Bend one knee, lifting that foot's heel off the ground. Keep the other foot flat on the ground and your knee, hip and back straight. Lean forward, bending your ankles and elbows, until you feel the extended calf tighten. Hold for up to 20 seconds, then relax. Alternate from leg to leg and repeat three times with each leg. This strengthens, stretches and works out pain in the calves and Achilles tendons.

Ankle Pulls ►

You'll need a towel for this stretch. Lie on your stomach with one leg straight and the other bent at the knee, pointing toward the ceiling. Loop the towel or strap around your bent leg and hold the ends with your hands, behind your back. Curl your neck and shoulders upward, and attempt to straighten your bent leg against the tension from the towel until the thigh is taut. Hold for 20 seconds, then relax. Repeat three times, then switch legs and repeat. This exercise is good for the thigh muscles.

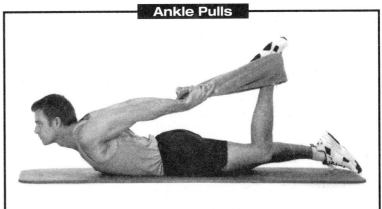

Ankle Pulls

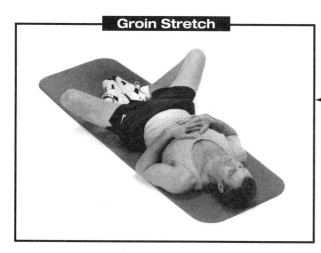

Groin Stretch

◄ Groin Stretch

Lie on your back with the soles of your feet touching firmly. Let your knees and hips relax and hold the position for 40 seconds. This relaxes the body and helps prevent groin pulls.

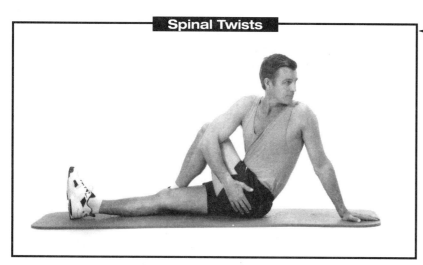

Spinal Twists

◄ Spinal Twists

Sit with your right leg straight. Bend your left leg so it crosses over the right and your foot rests on the outside of the right knee. Bend your right elbow, resting it on the outside of your upper left thigh. Let your left hand rest on the floor behind you. Slowly turn your head to look over your left shoulder while rotating your upper body toward your left hand and arm. Hold for up to 20 seconds, then stretch the other side. This is good for the hips, back and rib cage and reduces or prevents back and hip pain.

Strength Training

Finally, Coates suggests you supplement your running workout with appropriate strength training—with weights. "Appropriate" means a good overall workout, he says. It also means experimenting a bit and finding what works for you.

"The biggest thing with strength training is that you need to listen to your body while you're running," says Coates. "You know when you're creating a muscle imbalance and trying to run with it. You don't feel biomechanically fluid anymore. Or if you feel you're carrying around extra baggage, your upper body is feeling bulky, you're probably overdoing it.

Lift like you're a runner; don't lift like you're a lifter. You're always looking at lifting through a runner's eyes. You're not looking at lifting to get so many more pounds on the bench and so many more pounds on the arm curl and to flex in front of the mirror. The program that works is the one that makes you feel good when you're out running. You find it on your own. Pick a sound overall program, and with a little bit of trial and error, find what works for you."

There are a few specific strengthening exercises

for runners that Ken Sprague, coach and strength trainer, owner and operator of the original Gold's Gym and author of *Sports Strength* recommends.

"Some strength training can help runners avoid injury," says Sprague. Most runners, he says, experience at least one relatively serious injury a year.

The exercises he recommends can be done with free weights or with gym equipment. For each exercise do two sets, ten reps per set, at 65 percent of your one-rep maximum, two days per week.

Sprague's program for runners includes:

- Dumbbell lunges for hip and leg thrust
- Dumbbell step-ups and step-downs for hip and leg thrust
- Leg curls to prevent hamstring injuries
- Rumanian dead lifts for torso stability
- Bench press with close grip to improve arm drive
- Toe raises with seated leg press machine for ankle extension

Then there are two more—the pull-up (it helps with upper-body pull) and a different type of leg raise.

Pull-Ups

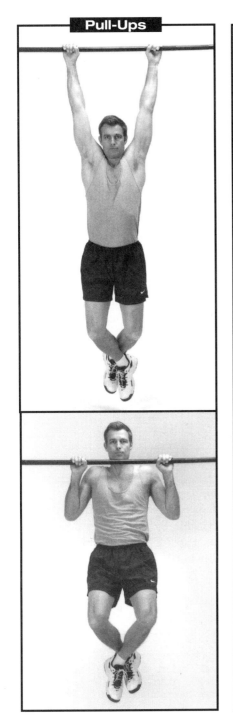

Leg Raises with Dumbbells or Ankle Weights

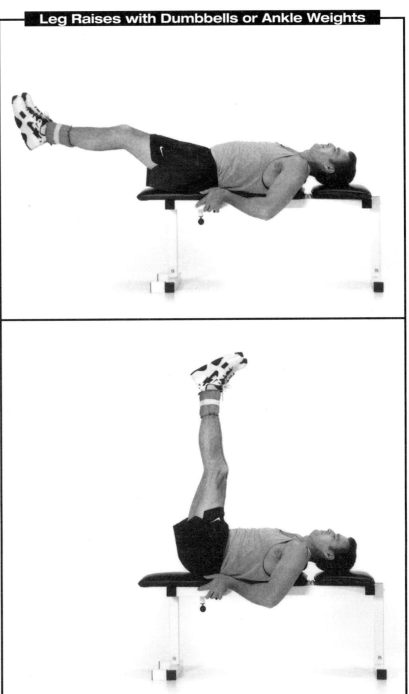

Pull-Ups ⬆

Hang from a chinning bar with your palms facing forward, hands about 18 to 20 inches apart, arms extended. Your feet should be about six inches off the floor. It's okay to cross your feet or bend your knees; just don't kick your legs.

Pull yourself up until your chin clears the bar. Slowly return to the starting position so your arms are again fully extended.

Leg Raises with Dumbbells or Ankle Weights ⬆

Sit on a bench. Stand a low-weight dumbbell between your feet, holding your feet together, so that they can comfortably lift it. (You can increase the weight as strength develops.) Lie on your back, and then extend your legs, your feet holding the dumbbell.

Raise both legs together, keeping them as straight as possible (it's okay to bend your knees at first until you attain the necessary flexibility to stretch your legs straight). When properly done, your feet will be directly above your hips, with your legs at a 90-degree angle to your torso. Slowly lower your legs to the starting position. Do two sets of 8 to 12 reps.

If you don't trust your feet to hold a dumbbell, you can use resistance tubing or ankle weights.

Swimming

Peak Points

- **Focus primarily on form.**

- **Swim with your whole body, not just your arms and legs.**

- **Mix weight-room training with in-pool exercises for maximum performance.**

Think of the pool as a liquid gym—a damp and dynamic circuit trainer that works out every major muscle group, plus your heart and lungs, often all at the same time.

Whether you swim for sport or for exercise, the big challenges to aquatic action are probably more cardiovascular than muscular. "Swimming is a very aerobic sport," says John McVan, aquatic specialist at Iowa State University in Ames. "It's certainly a good workout for the arms, legs, back, chest, torso and so on, but you have to build up your heart and lung capacity to be really good."

Mastering the Water

We'll tell you what exercises will make you a better swimmer in a bit, along with how to use your pool as a workout tool. But when it comes to swimming at your peak level, first and foremost is the issue of technique.

"Most people don't know how to breathe, don't know how to distribute their weight in the water and don't know how to make themselves more hydrodynamic—how to be more slippery in the water," says Terry Laughlin, director of the Total Immersion adult swimming camp in Goshen, New York. "You could be the strongest man in the world, but if you don't have good technique and form, none of that muscle will do you the least bit of good."

Here, then, are some tricks from our experts to being smoother, sleeker and faster in the water.

Swim with your body. The first step to being a better, stronger swimmer is accepting that everything you learned in your old swim classes at the Y is probably wrong. For starters, stop thinking of your arms and legs as the things that propel you through the water.

"Think of swimming as an all-body exercise. Your power is not in your arms and legs, it's in how you position your whole body, how you can make it faster and sleeker. Your arms are important, but they account for about 10 percent of what can make you a good swimmer," says John Troup, Ph.D., former director of medicine and sports science for the U.S. Olympic Swimming Team.

Swim downhill. Your lower body is heavier and denser than your upper body, so your legs drag. If you try to compensate by kicking harder, you'll just exhaust yourself. Instead, Laughlin suggests, lean on your chest as you swim. This will keep your hips and legs near the surface, he says. You should notice your hips and legs feeling lighter, as if the water were supporting more of your body weight.

Swim taller. Stretching your hand forward before pulling makes your body longer, allowing it to slip through the water more easily, says Laughlin. If you use your hand to lengthen your body line rather than using it to push water back, you'll

Proper Stroke Form

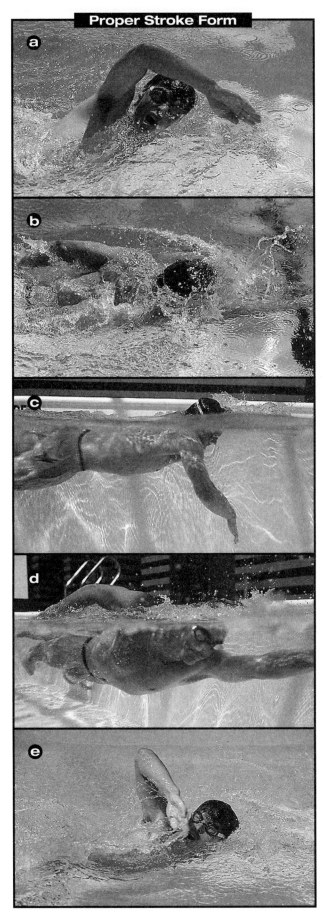

contribute far more to your speed. As each hand enters the water, reach out before starting your pull. Don't rush the motion, Laughlin cautions. Your hand should reach forward at the same speed your body is moving forward.

Get power from your hips. It's your hips, rather than your shoulders, that are your engine. Roll them from side to side to make your stroke more powerful and rhythmic. When you begin to pull, use your arm and shoulder muscles to hold onto the water as your body roll pulls you through the water, says Laughlin. You should feel your stroke rhythm in your midsection as it rolls back and forth rather than in your arm turnover.

Rotate your breathing. When you've mastered swimming on your side, think about how you're breathing, too. Roll your body to the side, and breathe as you do. If you breathe by turning or lifting your head, your legs will sink and break your trim swim form.

Perfect your stroke. Keep in mind that your arms are major players in what propel you effectively through the water. You'll want to spend some quality time working on that stroke so you're not "hacking"—chopping your way inefficiently across the pool. "You might feel like you got a good workout after something like that, but in a practical sense, it's no way to swim," explains McVan. According to our experts, this is:

a Entry. Watch where your hand enters the water—ideally, say swim experts, you want it entering the water about 8 to 12 inches short of your full arm extension. Don't extend your arm, though, until after it's in the water. Position your hand at about a 30-degree angle to the water, palm facing away from your head.

b Down sweep. With your hand in the water, now is the time to fully extend your arm. Your shoulder should come down into the water, too; this will help you rotate your hips and shoulders and help give your body the efficient corkscrew spin you want.

c Inward sweep. Turn your hand so your fingers start coming back toward your body. You'll be bending your arm now, so keep your elbow up and pull your hand back toward your waist.

d Up sweep. Once your hand passes your lower ribs, push back with the heel of your hand. Now rotate your wrist so your little finger is the first one to leave the water.

e Recovery. Your arm is out and ready for the next stroke. Try to keep it relaxed. Raise your elbow up out of the water and let your forearm dangle from it as you swing forward into the water again. Don't windmill—raising your arm straight over your head. That will only slow you down.

Powering Up for the Pool

Swimming requires as much explosive power as it does endurance. "Unless you use it as a form of exercise where you're simply swimming laps, swimming is a sport that requires a lot of explosiveness if you're going to get good at it," says Dr. Troup.

You can build that strength on dry land, suggests Dr. Troup, by using weights as well as rubber stretch cords to help you do additional resistance training. (Gyms and fitness stores may carry rubber stretch cords; price varies from around $10 for a simple tube with handles to over $50 for a more elaborate kit.) But some of the best training you can give yourself will be through drills in the water. Here are a few conditioning ideas from our experts that incorporate the best of both worlds.

Weight Lifts

Shoulder Exercises

Your shoulders are important because they help control not only the power of your arms but also their form as you slice through the water. Where shoulders are concerned, you don't want to build up huge amounts of muscle, but you do want to be toned. In addition, you want your major joints limber and ready to help propel you through the water. Shoulder exercises will do both, according to Dr. Troup. The inclined bench press will work your shoulders, arms and chest. You should also do upright rows and lat pull-downs to target your shoulder muscles exclusively.

Abdominal Exercises

The stronger your abdominal muscles are, the quicker you'll be able to maneuver the rest of your body when you swim. "The abdominals are key, because they help you move your hips and legs, and they keep you turning through the water," points out Dr. Troup. To keep your abs in top form, you should do various forms of crunches; good ones include regular, raised-leg and oblique.

Stroke Drills ➤

To improve your stroke, Laughlin suggests swimming laps by stroking with only one arm, while keeping the other straight out in front of you. Or do catch-up drills: Keep your right arm outstretched all the way through the left arm's movement. Then, when you've brought your left arm forward and it starts to cover your right, stroke with your right arm.

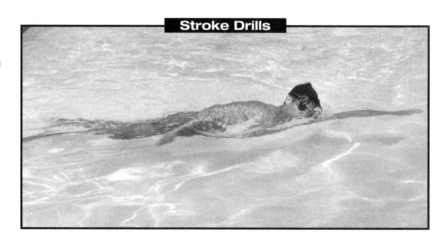

Stroke Drills

Kick Drills ➤

One of the best swim drills to help you find your balance in the water is to swim laps by kicking only. Put your arms straight out in front of you and kick (it's also a great leg exercise). Concentrate on where your balance is. Breathe by moving your chin forward and lifting your head up slightly. This will momentarily put you off balance, so work to "press the buoy" (the spot in your upper chest where your buoyancy resides) quickly to find your balance again as soon as possible.

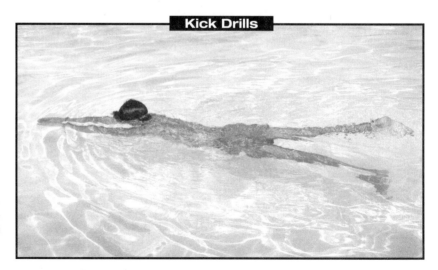

Kick Drills

Cross Jumps

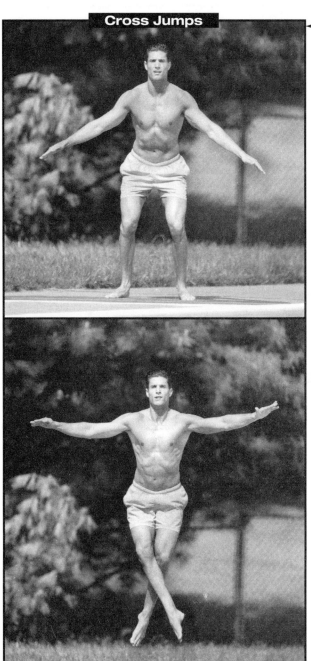

◀ Cross Jumps

Underwater explosive exercises and routines work wonders on otherwise landlocked legs, says McVan, who designs aquatic aerobics classes. This jump is great for working the side and front of your thighs as well as your glutes, all important muscles for helping you dive and move through the water. Start by standing in water up to your waist, your feet shoulder-width apart, knees slightly bent, hands at your side.

Now jump straight up, crossing your right leg in front of your left as you jump. As you start to come back down, return your feet to the starting position. Repeat, this time crossing your left leg in front of your right. (For clarity, the accompanying photos were shot out of water.)

Split Jumps

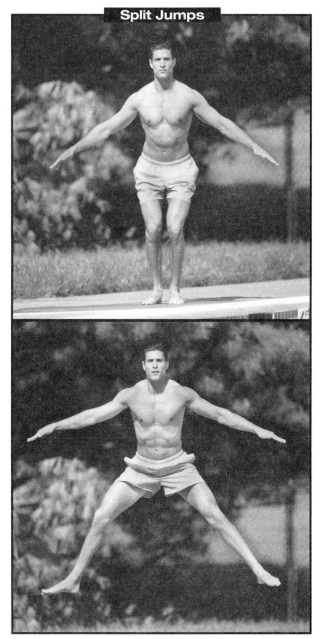

Split Jumps ▶

This jump also works most of your upper-leg muscles, including the muscles on the inside and outside of your thighs. Start by standing in waist-high water, your feet together, knees slightly bent and arms extended from your sides for better balance.

Jump straight up, and extend your legs out to the sides as you leap. Return to the starting position.

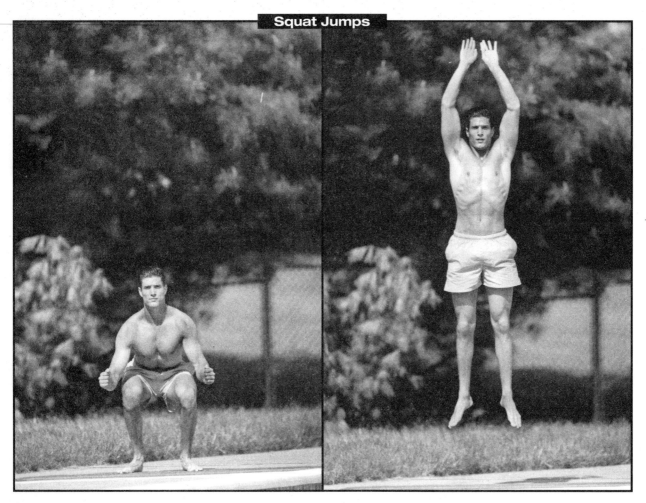

Squat Jumps

Squat Jumps ▲

This is another leaping exercise for your quads and glutes. Stand in waist-high water, your legs about hip-width apart, arms at your sides. Squat down so your butt is parallel to the pool floor.

Pushing off from your heels, leap straight up. As you come back down, try to land on your toes, then the balls of your feet, then your heels. Return to the squatting position and repeat.

Note: As you get stronger, you can move all of these exercises into chest-high water, just to make the jumping a little harder.

Stopping Pain at a Stroke

One of the greatest things about aquatic exercise is that it's both hard and easy—easy on the joints, that is.

"Because swimming is not a weight-bearing activity, it doesn't cause as much stress on joints as other exercises," points out John McVan, aquatic specialist at Iowa State University in Ames. "Although swimming is an excellent sport for everyone, it's especially good for people who have back pain or arthritis." As McVan points out, either condition usually forces men into a more sedentary existence, which only makes their joint and back pain worse. "Swimming, on the other hand, will get these men mobile, get their blood flowing and take some of the strain off their injured joints while they're doing it."

Acing Aquatic Ailments

Swimming may be a great way to get your exercise, but it's also a sport fraught with some unusual hazards. Here's a short list of potential pool-borne perils and ways you can beat them so they won't keep you out of the water.

Swimmer's Ear

Cause: This is an infection of the outer ear and ear canal caused by chronic exposure to moisture. Soggy skin in the ear canal allows bacteria and fungus to penetrate the skin and cause pain, swelling, itching and a plugged feeling. In severe or untreated cases, it can lead to dizziness, deeper ear infection and hearing loss.

Remedy: Prevention is best—use earplugs to keep your ear canals dry. If water gets into your ear, tip your head to the side and down, pull outward on your ear and drain the water, suggests David R. Nielsen, M.D., chairman of the Professional Relations and Public Education Committee of the American Academy of Otolaryngology/Head and Neck Surgery. If you don't have a history of a perforated or ruptured ear, you can try over-the-counter ear drops, he suggests. These are usually made from alcohol and acetic acid. You can also make your own by mixing equal amounts of rubbing alcohol and white vinegar.

Swimmer's Eye I

Cause: Eyes can get sore and bleary from chlorinated water.

Remedy: Invest in a pair of padded swimmer's goggles, suggests Paul F. Vinger, an ophthalmologist from Concord, Massachusetts, and eye medical consultant to the U.S. Olympic Committee.

Swimmer's Eye II

Cause: This affects contact lens–wearers only. Pool water can cause contacts to dry out and stick to your eyeballs.

Remedy: If your lenses get stuck, don't try to pry them out, warns Dr. Vinger. Instead, wait 30 minutes after getting out of the pool or rehydrate your contacts with saline solution before taking them out.

Swimmer's Hair

Cause: Chlorine from pool water turns your hair brittle and, in some cases, discolors it, giving your coif a greenish tint.

Remedy: To help reduce the damage from chlorine, wash, rinse and condition your hair immediately after getting out of the pool. Meanwhile, avoid direct sunlight, which intensifies the effect of the chlorine, says Gregory Miller, head of the color department for Vidal Sassoon in New York.

Swimmer's Teeth

Cause: Chemicals in gas-chlorinated water erode tooth enamel. This can lead to discoloration and chipping over time. (This usually affects fitness swimmers, people who swim at least once a day.)

Remedy: Keep your mouth shut in the water, except to breathe, suggests Steven J. Filler, D.D.S., associate professor at the University of Alabama at Birmingham.

Turning On the Water Works

Now that you know the particulars of powerful pool performance, you'll want to put them all together for a total water workout. "Working out with water is just like working out with weights. You don't want to dive right in and start doing laps until you drop. You want to start with a five- or ten-minute warm-up, then do several different drills or aquatic exercises. Then you'll want to have a cooldown phase," says McVan.

Unlike a weight-based routine that would build only strength, your water workouts should focus mainly on building technique and improving heart and lung capacity, with a few explosive exercises thrown in as well. To build your own aquatic exercise routine, follow our experts' suggestions below. If you decide to do a regular swimming workout, keep it to every other day. We've broken the exercises up Chinese-menu style—just pick one from each section.

The Warm-Up

In and Outs

From a diving board or the side of the deep end of the pool, enter the water via a feet-first jump, cannonball, dive or even a jackknife. Then swim to the nearest ladder, climb up, walk briskly to your original entry point and begin again. After about six to ten repeats, you'll have elevated your heart rate, unknowingly worked on "body-streamlining" and experienced a little unconventional water fun to boot, says McVan.

Press Your Buoy ➤

This is a good warm-up for beginners. Spend five minutes trying to find your balance by kicking facedown in the water and pressing the "buoy." (To remind you: That's the spot in your chest where your buoyancy resides.) Breathing will cause you to get off-balance each time you raise your head to inhale. As part of the exercise, work to recover your balance as quickly as possible after each breath.

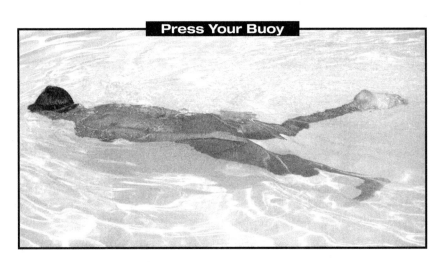

Press Your Buoy

In-Water Jump Drills

Do a series of the cross jumps, split jumps and squat jumps described above—roughly five to ten each. "Don't overdo it—this is only a portion of your pool training. You don't want to tire yourself out too soon," says McVan.

The Workout

Laps

When most people think of fitness swimming, this is the exercise that leaps to mind. "There are a lot of people who enjoy—and get a lot of benefit from—swimming laps," says McVan. Swimming laps can be a good way to benchmark your progress. You ought to be able to swim at least 18 laps nonstop, says Laughlin. "That's a bare minimum for fitness swimming," he says, and adds that a lot of people can't do it. If you're one of them, make it a goal to work toward.

Stroke Drills

Spend 20 to 30 minutes doing the stroke and kick drills mentioned above. Ideally, don't do one drill to the point of exhaustion, or all of them one after the other. "The point of a stroke drill is to learn proper technique and, once you've learned it, to hone it," says Laughlin. Stick with two drills per workout—one stroke drill, one kick drill—for 10 to 15 minutes each.

Pool Games

One option for a pool workout is to build your warm-up and cooldown around an aquatic group activity, such as an aquatic aerobics class or a game of water polo. McVan suggests calling your local health club or nearby college. "If they have an indoor pool, odds are they have a year-round program of events and activities. You can usually get involved for a nominal fee," says McVan.

The Cooldown

Tread Water

To cool down after your workout, spend a few minutes easily treading water. Try not to touch the bottom of the pool.

Balance on Your Back

Practice balancing on your back—press your head and shoulder blades into the water, tuck your chin slightly, keep your head still and keep your knees and toes below the surface. Breathe normally.

Slow Strokes

Do a couple of slow laps from one end of the pool to the other. As you swim, count your strokes. You should aim to swim each lap in 20 strokes or less. If you can't do this, spend more time on the stroke drills.

Breathing Exercises

As you swim your cooldown laps, practice rolling and breathing—breathe first on one side, then on the other.

In-Line Skating

Peak Points

- **Keep your torso muscles strong for better balance.**

- **Focus on strengthening leg muscles—especially the inner thigh and quadriceps.**

- **Build your heart and lung power for better skating stamina.**

Remember the roller rink of your junior-high days? You strapped on the old four-wheel skates and slid onto the circular concrete plateau, staggering and swaying like a fast-moving drunk. Your mind wasn't on having fun; it was on how not to take a spill and wake up sore the next day.

The same principle applies to rollerskating's newest incarnation, in-line skating. Skates have gotten lighter, faster and more aerodynamic. It's not likely we can say the same about you, particularly compared with when you were 12. Sure, skating itself will help you develop the muscles and skills you need to improve. But to become a good skater fast, you need to get your body prepared.

Studies show that an in-line skating workout burns about 550 calories per hour—more if you are going uphill. That's a lot of calories, making in-line skating intensely aerobic. To handle the exertion, you'll need a strong heart and a large lung capacity.

It also means needing solid inner-thigh and groin muscles for the constant side-to-side motion of skating. That means having good calf and lower-leg power for all the curb-hopping, manhole-dodging, pedestrian-swerving acrobatics you'll be doing. Finally, it means having firm abdominals and a good lower back to help you maintain the proper skating position.

The Core Routine on page 121 is sufficient to prepare you for some of the rigors of life on a roll. But if you want to achieve the kind of grace and power you've envied in the hot dogs who burn by you in the park every weekend, you'll need to add a powerful lot of aerobic exercise to your workout schedule, says Joel Rappelfeld, in-line skating instructor from New York City and author of *The Complete Blader.*

More than that, he says you'll need to target the torso and leg muscles that will not only keep you moving forward fast but that will also help keep you on balance.

A Rolling Resistance Regimen

Although the best way to be a better skater is—what a surprise—to skate as much as possible, you can also improve your skating form by doing regular off-wheel stretching and resistance training.

"You don't have to be muscle-bound to be a good skater," says Rappelfeld. "But you have to work on the muscles that are going to propel you and help you to control your motion while you're moving." The flipside to strength building, though, is flex building. "Being able to relax your muscles and being flexible are absolutely key for good skating. If you're tight while you're skating, you'll pull a muscle or fall or both," says Rappelfeld.

Here are some basic lifts—make them part of your regular workout, which means doing them at least three times a week, says Rappelfeld. We've also included some stretches, which you should also do three times a week and just before you go skating.

Reference Points

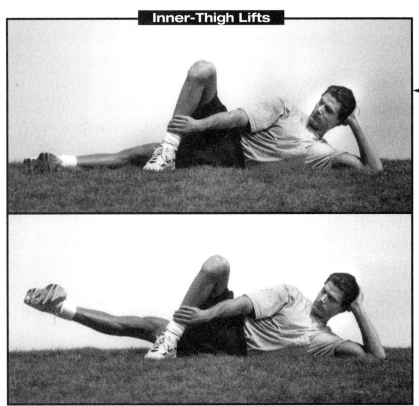

◄ Inner-Thigh Lifts

This lift, with or without ankle weights, helps work the muscles that keep your legs parallel while you skate.

Lie on your left side, left leg straight, right leg bent, foot in front of your left leg, flat on the ground. The side of your left foot should be facing the sky.

Now lift your left leg straight up, about eight to ten inches off the ground. Hold for a count of two, then lower. Keep your left foot flexed as you lift. Do 8 to 15 reps, then switch sides.

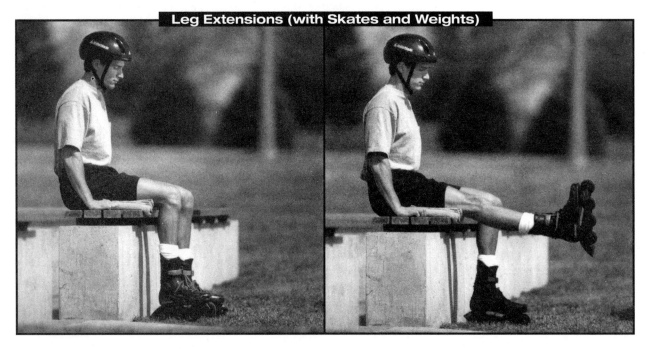

Leg Extensions (with Skates and Weights) ▲

These are like leg extensions you've probably done in the gym, only this time you're doing them with the weight of your skates as resistance. "Working out with the equipment on will get you used to the feel of it. The more comfortable you are, the better you'll skate," says Rappelfeld. For added resistance, add ankle weights.

Sit on the edge of a chair or bench, with your legs bent and hanging down freely. Place a pillow or towel under your right knee to raise it slightly and absorb pressure.

Slowly lift your right leg, straightening it as you lift, but not quite as far as a fully locked knee position. Do 8 to 15 reps, then switch legs.

Blading Basics

At last count, roughly ten million American men were strapping on skates and taking them for a spin—chances are you were one of them. But whether you were renting them for an afternoon or shelling out over 200 bucks for your very own pair, you may not have taken the time to get proper instruction.

"Most guys just go out there and roll around, trying to teach themselves. This is how you get injured or develop bad habits," says Joel Rappelfeld, in-line skating instructor from New York City and author of *The Complete Blader*. If you're strapping on blades for the first time, the smart thing to do is to get a lesson. Your local skate shop should have a listing of upcoming lessons and workshops. Pick ones led by instructors who are accredited by the International In-Line Skating Association, he says. And lesson or no, he cautions that you shouldn't skate one step without proper protection—helmets, knee and elbow pads and wrist protectors.

Meanwhile, here are a few basic tips to keep you looking dignified from the first time you strap on the skates.

Take a fall. Like martial arts, in-line skating is predicated on the notion that sooner or later you're going to end up on your hinder. Trust us, it will happen. So practice taking a plunge. "Ideally, try to fall forward—falling backward can really do a number on your spine. And the more you fall, the more confident you'll be as a skater because you'll see that the safety equipment really does work," says Rappelfeld.

Get on your knees. Of course, one way to limit the number of times you let gravity have its way with you is to stay in your most stable position. "When you're on skates, that means leaning forward with your hands on your knees," says Rappelfeld. If you feel like you're about to fall, the hands-to-knees position will stabilize you.

Know when to stop. More important, know how to stop. "Practice with that brake—it's usually on the back of the right boot," says Rappelfeld. Start with your feet parallel, then roll your braking foot forward while bending your non-braking leg. Lift the toe of the braking foot and force the brake down by extending your braking leg further in front of you. Note that some skates are coming equipped with a new braking system that doesn't require lifting the toe; be sure to know what type you have before going down a hill.

Rock and roll. The easiest way to start rolling from a standing stop is with your feet parallel. "Then, start walking like Frankenstein," says Rappelfeld. Rock back and forth from side to side, shifting your weight from your left leg to your right. "Point your toes out, and you'll start moving." Then put your feet in a parallel position to roll, he says.

Warm Up

The key to being a skater par excellence is to be loose and flexible, ready to react to anything that may cross your path, says Rappelfeld. Since your legs will be doing most of the work, be sure to pay special attention to them with hamstring and thigh stretches as well as lunges for the inner thighs. Finally, since groin pulls are a real danger with skaters, be sure to do butterfly stretches or other similar groin stretches.

Abdominal Exercises

As you've probably figured out by now, your abdominal and oblique muscles are your power base for just about every sport you enjoy—skating is no different. "They help you turn, they help you push off when you skate, and they help center you," says Rappelfeld. Keep doing those crunches, and for the obliques, be sure to throw in some crunches with twists.

How to Have a Stroke

The most important move to learn in skating is proper stroking, says Joel Rappelfeld, in-line skating instructor from New York City and author of *The Complete Blader*. It's the move that gets you gliding across the asphalt. Here's how to do it.

❶ Stand with your knees and waist bent and feet parallel to one another. Lean slightly forward so your nose, knees and toes are lined up with one another.

❷ Turn your right foot to a 45-degree angle. Now push directly out to the side with your right foot. As you push, shift your weight to the left foot. Lean in the direction you're moving.

❸ After you've pushed off, bring your right foot back up so that it's rolling parallel with your left foot.

❹ Repeat the push-off with your left foot.

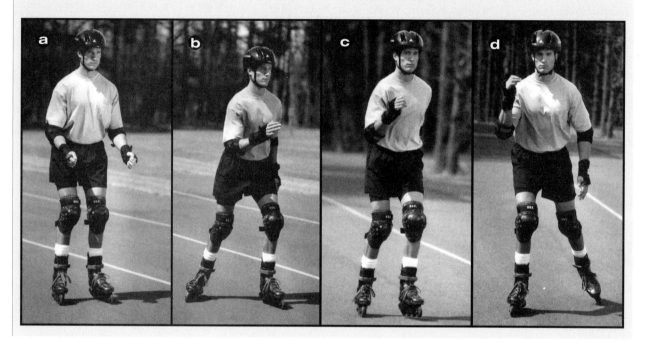

Slide Aerobics

To improve your cardiovascular fitness and your skating muscles at the same time, try to do at least a half-hour once a week of slide aerobics—where you slide back and forth on a vinyl sheet, replicating the swaying motion used in skating. "It's one of the best workouts around because it so closely mimics skating—you use the same muscles, too," says Robert King, fitness trainer at the Vail Athletic Club in Colorado.

Most health clubs sponsor at least one slide aerobics class a week. Or you can buy your own slide for anywhere between $25 and $70 and do the workout at home.

The Next Level

At first, skating is going to be a trial-and-error proposition for you. But as you get more comfortable in your skates, you're going to want to up the ante a little bit. "The better you get at skating, the less of a workout it becomes. So you constantly have to challenge yourself to do better, harder things," says King. Here are some tips for you high rollers out there.

Sculling

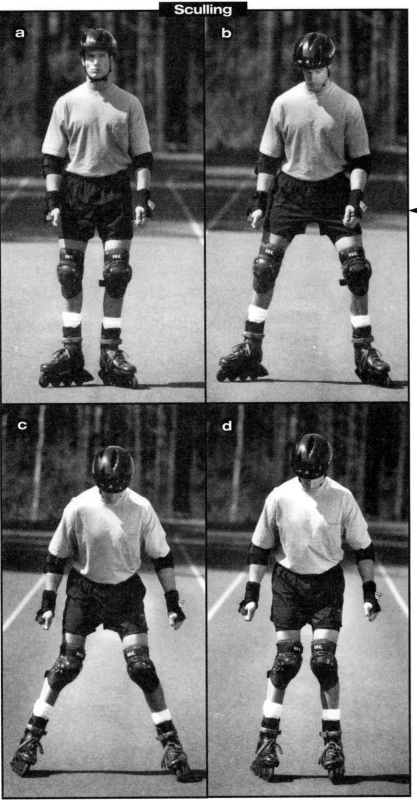

◄ Sculling

For novices and advanced players, sculling is a universally great exercise. Not only does it allow you to practice and improve your control on wheels but it's also a good inner- and outer-thigh muscle exercise for all skaters. Here's how to do it.

Ⓐ Stand upright, heels together, knees slightly bent, feet at about a 45-degree angle.

Ⓑ Using the inner edges of your skates, let both skates roll out away from each other, until your feet are just beyond shoulder-width apart. You should start to roll.

Ⓒ As you roll forward, pivot both heels and point your toes in.

Ⓓ Slowly start to pull your feet together until they're almost together.

Pivot your heels and point your toes out and begin the outward motion again.

Note: The wheels of your skates should never leave the ground.

Skate Keys

Remember these key points when you're skating, suggests Joel Rappelfeld, in-line skating instructor from New York City and author of *The Complete Blader*.

- Always wear safety gear—including helmet, elbow and knee pads and wrist guards.
- Skate on the right, pass on the left.
- Avoid heavy traffic.
- Be alert for road hazards like car doors flying open in front of you as well as cars pulling out of parking spots, driveways or intersections.
- Avoid water, oil and sand.
- Don't wear headphones.
- Yield to pedestrians. You never know when you might be one yourself.
- Don't forget to have a good time.

Foot Drills

First-time and self-taught skaters often develop the bad habit of skating with their feet shoulder-width apart or wider. "That's okay if you're a beginner, but as you get better, you should wean yourself off of a wide stance," says Rappelfeld. It only tires out your hips and thighs.

The key to getting better is to get your feet together, says Rappelfeld. "The wider apart your feet are, the less power you'll have in every stride you take," he says. To practice closing the gap between your skates, consciously bring your feet together about every third stroke and coast that way for a moment. "Gradually reduce the interval from three strokes to two, then to one. Pretty soon you'll have your feet closer together without even realizing it," says Rappelfeld.

Stride Drills

As you get more confident and want to take things faster, remember this: The longer the stride, the further the glide.

"Bring your body position lower, bend your knees more, and your strokes will become longer. Just imagine the body position of a speed ice skater," says Rappelfeld.

Uphill Drills

As you get better on your skates, the benefit you'll get from skating will start to level off. The instinctive answer is to speed up your skating, but that could expose you to more danger and not increase your workout by all that much, says King. So instead, skate uphill. Do this as a drill exercise, like the skating equivalent of running stadium stairs. "Power up the hill, then walk back down on the grass as a rest between each drill," says King. Do five to ten drills each time you go skating. You'll notice big increases in your speed and power when you're back on level ground.

Pole Drills

To get your upper body into the workout, break out the ski poles and use them. This is not a crutch for novices, either. "Sure, they can help the beginner keep his balance. But they're also great on hilly terrain, and they get your upper body into the workout," says King. As King explains, planting poles and pushing off with them can burn more calories than skating alone. For safety's sake, use blunted poles specifically designed for non-snow use, such as Exerstriders. Or cap your pole points with styrofoam or cork, or use special caps available where blading accessories are sold.

Baseball

Peak Points

- **Strengthen arm and shoulder muscles to prevent overuse injuries from throwing and hitting.**
- **Do running and sprinting drills to get legs and hips used to the stop-start action of the game.**
- **Start a regular stretching program before the season starts, and continue it until the season ends.**

It seems like we men of America came from the womb knowing how to play baseball. Deep in the memory of every muscle in our bodies, it feels like there's pre-programmed instruction on how to swing, catch, throw, slide; even how to pound the mitt, kick the dirt and tug the hat. We know that the moment we step out of the dugout, our bodies will summon those ingrained skills and we will instantly be ballplayers.

If you agree with that statement, then you have already fallen victim to the greatest enemy of the casual ballplayer—nostalgia.

"Just because he played *as* a kid, every guy thinks that he can go out there anytime and play ball *like* a kid—and that's what will injure him," says Jim Rowe, a certified athletic trainer and head trainer for the Boston Red Sox.

There is hope for you, and hope for the young champion ballplayer that's still inside you. First, you need to transfer all your old baseball and softball skills from the memory of your 12-year-old self to the physical reality of an older, bigger you. As a kid, you didn't need to do much preparation. As an adult, your body needs pre-training, pre-game stretching and—you knew this was coming—a weight-training regimen. That weight training isn't just to give you strength at the plate or speed in the field, it's also to protect your body from the ravages of the sport.

Building Strength in the Field

"Baseball and softball are very hard on the body—you don't recognize that as a kid," says Rowe, who also serves as physical trainer for the Red Sox Fantasy Camp. "Before guys come to the camp, I try to remind them what baseball is all about. There's lots of stopping and starting, which is hard on the hips, thighs and knees. There's lots of throwing, which is hard on the arms and shoulders, and lots of swinging, which puts a strain on your whole body."

Whether you're a Little League coach or a player on the company softball team, you'll benefit from these pre-season and in-season training tips. They'll get your body used to the physical demands of the sport and help you make the most of your time in the field. Play ball!

Play catch. One of the simplest training

Reference Points

Peak Hitting Points

When you step up to the plate, bear in mind these key elements of form. Perfect them, and you'll get that ball downtown without swinging yourself into a sports injury, according to Cecil Whitehead, 1990 National Softball Player of the Year, now athletic director for the city recreation department in Valdosta, Georgia.

1. Hands: Grip the bat so your middle row of knuckles on both hands lines up. When you're preparing to swing, you should hold the bat so your hands are shoulder-high, away from and to the rear of your body.

2. Arms: Extend your arms as you make contact, not before. Make sure you swing through the ball. On follow-through the bat should wrap around your front shoulder.

3. Hips: The key to a powerful swing. As you swing, turn your hips toward the ball—when you connect, your belt buckle should be facing the pitcher.

4. Legs: Initially, most of your weight should be on your back leg, your knees slightly bent. As you swing, you'll transfer your weight to your front leg—when you connect, your front leg should be fairly straight, your back leg bent.

5. Feet: Stand with your feet shoulder-width apart. Your back foot should be flat on the ground, supporting your weight. As the ball comes at you, point your front foot toward the pitch. When you swing, pivot on the ball of your back foot and the heel of your front.

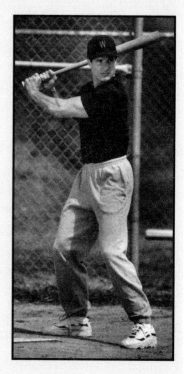

exercises is also one of the best. "Just playing catch with someone is a tremendous benefit. It gets you loose for the game, helps you improve your speed and aim, and improves your eye-hand coordination," says Cecil Whitehead, 1990 National Softball Player of the Year, now athletic director for the city recreation department in Valdosta, Georgia.

But there's a catch to catch, an actual training program you should follow, says Rowe. Start slow—play catch for about 20 minutes, three times a week. Stand about 50 feet apart. Start out lobbing balls to one another—just throw in long, slow arcs. Each week, increase the distance by about 10 feet, until you're 100 feet apart. As you get further apart, you'll have to throw the ball a little harder and a little better. "Just take your time," cautions Rowe. "Don't step out the first day and try to throw it 100 feet."

Sharpen your vision. To hit or field well, you need to keep your eye on the ball, so you need sharp visual abilities.

"You can't improve your vision, but you can improve your dynamic visual acuity, which is the speed at which you see the ball and react to it," says Paul Planer, O.D., optometrist and author of *The Sports Vision Manual.* To help you track balls better, write some letters or numbers on an old ball or beanbag and play catch with a teammate. As you're about to make the catch, focus on the ball and look at the letter or number. After you catch the ball, call out the last letter or number you see.

Round the bases. Baseball and softball put a special demand on the leg joints and muscles. At any given moment, you could have to go from a standing start to an all-out sprint, whether you're trying to shag a fly or steal a base. "That stop-start action really stresses the whole lower body," says Rowe. He recommends sprint drills and running to help pre-train your body. For example, run for a few minutes, then do 30 seconds of all-out sprinting; then run for a few more minutes, then sprint.

Also, you can go to the ball field and run the bases—each trip around the diamond is one lap. Alternate slow laps with sprint laps. "This gets you used to the field, to making fast turns around the bases," says Rowe. As a warm-up, do five to ten laps before each game, or go on off days when the field is empty and do a longer base-running drill.

Be shifty. An essential part of hitting, long-distance throwing and powerful pitching is being able to shift all your weight into the swing or the throw. Do shift drills before a game.

Start with all your weight on the heel of your back foot, then slowly roll forward, shifting the weight to your hips. As you do this, step slightly forward on your front foot. Transfer your weight to your front heel then, finally, to the ball of your front foot. It may look silly, rocking back and forth like that for a few minutes, but you'll see the benefits on the field.

Peak Fielding Points

When you're shagging flies or snagging grounders, the smoother your fielding, the faster you can get the ball in, and the better your chances of making an out. Next time you put on your glove, review these key points in your fielding form.

1. Head: Make sure you field the ball above and in front of your head—you shouldn't have to catch the ball above and behind your head.

2. Throwing arm: Make sure you catch with two hands so you can get the ball immediately into your throwing hand. Hold the ball in a two-fingered grip. As you throw, follow through so your hand comes down past your front knee.

3. Catching arm: At the same time that you catch and pass the ball to your throwing hand, the elbow of your catching arm should move forward and point toward the target.

4. Legs: As you're preparing to throw, keep your weight on your back leg. Your front foot should be pointing in the direction you're throwing. As you're throwing, take a step forward, shifting your weight to the front.

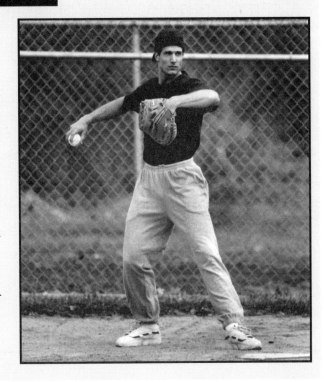

"It could help your balance and get you prepared to use all your weight for a swing or throw—without tearing a muscle in the process," says Rowe.

Watch weighted bats. For years you've seen the big-leaguers in the on-deck circle swinging bats with weights on them, preparing for their moment at the plate. Well, this is one example you don't want to emulate.

A weighted bat can actually throw off your timing, says Rowe. More important, you have a weight at the end of a long bat that your arms are swinging. "You don't realize it, but you're putting tremendous strain on your shoulder and arm joints," says Rowe. Don't strike yourself out before you step up to the plate. When you start warming up, use just the bat you're planning to hit with.

Stepping Up to the Plates

To increase your power on the field and protect your body from the ravages of play, you need to start your weight training at least a month before the season starts.

"If you're a very serious player, you should be training year-round, obviously. But if you at least give yourself a month or two and work on flexibility and strength training for the muscle groups that will take the most punishment, you'll really get a lot more out of the season. You won't feel nearly as sore after a game, and your performance really will improve,"

says softball champ Whitehead. "It used to be taboo to work out with weights, but now there isn't a serious player who doesn't do it." Step up to the plates—the weight plates, that is—and get cracking. Use our Core Routine on page 121 as a basis, then add the following:

Stretches

Before a single player shows up at the Red Sox Fantasy Camp, trainer Rowe makes sure everyone has a copy of his stretching routine for players. "After the camp, it's the one thing I hear over and over. Guys are limping around, wishing they'd spent more time stretching before they came," he says. At least a month before the season starts, establish a stretching regimen—three times a week. Hold each stretch for 20 to 30 seconds, and if you have time, do several reps of each stretch. You'll find a full sequence of stretches in Flexibility on page 32. You should also do these.

- Shoulder shrugs without weights.
- Trunk twists: Hands on hips, feet shoulder-width apart; rotate your body from left to right. Don't jerk or bounce—do slowly and smoothly, holding at the farthest point.

Empty-Can Raises

Any sport that involves swinging is going to be tough on the shoulders. Baseball and softball are even harder on shoulder and arm joints because of all the throwing and pitching your arms are required to do.

"You don't want to bulk up your arm muscles, because that can affect your ability to throw the ball with precision," says Rowe. But you do want to get the joints used to your impending activity.

A good exercise is the empty-can raise, in which you raise and twist your arm at the same time, as if you're emptying a can (the motion is explained in full in Racquet Sports on page 216). Never use more than a five-pound weight for this. Do three sets of 8 to 12 reps.

Grip Exercises

Whether you're choking up on the bat or aiming the ball for your cut-off man, you'll need a reliable grip. "Most weight-training exercises for the arm automatically work the hands and strengthen the grip," Whitehead points out.

You might also want to keep a tennis ball, rubber ball or exercise putty by your desk at work. Use it a couple of times a day for each hand—do 50 squeezes per hand.

Wrist Rolls

In baseball and softball, a key to powerful hitting is your ability to "snap" your wrists the moment you connect with the ball. "The greatest hitters have quick wrists and strong forearms," says Rowe. Follow their lead and add wrist rolls to your workout.

Abdominal Exercises

Your abs and obliques hold everything together. "They need to be strong when you twist for a swing or throw," says Rowe. Do sidebends with dumbbells and oblique crunches.

Leg Exercises

In addition to running and sprinting drills, be sure to do plenty of leg exercises, especially leg presses and lunges. Also, do some leg curls to help strengthen the hamstrings along the underside of your thigh. "That's an often neglected area, and it comes into play when you wind up and throw or swing," explains Rowe. "I've seen pitchers pull their hamstrings from pitching because they put their whole body into the throw, and their hamstrings weren't up to the stress."

Basketball

Peak Points

- **Strength-train with weights.**
- **Develop agility and jumping capacity with both legwork and footwork.**
- **Strengthen fingers, wrists and forearms for precise ball-handling.**

You want to shoot further, quicker and with pro precision.

You want to sprint faster.

You want to grab the rebound, pivot and pass in a split second.

You want to heighten your jump.

You want deadly accuracy and speed when you dribble and pass.

You want to increase your endurance and stamina so you can keep up with, and even outperform, your basketball buddies and, especially, the competition, as the clock ticks past 30, 40 minutes. This is a game where you move, move, move. You scurry here, you sprint there, you block, you chase, you grab, you run, you jump, you shoot, you score. Basketball is not for the meek. You know that.

If you regularly play full-court ball, you're probably in pretty good aerobic condition. But if you're not strength-training, you're only playing at a portion of your potential.

Why Strength-Train

To play better basketball, you need to work with weights. All the big guys do. You can use the machines at the gym or use free weights at home. But you'll never know what kind of basketball you can really play until you've done a strength program.

Why? Listen to Ken Sprague, coach and strength trainer, owner and operator of the original Gold's Gym, author of *Sport's Strength, The Gold's Gym Book of Strength Training* and other similar books, and a physical monster of a man who trained alongside Kareem Abdul Jabaar when Jabaar was playing pro.

"The stronger someone becomes, the more power he produces at a given moment," Sprague says. "Basketball is a real contact sport, so the stronger the player—especially inside players, forwards and centers—the better. Strength becomes integral to your game.

"Reaching for a ball on a rebound is a good example," Sprague continues. "The stronger fellow is going to pull that rebound away from a weaker fellow. Also, strength extends the effective range of your shot. If you can make the shot with only 50 percent of your strength instead of, say, 100 percent, then you have a lot of strength left that you can apply to controlling the ball."

The General Program

Here are the objects of the program Ken Sprague advises.

Reference Points

- Increase your leg and hip thrust
- Boost your upper-body thrust
- Raise your upper-body pulling power
- Strengthen your knee's lifting power
- Strengthen your torso so it can twist and turn smoothly and better stabilize your body
- Build stronger back and ankle muscles
- Improve your ball control

Underlying most of these exercises, says Sprague, is increased power for jumping. All the leg, thigh and calf work obviously adds power to your jump. But so does some hip and spinal work accomplished with box jumps and Rumanian dead lifts. These give you power to snap your back straight and thrust your hips forward explosively during the jump.

Nobody minds the fashionable ripples achieved from abdominal work. The program's crunches give you clean-cut, muscular abdominals, which serve to stabilize your torso upon landing. So there's your free bonus: abs of steel.

This is a program you stick with year-round, in-season and out, though you vary its intensity. You quickly lose the edge and strength gains if you lay off the program when you're not playing, says Sprague.

Sprague advises using a periodization program for maximum benefits during the off-season. To spark your memory, that's a program of altering your weights and rep count constantly. It's described at length in Basic Fitness on page 118.

In season, balance court time with gym time, but be sure to get in two weight-lifting sessions per week, doing two sets of ten reps at 65 percent of your one-rep maximum, Sprague says. And be sure to schedule at least two days' rest time before a game, he says. Otherwise, you'll overtrain and actually lose ground.

The Exercises

These are the specific strength-training exercises Sprague recommends for basketball players. Pencil out these 11 exercises into a periodization program as outlined on page 120, and you'll have your exact off-season ongoing workout routine.

- Squats, for leg and hip thrust
- Dumbbell lunges, for leg and hip thrust
- Box jumps, for leg and hip thrust
- Leg curls, to strengthen hamstrings and protect from injury
- Bench press (narrow grip), for upper-body thrust
- Pull-ups, for upper-body pull
- Rumanian dead lifts, for back extension
- Straight-leg raises, for knee lift and torso stabilization
- Grip strengtheners, for ball control
- Toe raises, for ankle extension
- Crunches, for ab strength and torso stabilization

Beyond Strength Training

Obviously, all that strength won't do you much good if you don't have the heart and lung conditioning to apply it over and over and over, hour after hour of Saturday pickup ball. It's often the best-conditioned player who wins the game with the last-second breakaway layup, you know. So to have the stamina you need to be a true basketball master, you'll need to be in top aerobic shape, says Allan M. Levy, M.D., a long-time sports doctor for major teams, partner at the Sports Medicine Center in Fort Lee, New Jersey, and co-author of the *Sports Injury Handbook*. That means an ongoing program of running, bicycling or whatever your aerobic pleasure, preferably with three vigorous sessions per week. Dr. Levy recommends running. Once you can comfortably run three to five miles several times a week, you should add in sprints or interval training. Wind sprints develop the endurance and explosive bursts of speed that come in so handy in basketball.

Also, the amount of twisting, turning, pushing and shoving that occurs in a basketball game means flexibility is crucial to avoid injury, says Dr. Levy. Before any workout and before and after every game, go through a basic stretching routine that covers all parts of the body. Do some warm-up work first, though, before stretching. We offer some great warm-up routines later.

Finally, all that strength and stamina will be wasted if you don't develop good ball-handling skills. "At its best, basketball is a game where five players move the ball as a team," says Hal Wissel, doctor of physical education, director of player personnel for the New Jersey Nets and author of *Basketball: Steps to Success*, an excellent training guide for the sport. That means great passing, smart dribbling, good peripheral vision and much more. Here are some drills from Dr. Wissel and others to get you on your way to hoop mastery. The ball-handling drills will strengthen your fingers and forearms as well.

Carioca Drill

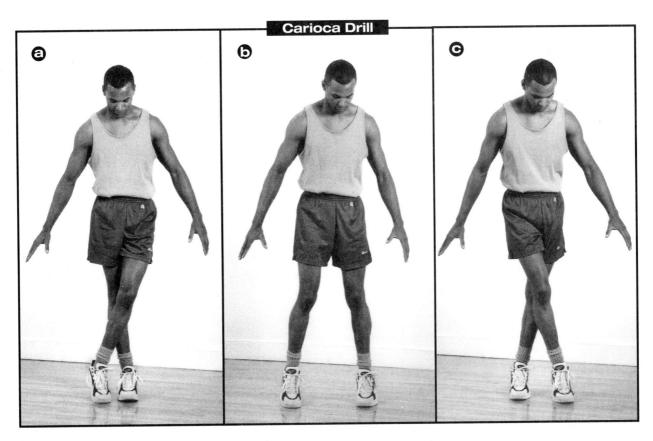

Carioca Drill ▲

This foot drill, suggested by Dr. Levy, develops side-to-side agility and strength. Cross one foot over the other, again and again and again, moving quickly from side to side of the court.

Box Hops

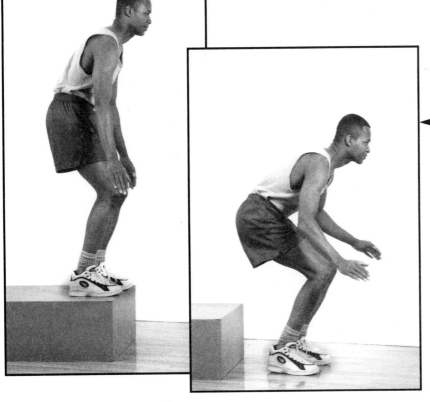

◄ Box Hops

Do this with a bench or a box to build your jump. Stand on the box, with your knees bent and your feet about a foot apart. Jump forward to the floor or ground, bending your knees when you land. Spin to face the bench or box and jump back onto it, deeply bending your knees again. At this point you'll be facing the opposite direction than when you started. Repeat to exhaustion.

Shoot and Dunk Like a Pro

The *swish* of a ball sailing through the net is much more satisfying than the *boing* of a ball hitting the rim or backboard. Here are streetball world champ David Jensen's secrets for perpetual swish-hood.

• Face the basket. "Get your chest and feet square with the basket," he says. It may not look fancy, but it works.

• Favor one hand. Both hands bring the ball up, but get your weak hand off the ball before you release. That's the southpaw hand if you're a right-hander. You have better control and speed when you use your dominant hand.

• Let the wrist do the precision work. Release from the wrist. Let the ball roll from your fingertips, slipping off the index and middle fingers last. If you're shoving the ball with your arms, you don't have much precision. Think wrists, fingers.

Then there's the matter of the dunk.

Here we defer to Chip Sigmon, Charlotte Hornets strength and conditioning coach. His advice? Well, it's what a big part of this chapter is all about: strength training and jumping work.

• Powerful legs. Obviously, you need great leg muscles for jumping. You get that from squats and lunges and leg presses.

• Powerful shoulders. Upper-body work, especially shoulder-strengthening routines, add a lot of zip to your jump, says Sigmon. They help pull your arms and the rest of your body upward. He recommends upright rows and military presses.

• Jumping drills. Sigmon recommends a box jump similar to the one we describe. Another exercise he recommends is the rim jump. Pick a spot on a wall, or a tree limb, about six inches higher than you can reach. Jump up and try to touch it with your dominant hand. When you land, immediately spring back up with another jump and try to slap the spot with your other hand. Keep alternating hands, and do two sets of ten jumps each. As you improve your ability, raise the target spot and keep at it, he says.

• Practice, practice. First from underneath the rim, later with a running start. Use both feet to push off, and extend your legs, back and arms fully through the jump, he says.

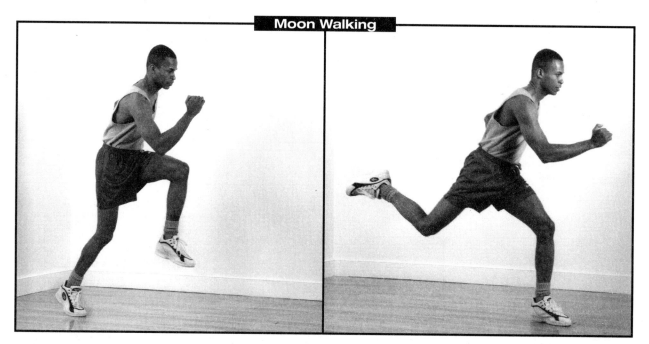

Moon Walking ▲

Leap your way up and down the court several times in smooth, giant, bounding steps, as though playing on the moon, free of the Earth's gravity, says Dr. Levy.

Ball Handling

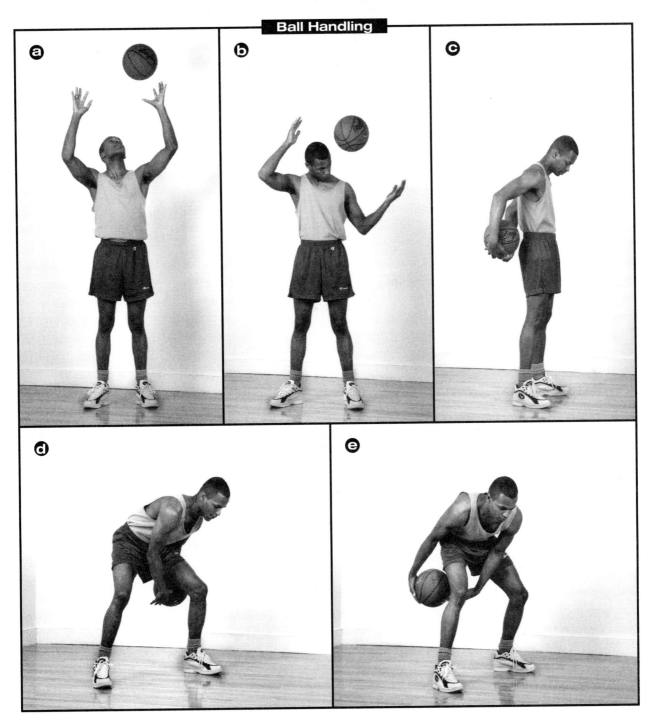

Ball Handling ▲

This warm-up from Dr. Wissel consists of passing and catching the ball, going from one hand to the other. There are six basic moves here.

- ⓐ Over your head
- ⓑ Around your head
- ⓒ Around your waist
- ⓓ Around one leg
- ⓔ Around the other leg
- ● Figure eight through your legs

Begin with your body in balanced stance. Pass and catch the ball from one hand to the other forcefully by flexing your fingers and wrists, Dr. Wissel says. Do a complete follow-through on each pass, pointing your passing fingers at your catching hand, he says.

Again, practice each of these moves ten times in one direction, then reverse direction and do ten more. Your goal is to get through all six parts, both directions, in three minutes with a maximum of three errors.

How Shaq Does It

Basketball superstar Shaquille O'Neal swears by strength training. He does crunches, followed by weighted sit-ups, seated leg tucks and lumbar extensions for 20 minutes three to four days a week. The ab workout saves his back as he charges his 300 pounds around the court, he says. Before he incorporated the ab routine into his workout, he sometimes had back problems. But he adds, "Not anymore."

O'Neal's legwork involves time on a leg-press machine and five to ten minutes of strides across the court—like the exercise we teach in this chapter called moon walking; he also does sprints throughout practice to develop and maintain speed.

And stretching gets top priority. "I stretch at least 20 minutes every day, no exceptions," he says. He focuses on stretching his legs, back and shoulders, improving range of motion and, thus, revving up more power.

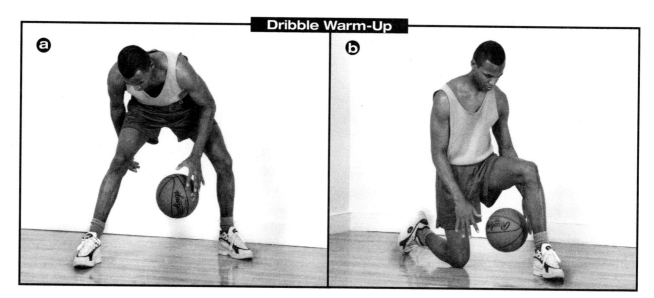

Dribble Warm-Up

Dribble Warm-Up ▲

This five-part warm-up develops the dribbling ability of both hands. Here are the steps, according to Dr. Wissel.

● Crossover. In a balanced stance, change the ball from one hand to the other, dribbling it below your knees and not wider than your knees. Keep your nondribbling hand up as a guard, and change the position of your feet and body to protect the ball. Alternating from left to right and right to left, complete 20 repetitions.

❷ Figure eight. Dribble the ball in a figure eight from back to front through the middle of your legs. Change from one hand to the other after the ball goes through your legs. After ten repetitions, change direction and do ten more.

❸ One knee. Continue to dribble the ball as you kneel down on one knee. Starting in front of your knee, dribble around to one side and under your raised knee. Change hands and dribble behind your back leg. Again change from one hand to the other and continue to the starting point in front of your knee. Dribble in a figure eight for ten repetitions in one direction; change directions and do ten more.

● Sitting. Continue to dribble as you sit down. Dribble for ten repetitions on one side. Raise your legs, dribble the ball under them to your other side, and dribble on that side for ten repetitions.

● Lying down. Continue dribbling as you lie down on your back. While lying down, dribble for ten reps on one side. Sit up, raise your legs, dribble the ball under your legs to the other side, lie down and dribble for ten more reps.

Two-Ball Dribble

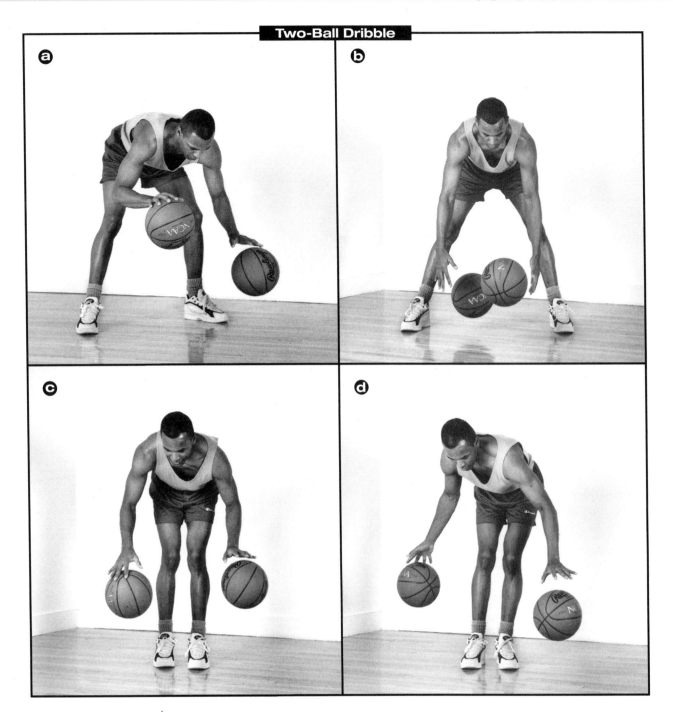

Two-Ball Dribble ⚔

Dribbling two balls at once is tough but fun. There are six parts to this approach, suggested by Dr. Wissel.

● Together. Dribble two basketballs below knee level simultaneously.

❷ Alternate one up and one down. Dribble two basketballs below knee level simultaneously, so that—you guessed it—one is up when the other is down.

❸ Crossover. While dribbling two balls low and close to your body, cross them back and forth, changing them from one hand to the other. Alternate which hand reaches in front.

❹ Inside-out. An inside-out dribble is a fake change of direction. Dribble the two balls to the sides of your body. With one, start a dribble toward the front of your body, but then rotate your hand over the ball to dribble it back to your side. Do it with one ball at a time, and then with both.

● Through your legs. Dribble first one ball, then the other, and then both balls through your legs.

❻ Side-pull forward and back. Dribble a ball at each side of your body. Then dribble them backward and forward, using your fingers and wrists as though pulling them back and forth.

Golf

Peak Points

- **Stretch, stretch, stretch before every round to avoid injury and to have a fluid swing.**

- **Work on your abdominal muscles to stabilize your swing and protect your back.**

- **Do strength training, concentrating on wrists and legs, to add speed and power to your swing.**

For too long, golfers got no respect. Mention that you golfed to a nonplayer and you'd inevitably get teased about the ugly plaid pants that had to be hanging in your closet.

But things have changed. Golf is getting more and more popular. Nearly everybody who tries it likes it. Golf, people are realizing, is a fun, challenging game of skill, played in a truly beautiful setting. Respect has arrived.

But the respect only goes so far. For example, don't try selling golf as great exercise. Carrying a full golf bag for 18 holes, well yes, that's very good for you. But the actual game, taking up to six hours to hit the ball less than 150 times (let us hope), with at least half of those hits being putts or chips, is not exactly a day at the gym.

The irony is that for a sport that offers such limited exercise potential, it also carries high injury potential.

A golf swing puts extraordinary torsion ("torsion" is a twisting or wrenching force) on your back and spine—up to eight times your body weight during a swing, says Allan M. Levy, M.D., sports doctor to the stars, partner at the Sports Medicine Center in Fort Lee, New Jersey, and co-author of the *Sports Injury Handbook*.

Also, every golf swing is in the same direction. What muscle building it does is lopsided. And if you aren't warmed up and flexible, the sudden swift torsion is jarring. It's likely to tax and strain muscles leaving you, at the least, uncomfortable the next day, says Dr. Levy. In particular, players often suffer lower-back pain from the constant one-direction torsion, says New York City chiropractor Joseph Askinasi.

Working Out for Golf

Practice improves your skills, but a powerful swing and a pain-resistant body require workout time away from the course. To be your best at golf, you'll need general conditioning and golf-specific strength building. It's what the pros do.

"Muscles from the head to the toe are involved in a golf swing, and a long drive requires strength," says Ken Sprague, coach and strength trainer, owner and operator of the original Gold's Gym and author of *Sports Strength*. "The strength with which you hit the ball contributes to its speed,

A Pro Trainer's Top Tips

Randy Myers, head trainer at the PGA National Resort and Spa in Palm Beach Gardens, Florida, works with more than 40 touring professionals. What they do, you should do, he says. And the biggest thing they do that he doesn't see recreational golfers doing?

"Stretching," he says. Stretch before and after a round. And "instead of sitting around drinking beer on the 19th hole, find a place where you can at least get crossover stretching—trunk rotation—for the lower back," he says.

"What's amazing about golf," says Myers, "is that if you're a golfer, you'll spare no expense to buy the clubs that Greg Norman uses or the wedge that Fred Couples uses." But, he says, there's more to Norman's and Couples's games than good equipment. "These people are also doing conditioning activities—stretching and different things. And if Greg Norman is doing stretching, you should be, too."

Myers also develops strength-training programs for his players—exercises with weights like we recommend within the chapter. And he offers an insider's exercise tip. "You heard it here first: The best upper-body conditioning exercise for golf, bar none, is an inclined push-up. I'll tell you why. It strengthens the upper chest and mid-back, keeps you in a good postural position and also gets extension for the biceps and forearms."

What equipment do you need? A desk, a sturdy table or a bathtub. An inclined push-up is simply a push-up done on an incline. You plant your hands on the edge of the furniture instead of the floor.

"I've worked with Corey Pavin," says Myers. "When he travels, he often does dips or inclined push-ups on his desk or on a bathtub. And that's really a part of his upper-body conditioning when he's playing events."

---

which in turn determines how far the ball travels down the fairway."

Just as important, trainers put a tremendous emphasis on flexibility, flexibility, flexibility, notes Dr. Levy. Pro players, he says, spend 45 minutes warming up and stretching before they tee off. Flexibility is your best defense against back injury.

And provided you have the verve to forgo the golf cart, you'll need some endurance training so you won't be huffing and puffing by the 18th hole. Walking 18 holes on a golf course is well over four miles, say DeDe Owens, Ed.D., and Linda K. Bunker, Ph.D., in their book, *Golf: Steps to Success*.

If your partners will chug along, you can turn the distance to your advantage and actually transform golfing into a minor workout, says Sprague.

"Carry your own clubs and move as rapidly as possible from tee to the ball to the next tee. That's a practical way of working on developing the stamina specific to the game," he says.

What to Do

Our Core Routine on page 121 is a good starting place for general strength training for golf. The only area you really don't want to build excessively is the chest, says Sprague. Too much bulk there will interfere with your swing.

Here is what golfers need to pay particular attention to and why, according to Dr. Levy.

Leg Exercises

Long, tall players have a natural advantage in golf because the power of the swing comes from the legs.

For a powerful swing, strengthen your legs with toe raises, leg extensions and leg curls.

Obliques Exercises

Remember? The obliques are the muscles on the sides of your belly that help twist your torso and support your back. They are crucial in golf for hitting power and accuracy, and for protecting your back during strong swings. Do exercises such as oblique crunches and oblique twists. Also do exercises to strengthen your torso-folding abs muscles, such as crunches.

Shoulder Exercises

To improve and support your swing, build your shoulder muscles with side lateral raises and shoulder extensions.

Wrist and Forearm Exercises

Here we're not talking power, but accuracy and precision. Strong wrists and forearms translate into greater club control and, thus, more accurate shots. Develop them with forearm curls, reverse forearm curls and wrist rolls.

Also, palm-up and palm-down elbow stretches lengthen the extensor and flexor muscles of the wrist so you can avoid a form of tennis elbow to which golfers are prone. Finally, Sprague recommends using a grip strengthener to develop hand strength.

The Pre-game Routine

You arrive at the course at 7:40 A.M. and have 20 minutes to tee time. You a.) get a small bucket of balls and start whacking, b.) get some scrambled eggs and coffee or c.) do a thorough warm-up and stretching routine to get your body ready.

You know the answer. Convince yourself. Here's how to proceed.

First, you warm up. The object of warming up for golf, says Dr. Levy, is to get blood flowing in the muscles before subjecting them to stretching and tension—not necessarily to get the heart pumping hard. Just two or three minutes of warm-up is all that's needed, he says.

It's an important step, says Dr. Levy. Don't skip it. Warm up with jumping jacks, running in place or walking vigorously for a few minutes.

Next, you stretch. Here's an on-the-course stretching routine, adapted from the recommendations of Dr. Owens and Dr. Bunker in *Golf: Steps to Success*. You'll need your driver for some of these.

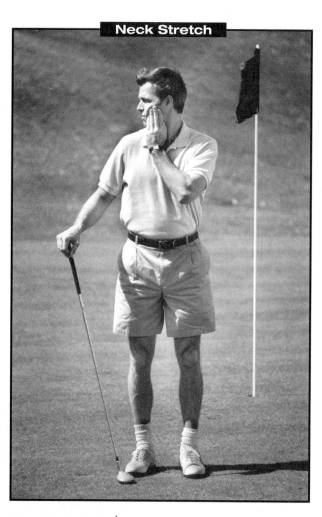

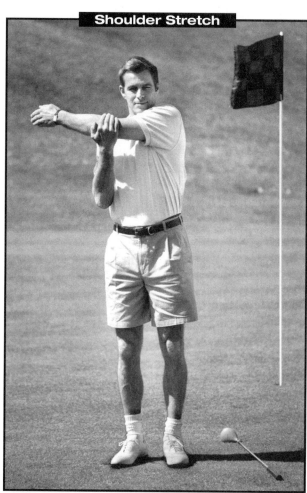

Neck Stretch ▲

Stand straight and relaxed. Rest one hand on a golf club, whose head (or handle) is resting in front of one foot. Turn your head and neck to the golf-club side of your body. With your other hand, gently push against your jaw so your chin touches your shoulder. Hold for 15 seconds. Relax, and switch sides. Do it a total of six times in each direction.

Shoulder Stretch ▲

Stand with your heels close, toes pointed out at a 45-degree angle. Draw your left arm across your chest at shoulder height and, with your right hand on your left elbow, gently pull your arm closer to your chest. Hold the stretch for ten seconds, then reverse arms. Do a total of six for each arm.

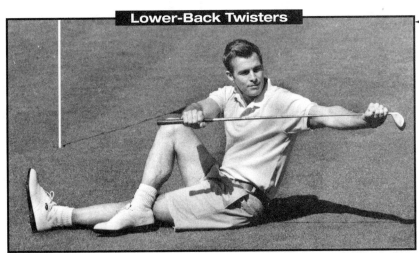

Lower-Back Twisters

◄ Lower-Back Twisters

Sit on the ground with your legs stretched in front of you. Bend your right knee and put your right foot on the ground outside your left knee. Grasp a golf club, hands on each end, hold it at shoulder height and turn to the left as far as is comfortable. Hold for a count of ten. Do this six times. Then reverse positions and repeat the same number of times on the other side.

Couple this stretch with one of the next two standing stretches for the back, suggests Dr. Bunker.

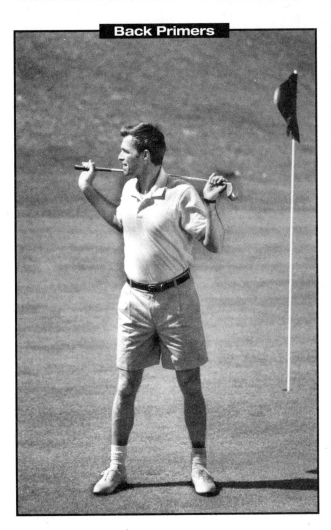

Back Primers

Side Twisters

Back Primers ▲

Place the club behind your neck, across your shoulders. Hold it at each end. Keeping your hips facing forward, twist your shoulders—torso and upper body—as far as is comfortable in one direction, hold for 15 seconds. Then twist in the other direction and hold. Do six on each side. Don't just rock back and forth, warns Dr. Levy. That actually tightens your muscles. Twist, hold and stretch.

Side Twisters ▲

Stand with your feet slightly apart. Grasp the golf club midway up the shaft with both hands, and lift your arms straight up in the air. Bend your upper body to your right as far as is comfortable for a count of ten, and then to the left for the same time. Do six reps on each side.

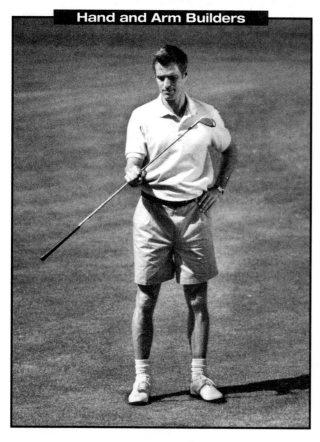

Hand and Arm Builders ⬆

Stand with your legs shoulder-width apart, arms close to your body. Grip the club in the center of the shaft with your right hand and bend your elbow so your forearm and palm are parallel to the ground. Rotate your wrist a half-circle to the right, then back to center. Do ten, then switch hands and repeat, rotating your arm to the left. Do six sets of ten repetitions for each arm.

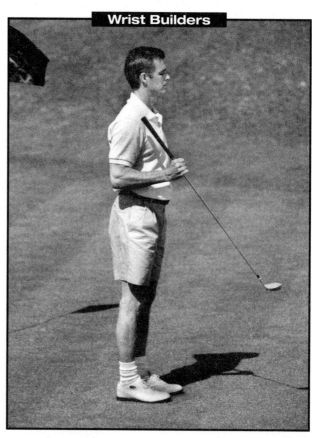

Wrist Builders ⬆

Stand with your legs shoulder-width apart, arms close to your body, one arm bent at the elbow so your forearm is parallel to the ground, but with your palm facing inward. Grip a club in the middle of the shaft so its ends point up and down. Gently rock it forward and back a few times, then switch arms and repeat.

Leg Stretcher ▶

Stand with your right foot crossed over your left. Holding a golf club at the ends, bend gently forward, relaxing your upper body and letting the club reach as close to the ground as is comfortable. Hold for ten seconds. Repeat six times. Then reverse the foot position and repeat six times.

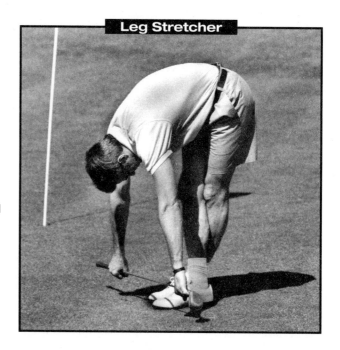

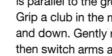

Taping Yourself

Want to play better golf? Watch TV. That is, watch *you* on TV.

It's the advice of former bank chief executive Dick Noel, who shaved his handicap in half in two seasons with this and a few other tricks we'll let you in on.

Another of Noel's tips comes first, before watching TV: Buy a rubber golf mat and set it up in your backyard. Then unwind each evening hitting plastic golf balls—the kind that won't take out your neighbors' windows. So what if they're toys? The swing is the same. So is the slice and hook. Fifteen minutes a night, each work night. That's Noel's prescription.

Now, time for the TV. Almost.

First, set up a video cam next to the practice mat to record your swings. Tape yourself once every couple of weeks. Indicate to the camera when you hit a good shot.

Now watch TV. You'll probably see some things you don't like. And you'll fix them. Because a picture is worth a thousand words.

Noel also recommends comparing your best swings to that of a great pro teacher on video. He likes *Golf with Al Geiberger* from SyberVision.

Other tips?

• Play with people who are just a bit better than you, Noel advises. This keeps you on your toes.

• Hit the links by 6:45 A.M. a couple of days a week. Play five or six holes, and play two or three balls each hole. Drop some balls in the traps and the deep rough. Playing the extra shots does wonders for your short game, Noel says. You're at work by 8:30, he says.

• Do a full-body weight-lifting routine and a stretching routine. We already told you this. Noel lifts Mondays, Wednesdays and Fridays for 45 minutes. He does 15 minutes of stretching on Tuesdays and Thursdays. Within three weeks, he saw the payoff. He was hitting balls farther and was more chipper after 18 holes.

For the Hard Core

Want to talk really serious golf muscles—the kind you only get in a gym? Talk to Sprague.

"It's not very common for golfers to be bodybuilders," notes Budd Coates, a trainer and exercise physiologist in Emmaus, Pennsylvania. Still, says Sprague, "specific strength training can really help your game."

Here's Sprague's specialized full-body training program for golfers.

Off-season, Sprague wants to see you in the gym two or three days a week doing the exercises below. Figure out your correct weight and rep levels using the periodization method described in the Basic Fitness chapter on page 118. In season, stick to two days each week and do two sets of each exercise, eight reps per set, using 75 percent of your maximum lift level.

• Dumbbell lunges for hip and leg thrust
• Dumbbell step-ups and step-downs for hip and leg thrust
• Oblique twists for strong torso rotation
• Upright rows for shoulder development
• Rumanian dead lifts for back extension
• Forearm curls for wrist and forearm strength
• Grip strengtheners for finger and hand strength
• Pull-ups for upper-body pull
• Crunches for a stronger abdomen

Racquet Sports

Tennis, racquetball, squash—as racquet sports go, each may be a totally different animal from the other, but your body doesn't know that. All your body knows is that you're in a playing zone that seems roughly the size of a postage stamp, doing enough explosive activity to fill a football stadium. You're charging, lunging, reversing direction in a split second, all the while using an oversized paddle to control a tiny ball with a series of swings that seems carefully calculated to rip your arm from its socket.

And you're trying to have fun all at the same time.

Fault-Free Fitness

Racquet sports are games of endless swinging and running, stopping and starting. That sort of work takes a major toll on muscles, not just in the thighs and feet, but also in the shoulders and upper arms.

"And the muscles are just the tip of it," says Todd Ellenbecker, P.T., clinical director of Physiotherapy Associates Scottsdale Sports Clinic in Arizona and a member of the U.S. Tennis Association's Sports Science Committee. "One of the real dangers of racquet sports is that they are incredibly hard on so many joints." Ankles, knees and hips pay their dues when you sprint, stop short and set up for your shot. Shoulders, elbows and wrists, though, have it even worse. You're trying to power the ball back at your opponent while maneuvering the racquet for aim and spin, says Ellenbecker. "You're trying to mix finesse with sheer strength, and your joints pay the price."

While perfecting your form can help you avoid a raft of joint problems, Ellenbecker says the real secret is mixing weight training and range-of-motion exercises. "The idea is to train your muscles and joints to move in certain ways so you won't injure them on the court." More important, strong muscles build a powerful cage of protection around your joints, which will keep you strong, fast and flexible through any rally. If you're an avid racqueteer, you'll want to add these exercises to your core workout.

Giving Tennis Elbow the Cold Shoulder

You don't have to play tennis to get the pain and swelling of tennis elbow. Heck, you don't even have to pick up a racquet.

This nagging injury, known by experts as lateral epicondylitis, can result from any overuse of the elbow. "You can get it from doing a lot of different activities," says Paul Roetert, Ph.D., director of sports science for the U.S. Tennis Association in Key Biscayne, Florida. But this elbow inflammation goes by its more common "tennis" appellation, not simply because "epicondylitis" is so darn hard to pronounce, but because so many amateur racquet-sports enthusiasts tend to use improper technique when they swing—especially when they use a one-handed swing. That improper form is what gets the elbow out of joint. So here are a few tips to keep from elbowing yourself out of the game.

Put your shoulder into it. Tennis elbow often occurs when, during a backhand swing, the player points his elbow toward the net, says Dr. Roetert. To avoid leading with your elbow, turn your shoulder toward the net and straighten your arm as you swing.

Avoid tension headaches. Sometimes, epicondylitis results from simply having the tension on your racquet too high, he says. A sporting goods store that strings racquets should be able to adjust the tension properly.

Be flexible. If your elbow is getting sore, maybe the blame lies not in the arm, but in the racquet. Dr. Roetert says a racquet made of stiff material won't absorb the shock of hitting a ball—and so the force travels down to your elbow. "If that's the case, I would strongly recommend going to a racquet that's made out of more flexible material, such as a composite racquet," says Dr. Roetert.

Shoulder Extensions

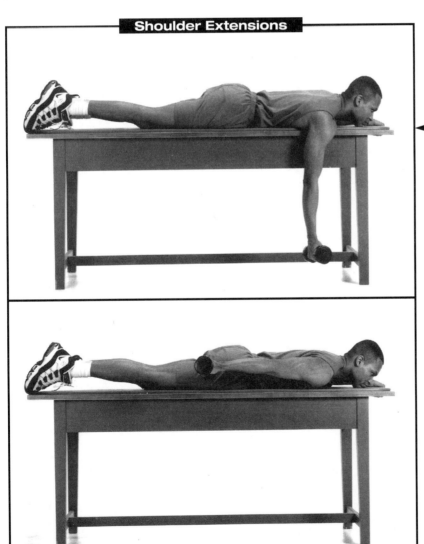

◄ Shoulder Extensions

Lifts like shoulder shrugs and seated or bent-over rows are great for racquet sports enthusiasts and should be part of your regular workout. You should also do this extension exercise, which works the muscles right at the top of your shoulder.

Lie face down on a table, with one arm hanging straight to the floor. Holding a light weight, or wearing a hand- or wrist-weight, point your thumb away from your body, your palm facing forward.

Now raise your arm straight back without bending your elbow. Stop at your hip—your arm should be fully extended. Lower and repeat for three sets of 10 to 15 reps, then switch arms.

Empty-Can Raises

Your serve wouldn't be much good without the rotator cuff, a powerful little bundle of muscle in your shoulder. Ellenbecker says most guys don't really work these muscles as much as they work surrounding ones. "That's bad, because you'll end up having an imbalance in your shoulder, and you can end up injuring—even tearing—the rotator cuff," he says. So pre-train that muscle bundle with empty-can raises.

Standing, hold a light weight (never more than five pounds) at your side. Keep your elbow straight and the thumb of the weighted hand pointing toward the ground.

Now slowly raise your arm to shoulder level at about a 30-degree angle to your body, as though you were emptying a can of tennis balls. Slowly lower, then repeat for three sets of 10 to 15 reps. Then switch arms.

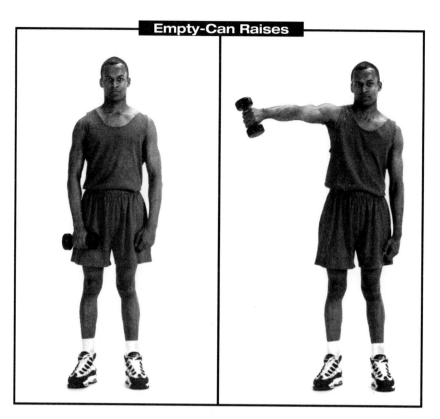

Empty-Can Raises

Back Extensions

Although your arms and shoulders do most of the work when you play racquet sports, you need a strong back to support every hit. "Most players tend to ignore the back, and as a result, they end up with underdeveloped back extensors, which is too bad," states Ellenbecker. Don't make the same mistake—make back extensions a part of your regular workout routine.

Obliques Exercises

Ellenbecker says crossover crunches, where you curl your trunk first toward one knee, then the other, will work the obliques, which are on the sides of your abdominals. "This supports your back and gives you more power for your swing," he says.

Neck Exercises

Super ballistic sports like racquetball require you to make a lot of fast direction changes as the ball bounces from wall to wall. Trying to keep an eye on that sucker can be as tough on your neck as on your arms and legs. "You're constantly swiveling your head around, following the ball, so it's probably a good idea to do some neck stretches before you play," says Ellenbecker.

Don't roll your head in a circle—that's the path to neck injury. Instead, tilt your head toward your left shoulder, hold for a moment, then tilt toward your right shoulder.

Wrist Exercises

Bolstering forearm and wrist power is key for any racquet-swinging sport. You can strengthen both areas with wrist rolls, says Dennis Van der Meer, founder and president of Van der Meer Tennis University on Hilton Head Island, South Carolina. To increase grip strength, you can do weight-plate finger raises as well.

Leg Exercises

You'll notice a significant improvement in your game if you spend some time working your lower limbs, too. "The best players in the world have hugely developed thigh muscles," says Van der Meer. "That's because you need that strength to push off and play at a very high speed." What's more, having strong leg muscles is going to help protect your knees and ankles, which take a good pounding on the court from all your stopping and starting.

So start with basic leg exercises—squats, lunges, extensions and curls. To toughen up the knee joints, cross-train with another aerobic sport, like cycling or running. Ankle stretches and toe raises will help keep the lowest part of your legs limber and ready for anything.

Weight Lifts to Avoid

Complex joints that they are, shoulders are easily wrecked from hours of high-speed serves and returns. To keep your shoulders strong and flexible, go easy on exercises like the overhead military press and the bench press.

"You may feel strong doing those lifts, but they're potentially damaging to the shoulder," says Ellenbecker. Do enough of them, and you'll not only hurt your game but you'll also expose yourself to shoulder tendinitis, a painful inflammatory condition of the tendon.

Full-Court Conditioning

"Every time you swing a racquet, you are doing some resistive exercises. So the more you play, the stronger you'll become," points out Van der Meer. That said, there are some extra toning tricks you should do to stay in shape. All you need to do them is your racquet, your duffel bag, a can of balls and, of course, a court.

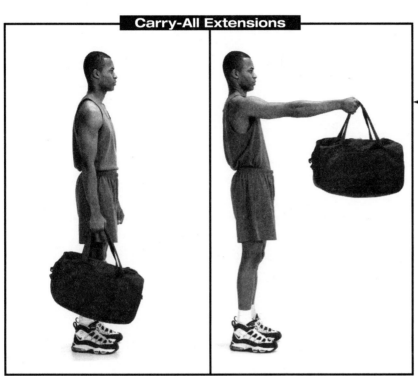

Carry-All Extensions

◄ Carry-All Extensions

That duffel bag with your change of clothes and tennis equipment is a lot more than deadweight—it's a free weight. Use it. Hold the bag in one hand, as though it were a dumbbell. Keep your arm straight, palm facing your side.

Now slowly extend your arm out from your body. Don't bend your elbow. Do 8 to 12 reps, then switch arms. This will strengthen your deltoids.

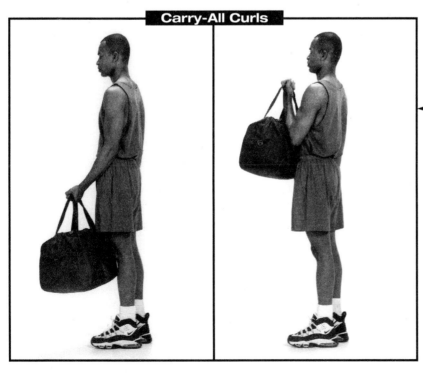

Carry-All Curls

◄ Carry-All Curls

For a quick biceps curl, hold your bag at your side, your palm facing front.

Now slowly lift the bag until your hand almost touches your shoulder. Lower and repeat for 8 to 12 reps, then switch.

"You'll limber up important arm and shoulder muscles that way," says Van der Meer.

Ball Squats

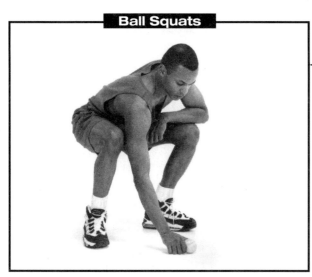

◄ Ball Squats

Your legs and groin can never be too flexible when you're playing. Van der Meer says you can keep them even more supple with something as simple as modifying the way you pick up a ball.

Instead of scooping the ball with your racquet, stand by the ball, feet shoulder-width apart.

Now squat down slowly to pick the ball up. Keep your shoulders and back straight and stay as upright as you can. You should feel the contraction in your quads. Snatch the ball, then return slowly to the starting position.

Ball Lunges

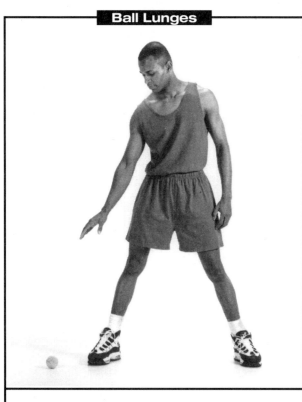

◄ Ball Lunges

You can modify that lunge you do in the gym for an on-court exercise between sets.

Position yourself so the ball is on your right side. Stand with your feet a little wider than shoulder-width apart, with your toes pointing away from your body.

Now bend your right knee, keep your left leg planted and shift your weight to the right side until your thigh is almost parallel to the court. Don't let your knee extend past your foot. Scoop up the ball and return slowly to the starting position. Switch sides next time you pick up the ball.

Ball-Can Lid Relays

Here's another tip for you tennis players: Get a ball-can lid and place it in the middle of the court. As you volley, run up and around the lid, then back to your starting position. "By the time you've completed the circle, the ball should have come back. Hit it and run around the lid again," says Van der Meer.

Baseline Sprints

While you're waiting around for your opponent to show up, increase your sprinting and explosive strength by doing this brief drill. Start in the middle of the baseline and sprint three yards to your left, recover back to the middle of the court and then sprint three yards to your right. Repeat several times.

For racquetball or squash, try sprints from the center of the room to each of the four corners and back to the center.

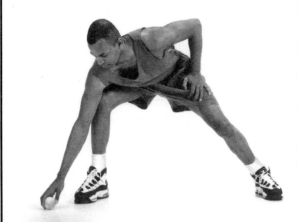

Skiing

You wouldn't think an activity that involved so much sliding and gliding could make muscles feel so stiff and ragged, but it can, especially if the activity in question is skiing. If you've spent any time on a cross-country or downhill ski trail, you know the kind of misery we're talking about—a bone-deep ache that not even the cool beauty of a snow-covered landscape nor the warm promise of an Irish coffee back at the lodge can erase.

"Most people feel the biggest burn on top of their thighs, in their quad muscles," says Robert King, an instructor at the Vail Ski School. King also designed and conducts a ski conditioning program at the Vail Athletic Club in Colorado. "But many skiers—even experts—don't often realize how hard skiing can be on other muscles, especially the hamstrings, the lower back and the abdominals."

Staying on Balance

It's precisely these areas of the body that yield many skiing-related injuries, agrees Lisa Feinberg Densmore, a former member of the U.S. Ski Team and producer of *Body Prep: The Ultimate Ski Fitness Video*. Take the hamstrings on the back of the thighs. If you don't exercise them as much as you work other leg muscles, you can create a strength imbalance that leads to muscle pulls in the back of the leg. That same imbalance can also cause a weak link in the muscular structure that surrounds and protects your knee.

"People who ski need to think in 360 degrees, all the way around the leg. When they don't, they increase their chance of ending up with a knee problem," says Densmore.

Moreover, because of the ever-changing demands of the skiing terrain, the sport can also be hard on the lower back and the abdominals, which bear the impact of skiing over jumps and moguls and also help you steer on the slope. "The stronger and more flexible those muscles are, the less chance you'll have of an injury. You'll also be a better, faster, more agile skier," says Densmore.

So you need to work on strength and flexibility to be a better skier, says Densmore, but it has to be the right kind of strength and flexibility. It has to be the kind that will allow your various joints and muscles to get you down to the bottom of the hill with a minimum of injury and a maximum of icy-cold, windchilled, adrenalin-tinged pleasure. To stay upright and injury-free, here's what our experts advise.

Work on lateral movement. As a preseason trainer, be sure to do plenty of sports and activities that emphasize side-to-side movement, suggests King.

"This really builds up legs and hips and helps train your body to move laterally," says King, who includes slide aerobics in his ski-training programs. If aerobics classes aren't your thing, Densmore suggests taking up sports like tennis or soccer, which also demand lots of sideways movement.

Strap on skates. To get your ski legs back under you in a hurry, get yourself a pair of in-line skates for the off-season. "It's one of the best activities going for skiers. It works the muscles you use when you carve a turn on skis, and it helps you keep proper balance for skiing," says Densmore.

Stretch, stretch, stretch. And when you're done doing that, stretch some more. "I don't mean a post-workout, five-minute stretch. I mean a whole flexibility routine where you're doing at least 20 minutes of stretching several times a week," says Densmore. "Skiing causes you to put your body in a lot of unnatural angles. If you want to be really good at it, you have to be flexible." Focus especially on your hips, thighs and groin as well as your lower back.

Conquering the Hill

Pre-season training is all well and good, but there's no substitute for perfecting your technique out on the trail, says King.

When you're on the slope, your main objectives are clear: You want to stay upright, you want to have control and, of course, you want to look good. "Proper form is the key," concurs Densmore. "Not only will it make you look graceful on skis but it will also keep you from falling, skidding out of control or pulling a muscle." Perfect some basics of ski form and you'll minimize your odds of becoming a human snowplow. Work on these essentials.

Stand up straight. For novice and intermediate downhill skiers, keeping their balance is a primary goal—and a primary challenge, says Densmore. This leaves a lot of skiers in a hunched-over, wide-stance position.

"Basically, you look like a gorilla on skis. And a lot of skiers start out that way because they feel comfortable and safe in that low position—that's where their balance is," observes Densmore. But if you don't take steps to correct this position, you'll actually be hurting your form in the long run.

"It's hard on the back, hard on the legs, and you don't look very good besides," she says. So make a conscious effort to stand up, keeping your skis shoulder-width apart. "The more you remember to stand upright in a relaxed position, the more natural it will feel. You'll be more graceful and fluid, too," adds Densmore.

Don't Do It

It's a time-honored exercise among athletes who prize strong legs. But if you ski, you'll want to avoid it—especially if you have knee problems.

It's called the wall sit or wall squat. Basically, you stand with your back against a wall and slowly slide down to a squatting position, using the wall as your support.

"The problem is that it mimics a position that's bad for skiing. Your weight and your balance are too far behind your knee," says Lisa Feinberg Densmore, a former member of the U.S. Ski Team and producer of *Body Prep: The Ultimate Ski Fitness Video*. Ideally, you want to do exercises that are going to improve your skiing balance, not take away from it. As a substitute, Densmore recommends regular squats or single-leg squats: Balance on one foot with the other slightly ahead of you and slowly squat down until your thigh is almost parallel with the floor (beginners can use a chair to help keep their balance). "It's safer on your legs, and it helps build balance and leg strength at the same time," says Densmore. Be sure to do both legs.

Know your pole position. For cross-country skiers, poles are part of the human engine that propels you forward, and you need only to keep them at your sides, planting and sliding, pulling, then pushing yourself ever forward.

For many downhillers, though, the theory of ski-pole positioning is less obvious. "Some beginners just think you only use poles to get up after a fall or to push yourself over to the lift," says Densmore. For Alpine skiers, though, poles are more than a form of damage control or minor locomotion—they're powerful navigational tools, helping you to steer and make high-speed turns.

"Using them effectively is all a matter of positioning and subtle movement," points out Densmore. "A lot of skiers wave them around or use too much upper-arm movement, and that will throw them off balance." Here are a few pole pointers Densmore recommends you remember the next time it's your turn.

1. Keep your arms slightly bent and hold your hands and poles comfortably in front of you. Keep your shoulders relaxed and your elbows about eight inches from your sides.
2. Plant the pole on the side you want to turn toward. A pole plant is no more than a flick of the wrist. Bend your wrist up and touch the pole just in front of your boot.

3. Ever so slightly, lift the ski on the side you want to turn toward as you plant the pole. This will make it easier to start a new turn.

4. As soon as you start the turn, unplant your pole so it won't rotate your upper body and cause your skies to slide.

Don't fight falls. Okay, sooner or later it's going to happen. The mogul you're taking decides to take you instead. Or some little kid suddenly veers into your path, and you must heroically divert into the ravine. As you head for the great white beyond, try to relax your body. One of the greatest causes of skiing injuries occurs not because we fall, but because of what we do to prevent falling, says Densmore.

If you're skiing and you feel yourself falling, just let yourself go. If you are in an uncontrollable fall and you can't stop your slide downhill, protect your head and try to get your feet downslope of your body, suggests Densmore. That way you will hit obstacles feet first. And if you're falling forward, cover your face and head and turn so you roll on your shoulders.

Training for the Trails

Sooner or later, if you want to conquer those black diamonds slopes or finish that circuitous cross-country trail with energy to spare, you're going to have to lift some weights to get that body in proper ski form. Here's your ski workout. Yes, it's heavily weighted toward legwork, but don't take that as a license to go easy on your upper body. "Shoulders, arms, back, abs—especially your abs—are all part of the equation. Don't leave them out," says King.

Shoulder Exercises

Your shoulders aren't just a handy place to drape your skis as you head back to the lodge. "You need them for planting and pushing off with your poles," says Densmore. Shoulder shrugs and upright rows will give you the power you need for on-trail maneuvering.

Quadriceps and Hamstring Exercises

As a matter of course, you should be doing exercises that strengthen not only the quads but also the hamstrings. In his specialized workout plan for skiers, Ken Sprague, coach and strength trainer, owner and operator of the original Gold's Gym and author of *Sports Strength*, recommends lunges and squats as well as leg presses.

Abductor and Adductor Exercises

Because of the lateral motion involved in skiing, Densmore says you'll want strong muscles on the inside and outside of your upper legs. Do outside and inside leg lifts either lying down or standing and using a weight machine with a pulley and a leg cuff.

Calf Exercises

Cross-country skiers, in particular, will want to build calf strength, since the calves take a lot of punishment during the forward sliding motion of that brand of skiing. Standing heel raises will build those muscles, Densmore says, plus they'll help stabilize your ankle, which makes it a good exercise for all skiers.

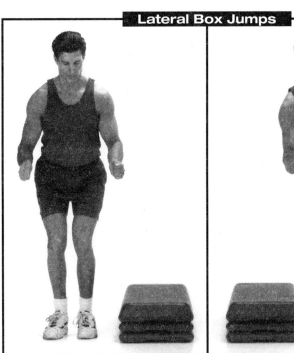

Lateral Box Jumps

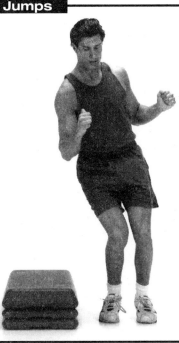

◄ Lateral Box Jumps

This is a variation on the old box jump, where you jumped on or over a box to build leg strength and explosive power. The lateral jump still builds leg power, but it also helps build ski-specific balance and coordination, says Densmore. Stand on the right side of a foot-high box, feet shoulder-width apart, knees slightly bent, hands held forward as though you were holding imaginary ski poles.

Now put all your weight on your right foot and jump to the left side and over the box. Position yourself so you land with your weight on your left foot. Pause a moment with your weight on your left foot, then leap back over the box to land on your right foot again. Do 20 jumps.

Tuck Jumps

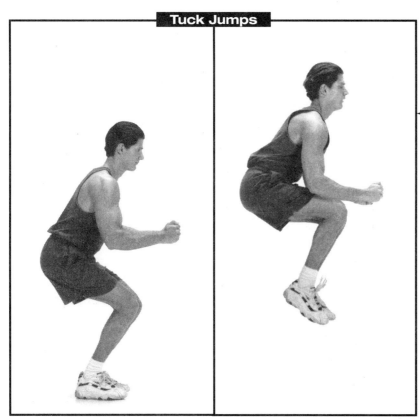

◄ Tuck Jumps

This classic jumping exercise helps skiers build both leg and abdominal muscle and power, Densmore says. Stand with your feet shoulder-width apart in a half squat, knees slightly bent, hands gripping imaginary ski poles.

Now jump straight up. While you're in the air, raise both knees up and try to touch them to your chest. Don't swing your arms for momentum. Return to the starting position and repeat. Do 10 to 20 jumps.

Football

If you're a big, beefy guy, chances are you were asked a hundred times while in school: "Play football?"

Strength and size, or the appearance of strength and size, spell football. It's a game of pumped-up monsters and chiseled speedsters smashing one another, chasing one another, sprinting like mad to catch, kick or bury a blimp-shaped piece of inflated pigskin.

If you were that big, beefy guy everyone wanted on the football team, and you actually decided to play, you'll never forget the boot camp your coach put you through. Because in football, there's no such thing as too much muscle, too much speed or too much attitude. You're out there to throw your weight around, act menacing and kick butt.

The converse also is true. You're out there to get your butt kicked. You can't avoid this in football. That's why it helps in part to be big and beefy. And that really underscores what a lot of the boot-camp training is all about. It isn't just to beef you up so you look threatening to the other side but also to limber you up and pad you out so you don't get injured while getting blocked, tackled and otherwise generally walloped. A big, beefy player sidelined for injuries is of no use to a team, says Ken Sprague, coach and strength trainer, owner and operator of the original Gold's Gym and author of *Sports Strength* and many related training books, and a weight lifter who trained alongside former L.A. Raiders Howie Long and the late Lyle Alzado.

So strength training, along with increasing skill and power, is a form of preventive medicine, says Sprague. And for those of us who weren't especially big and beefy to start with, it's essential if we're going to compete credibly, even in neighborhood weekend games.

For pro and amateur alike, the name of the game in football is "strength training, strength training, strength training," says Sprague.

The General Workout

Let's say you just want to play good weekend football. You're willing to tackle any position you're assigned, but you want to exhibit at least basic athletic competency. Then you need a core workout that builds strength for the five movements common to nearly all athletics and sports activities, says Sprague.

For each of these five movements, pick

one of the free-weight exercises you like, or alternate between them, suggests Sprague.

Upper-Body Thrust

You need this for shoving, blocking, throwing, reaching and even for pumping your arms when running. For optimum upper-body thrust, you need a strong chest, powerful arms and a fluid, conditioned shoulder girdle. We're talking pecs, deltoids, biceps, triceps, trapezius muscles. The recommended exercises:

- Bench press
- Dips
- Military press

Upper-Body Pull

Here we're talking about the upper back, biceps, chest, shoulders—latissimus dorsi, pecs and so on. This is the converse side of thrust. Good upper-body pull is the ability to grab a nimble ball-runner and drag him to the ground. It's the ability to use your arms to help dodge and dart and slip through the charging defense. Here are the best exercises.

- Pull-ups
- Bent-over rows

Back Extension

Is there anything you don't use your back for in football? Is a strong back better than a weak back? You bet. You need to build the muscles in the deep posterior group and the spinal erectors. Do one of the following exercises.

- Good-morning exercises
- Rumanian dead lifts

Jackknife

The ability to fold in the middle and spring apart, bend, turn, twist with power and precision depends upon abs. Abs, abs, abs. Necessary for running, for leg speed, for lunging, jumping, for rolling with the punches, for maximum throwing power and even for maximum leg power. Leg power doesn't reach the upper body without traveling through the middle— you don't want it dissipating in jelly. Your choices:

- Crunches
- Straight-leg raises

Leg and Hip Thrust

You need strong, conditioned hips and thighs— for power and stability, for turns, for speed, for resisting the pushes, shoves, slams. For shoving off. For kicking and running. Do one of these.

- Dumbbell squats
- Step-ups
- Dumbbell lunges

Other Needs

In addition to raw strength, you need three things to be great at the game.

- A conditioned heart so you have the stamina to play as hard in the fourth quarter as you did in the first. You get that from aerobic exercise, such as running, bicycling and swimming, says Sprague. As with nearly every routine in this book, try to get at least three aerobic workouts of 30 minutes each per week.

- Energy for short bursts of explosive power at any given time in a long game. Wind sprints help you achieve that. No matter what position you play, year-round you should incorporate daily wind sprints and aerobic running into your routine for leg-muscle explosive power and endurance, says Sprague.

- Flexibility to handle all the twisting, turning, bending and pushing you face in a game. If you can't bend easily in unusual directions, you are going to get injured, perhaps not the first time you are tackled or blocked, but soon enough. Always do a stretching routine after you're warmed up and after you've cooled down, advises Sprague.

Player-by-Player Programs

If you are serious about football, favor a particular position and want to be the best you can be at it, you need a specialized workout. Each of Sprague's specialized football workouts uses his Lineman Routine as a core, then adds exercises and emphasis where needed.

Here's how to tailor the program to the season.

- Off-season. The number of sets, number of reps and amount of weight all depend upon where you are in your periodization schedule, says Sprague. (See Basic Fitness on page 118 to learn how to structure such a workout.) Go through the whole routine two to three days a week.

- In season. Hold steady at two sets of each exercise, six reps each, at 80 percent of your one-rep

Smart Cross-Training

Football great Herschel Walker—a great believer in abdominal strength—has a secret football training tip.

Basketball.

That's right. In his book, *Herschel Walker's Basic Training*, which he co-authored with Terry Dodd, Ph.D., Walker revealed he plays basketball every day he's not playing football. And, he said, doing lots of twisting jump shots and layups gives him a great midsection workout that doesn't feel like work because it's so much fun.

That's one of the keys to great training, Walker says: Experiment with things that are fun.

Some other of Walker's training secrets—these for improving agility and endurance: jumping rope, taking karate classes and box-hopping.

maximum weight level, two to three days a week, Sprague recommends, or whatever your coach or trainer prescribes.

Now, here's what Sprague says you need to tailor the strength-building portion of the program to your position. Players other than linemen need to do the Lineman Routine as well as the exercises listed for their particular position.

Lineman (Core) Routine

- Military press for upper-body thrust
- Power cleans for upper-body pull. Power cleans are the old classic, in which you carefully raise a barbell from the floor up to your shoulders in one smooth motion. To do one correctly, stand with your feet about 16 inches apart and your shins touching a barbell in front of you. Grip the bar, bending so that your thighs are nearly parallel to the floor, your back straight, head looking forward. To start the motion, straighten your legs, raising the bar up to your thighs while keeping your arms straight. As your legs straighten, extend your hips forward, getting into an erect position. As your body straightens, keep the bar ascending by pulling with your arms and rising on your toes. When the bar reaches its highest point, bend your knees and catch the bar on your shoulders and upper chest.
- Rumanian dead lifts for back extension
- Crunches for jackknife
- Squats for hip and leg thrust
- Reverse trunk twists for torso rotation

Punters/Kickers

- Leg curls to prevent injury

Kickers need to pay particular attention to developing their quadriceps and abdominal and lower-back muscles, say Richard Mangi, M.D., Peter Jokl, M.D., and O. William Dayton in their book *Sports and Fitness Training.* The Lineman Routine works those areas, Sprague notes.

Centers

- Overhead triceps extensions for elbow extension
- Wrist curls for forearm and wrist strength
- Grip strengtheners for ball control

Quarterbacks

- Overhead triceps extensions for elbow extension
- Wrist curls for forearm and wrist strength
- Grip strengtheners for ball control
- Outside and inside shoulder rotations for preventing injury to shoulders
- Leg curls to prevent hamstring injuries

Running Back/Defensive Back

- Leg curls for injury prevention
- Dumbbell lunges for leg and hip thrust

On-the-Field Wisdom

You're strong, you're sleek, your body is prepared. But there's still something missing. Winning at football is not just about brute force and speed. It's also about fundamentals and using your head. Here are some basics to play by.

Tackle with your eyes. One of the most important things a defender can do is focus on his target, says Terry Shea, head football coach at Rutgers University in New Brunswick, New Jersey. "Great tacklers have great focus and concentration," he adds. Many missed and poor tackles are a result of shifting the eyes up to the ball-carrier's shoulders right before the hit. Maintain your focus on the middle of the runner's body, Shea points out. And use the sideline as an extra man to box in a runner, he adds.

Cover the receiver, not the QB. A tendency of many pass-defenders is to glance at the quarterback to see who he's going to throw to. "Defenders will take that peek right after the snap and thereby lose the cushion they had over the receiver," says Shea. In man-to-man coverage, concentrate on the receiver's shoulders and midsection; it's the best way to detect where he will be moving next.

Keep it at arm's length. When catching the football, receivers should extend their hands and elbows away from their body to make the catch, says Shea. "The last eight to ten inches of the ball's flight are very important. With your arms extended, you can follow the ball to the point of reception. With your arms tucked in, you greatly reduce your ability to follow the ball into your hands."

Run to glory. Use your energy to run down the field, not across it. "Make the defender miss you by the slightest of margins so that your downfield momentum is only slightly disturbed," Shea says. Too many runners expend energy making wide berths around defenders when they should be concentrating on running toward the end zone, he adds.

Don't lose it over special teams. It's common for a kicking team to run down the field in an uncontrolled mad dash, only to overshoot the runner. "On kickoffs, stay under control. Don't run down the field as fast as you can. Retaining the ability to quickly brake your speed allows you to maintain good balance and the ability to move laterally," Shea says.

Stand up straight. To avoid injury, stay upright when you're about to get hit, rather than tucking your chin to your chest. Also, ball-carriers shouldn't overextend their bodies as the defense arrives—it makes knees, elbows and necks too vulnerable.

Soccer

The world loves U.S. pro sports. The spectacle of football's Super Bowl, the tradition of baseball's World Series, the marvel of basketball's playoffs make great entertainment no matter what language you speak, what sports you play, what country you live in.

But for the United States to get true respect for its athleticism, it will need to field a great soccer team. And not because soccer is the sandlot game of choice in much of the world. It's because soccer is one of the hardest sports there is.

Soccer is a fast game—a heart thumper—that never relents. You block, twist, turn, skip, jump, kick and head the ball. But mostly you run, run, run.

In a 90-minute game, a player is likely to cover five miles or more of ground, says University of Pittsburgh varsity soccer coach Joseph A. Luxbacher, Ph.D., a former pro player, in his book, *Soccer: Steps to Success*. Some players may run up to ten miles in the same 90 minutes. Much of the running is in sprints—both short and long.

That's the running part. Soccer also is a full-body sport, says Ken Sprague, coach and strength trainer, owner and operator of the original Gold's Gym and author of *Sports Strength*.

Ask any soccer player after a game. There's not a muscle in their body that they don't feel has been twitched, stretched, tugged. Even the arms, which aren't used in play, get a workout—pumping as you sprint across the field, tossed this way and that to help you balance during agile turns and lunges.

To play this game well, there's no such thing as doing too much endurance, flexibility and strength training, soccer players and coaches agree.

In a bit, we'll offer a straight-ahead weight-room workout for those serious about building soccer muscles. But first, let's

look at a basic on-the-field training routine. It's built on the same five-step sequence as virtually every workout in this book. It should always be taken in order.

Warming Up

Get the body moving, the heart pumping, the blood flowing. This increases muscle temperature, improves reflex time and suppleness, and helps to avoid injury, says Dr. Luxbacher. He recommends a minimum of 10 to 15 minutes of warm-up for soccer players. Anything that gets you sweating should do the trick, but working with a soccer ball helps develop sport-specific skill at the same time, he says.

These three drills are great for getting the blood moving, says Dr. Luxbacher.

A Pro's Workout Secrets

U.S. soccer team legend Marcelo Balboa is aggressive on the field and even more aggressive when it comes to his training. The following are among his workouts.

• Daily bungee running. He ties a bungee cord to another player and tows him around the field for 30 minutes while dribbling, sprinting or running backward in 100-yard intervals.

• Daily weight-room lunges, squats, leg extensions to strengthen an injured knee, and weekly dips, curls, pull-ups and bench presses.

• Tennis, which provides great footwork, he says, and improves his reaction time.

• Mountain biking for two hours, twice a week, in the foothills near his team's Mission Viejo, California, training center.

• Nightly in-line skating, which builds the hips and thighs, he says, and is credited for his powerful kick.

• Sprints—series after series of 440-yard and 880-yard—once or twice a day, six days a week, year-round. The whole team does these.

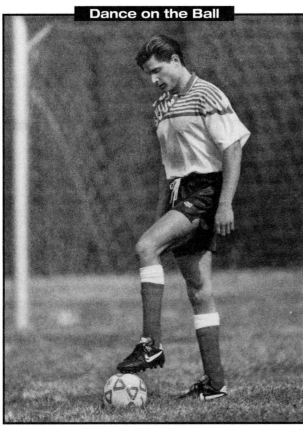
Dance on the Ball

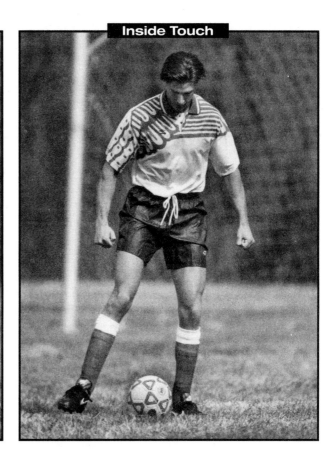
Inside Touch

Dance on the Ball ▲

The name of this drill describes what it looks like. Truth is, you barely touch the ball. Put it on the ground in front of you and barely touch the sole of one foot to the top of the ball, withdraw it quickly and place the sole of the other foot atop the ball, back and forth, quickly, for 30 seconds to a minute. This combines getting the heart going with a ball-control dexterity drill.

Inside Touch ▲

With your feet shoulder-width apart, tap the ball back and forth between your feet, using the inside of your feet, for 30 seconds to a minute. Do it as fast as you can. Rest and repeat.

Confined Dribbling

Limit yourself to a 10- by 20-yard area and start dribbling the ball slowly. Constantly change your speed and direction as you dribble the ball back and forth within the confines of the area. Keep the ball close to your feet. As you warm up, increase your speed. Do this for about five minutes.

Stretching

Once you're warmed up, go through a series of gentle, fluid flexibility exercises. Stretch your hamstrings and quadriceps, calves and Achilles tendon, groin, neck and back. See Flexibility on page 32 for a full-body routine and Running on page 181 for a selection of leg stretches. Dr. Luxbacher recommends static stretching—holding each stretch for 15 to 30 seconds—and doing two reps of each.

Dr. Luxbacher also offers this specialized back stretch using a soccer ball.

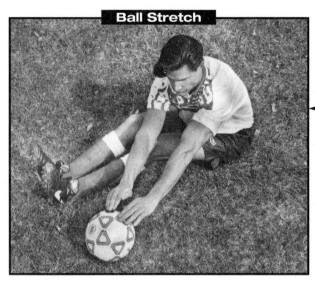

Ball Stretch

◄ **Ball Stretch**

Sit with your knees together, flexed. Slowly roll a soccer ball on the ground around your entire body, keeping both hands on the ball at all times. Roll it ten times in each direction.

Strengthening

Your strength-building routine will focus on your abs, legs, arms and chest. Try this on-field workout.

For the abs, Dr. Luxbacher recommends doing crunches. Do at least 10 and up to 30.

For the legs, here are two exercises Dr. Luxbacher likes. Do one or both in your workout.

For the arms and chest, nothing beats push-ups, says Dr. Luxbacher. You can do 10 to 30 regular push-ups or bent-knee push-ups. Or try Dr. Luxbacher's ball push-ups or walking push-ups.

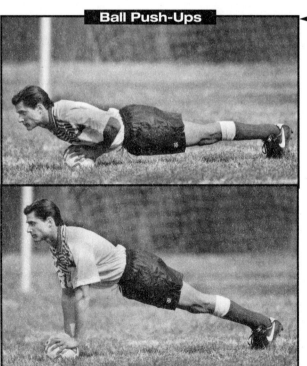

Ball Push-Ups

◄ **Ball Push-Ups**

This is a real upper-body strength builder. Get in a full push-up position, but with your hands on the top of a soccer ball. Support your body weight with your hands and toes and keep your legs and body straight.

Lift your body until your arms are straight, then slowly lower your body until your chest touches the ball. Without letting your body sag, do as many reps as you can up to 20 at first. These put a lot of pressure on your wrists; stop if you feel any pain or discomfort.

Step-Ups

Use a 12-inch-high bench or step-box from the gym. Face it and step up with one foot, then the other, and then step off, one foot at a time. Up, up, down, down. That's one rep. Do 20, rest, and then do it again.

Ball Hops

Keep your feet together and jump from side to side over a ball. Don't touch the ball. If you can't make the height, stand just in front or behind the ball and jump from side to side. Go as fast as possible for 30 seconds to a minute, rest, and then do it again.

The Art of the Header

Not every amateur soccer buff is eager to hit the ball with his head. The ball is not a sponge. And neither is the head. There's a real impact involved. And in hot and heavy competitive play, opponents sometimes crack heads while vying for the ball.

Pro player Marcelo Balboa admits, "I've been hit and dazed more times than I can remember. And that doesn't even include the times I've been sent to Never-Never Land." That doesn't stop him, though. Balboa claims he hits with his head more than 7,000 times each season.

In the optimistically titled *The World's #1 Best-Selling Soccer Book*, then pre-teenage players Ken and Steve Laitin explained how they taught friends to "head" the ball. View the process through children's eyes, and take childlike steps, and it doesn't seem so difficult. The Laitins' advice:

- Keep your eyes open and your mouth closed.
- Hit the ball; don't let it hit you.
- Hit with the center of your forehead.
- Don't dive and head a ball below waist height. You may get kicked in the head.

Sound advice, agrees former pro player Joseph A. Luxbacher, Ph.D., University of Pittsburgh varsity soccer coach and author of *Soccer: Steps to Success*.

Dr. Luxbacher notes that to become a complete soccer player, you need to develop a good "heading" technique, since the ball is in the air so much. In his book he adds these technique tips.

- Face the ball as it descends.
- Jump with two feet. While in the air, arch your upper back and tuck your chin toward your chest, keeping your neck firm and your vision on the ball.
- Time the jump so you connect with the ball at your highest point.
- Snap your upper body forward to give the ball velocity. The idea is to use your back and legs for force, not your neck.

And, to overcome the fear of hitting with your head?

- Put an adhesive-tape cross on the center of your forehead.
- Have a friend toss a beachball to you and practice hitting and directing it with the cross. As you gain confidence, move to a regulation-size ball.
- Practice heading a tetherball back and forth.

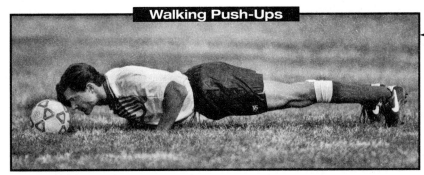

Walking Push-Ups

◄ Walking Push-Ups

While in push-up position (your weight should be on your arms and toes), nudge a soccer ball forward with your head for 20 or more yards, walking on your hands and toes. Keep your body rigid and off the ground.

Endurance

Soccer players need cardiovascular fitness to keep on keeping on in off-and-on bursts of activity for 90 minutes or so. While playing the game itself is a great endurance workout, there's more you can do than that. Dr. Luxbacher suggests two great endurance exercises, both of which help to have a partner for timing purposes.

Shuttle Runs

Place four cones along a straight line 5, 10, 15 and 20 yards out from the goal line. Race to the first cone and back, then to the second and back, and so on, as fast as you can. Your partner takes off as you return from the furthest cone and you rest. Do four to eight sets.

Cone Training

Put a cone 20 yards from the goal line. Starting at the line, dribble the ball around the cone and back as quickly as possible. Upon returning, pass the ball to your partner, who dribbles around the cone and then passes it back to you. Do 5 to 15 reps.

Wind Sprints

If you are in good condition already, do some timed running—a combination of running and jogging—once or twice a week to get to the next level. Here's the formula: Run at 85 to 90 percent of your top speed for one to two minutes, then jog for twice as long to recover—two to four minutes—then sprint again, and recover again. Four sprint-jog repetitions equals one set. Do two to four sets, says Covert Bailey, popular fitness writer and author of *Smart Exercise.*

Cooling Down

When the scrimmage, the running, the exercises are finally finished, don't just hobble to the locker room. As with all workouts, you need to cool down gradually. Part of this cooldown should be running through your stretches again. Do each stretch twice, suggests Dr. Luxbacher. This will help to prevent—or at least to lessen greatly—any next-day soreness.

Weight Lifting for Soccer

Finally, if you want to turn into a soccer monster, here's a weight-room workout devised by Sprague. In season, he wants you in the gym two days a week, doing two sets of 10 reps each at 65 percent of your one-rep maximum. Off-season, you'll work out three times a week, with the amounts and rep counts based on your own periodization schedule (this type of schedule is explained in Basic Fitness on page 118).

- Traditional squats for leg and hip thrust
- Dumbbell lunges for leg and hip thrust
- Pull-ups for upper-body pull
- Leg curls to prevent hamstring injury
- Rumanian dead lifts for back extension
- Military presses for upper-body thrust
- Leg raises with dumbbell or ankle weights for knee lift, kick and torso stabilization

In addition, do this exercise, which gives your body rotational strength.

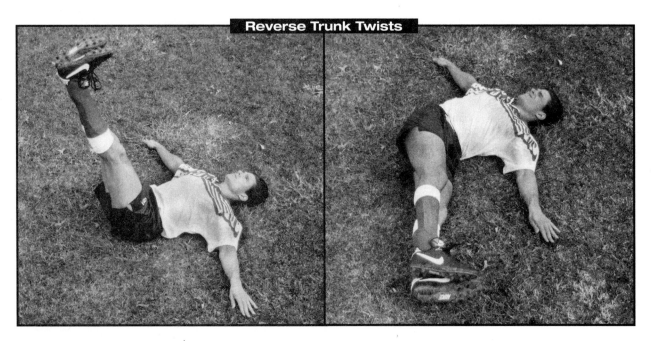

Reverse Trunk Twists

Reverse Trunk Twists ▲

Lie on your back, with your legs raised at about a 90-degree angle to the ground. Keeping your back as flat as possible, twist at your waist to slowly and gently lower your legs to the ground on one side. Then bring them back to center, and lower to the ground on the other side.

Beginners can start with their knees bent, feet flat on the ground, and should work up to having their legs straight up. Do two sets of 8 to 12 reps.

Hockey

Hockey pulls you in two directions at once. First, it's a sport of grace and coordination. Without that, you have no hope of using the long, thin stick to maneuver the short, fat puck across the slick surface—all the while trying to stay balanced on a pair of thin metal blades. As if that isn't hard enough, you're on a rink filled with other men trying to do exactly the same thing.

Which brings us to the second aspect of hockey: the checking, blocking, twisting, swinging and evading. Hockey is a brutal contact sport.

"If you're not crashing into something, you're in constant motion trying to get control of the puck. Or you're just trying to stay upright," says Edmund Connors, a certified strength and conditioning specialist in Hingham, Massachusetts, who has trained hockey players currently playing for the Boston Bruins, the New York Islanders and the Chicago Blackhawks. "Either way, you need to coordinate a lot of different types of exercises if you want to be any good at it. And that goes for the professional ice-hockey player as well as the guy who plays skate-hockey in the street," says Connors.

Being Slick on the Ice

Improving your balance, protecting your body against hard contact, building your leg and torso strength to skate well—these are the goals of hockey training.

"We train our players year-round. They get maybe three weeks off a year. Otherwise, they're constantly working on their hockey skills and conditioning," says John Wharton, head athletic trainer for the Detroit Red Wings and fitness consultant to the Dave Lewis Hockey Fantasy Camp in Fraser, Michigan.

As a casual player with a professional and personal life to lead, you can't do that, and you don't have to. "A man who does regular exercise for about a half-hour three days a week isn't going to have a problem playing hockey," Wharton says. Besides regular fitness training, you can increase your edge with a few tips the pros use.

Improve your balance. To help improve your sense of balance, Wharton recommends doing off-ice balance drills.

Stand on one foot with your eyes closed for as long as you can. Now try doing single-leg squats, flexing your knee to 90 degrees. Work up to 30 seconds, then a minute. As you get better, try to hop from leg to leg—30 seconds on one leg, 30 seconds on the other. "We have players do exercises in full equipment, just to get them used to their balance when they're wearing all their gear," says Wharton.

Get in-line. If your game is street hockey, then there's no excuse for you not to spend an hour on the in-line skates once or twice a week.

"And if you play ice hockey, it's still a very good training exercise," says Connors. "For the recreational player, nothing better mimics the motion and feel of ice skating." Besides straight skating, find yourself a quiet alley or cul-de-sac and set up some boxes and maybe even a net. "Build yourself a little obstacle course and run through it. Practice your stickwork. Every little bit helps," says Connors.

Hit the rink. Good as in-line skating is, if there's a year-round ice rink near you, use it.

"It's one of the most important things you can do," says Connors. "Skating is not a natural movement; you have to teach your body how to do it. If you don't teach it on a regular basis, your body is going to forget." Thereafter, each time you take to the ice, you'll likely spend half the game just getting your sea legs under you. "Instead, if you skate even once a week, you'll eliminate that problem," says Connors.

Play soccer. In hockey, your body has to get used to lots of lateral movement and quick direction changes. One of the best cross-training sports for that—and a terrific workout in its own right—is soccer.

"Many of our professional players actually play professional soccer in the off-season. It mirrors hockey in several ways—you have to work your way down the field, trying to maintain control of the ball while keeping away from players who are charging at you. It also uses the same muscle groups and energy systems as hockey. If you're training for hockey, this is just about the best sport you can do when there is no ice available," says Wharton.

Take a swing. There aren't many batting cages for hockey, but you can always hit the golf course.

"For the recreational player, golf wouldn't be bad. Of course in hockey, you can't swing your stick as high as you would in golf," says Connors. In fact, most sports that involve swinging a club or racquet are good cross-trainers, since they'll work your hips and abdominals. That will only increase the swinging power you'll need to get the puck out of there.

Take your medicine. To duplicate some of the dynamic action required in hockey, Wharton advocates working out with a 10- or 15-pound medicine ball. "It helps build the kind of explosive strength you

Stop-Gap Measures

Pucks, sticks, burly guys in close quarters, sharp skates, rough padding. In hockey, with all that jostling and swinging equipment, sooner or later someone's going to be spitting teeth.

In case that someone turns out to be you, you have two choices: Live life as a guy who smirks a lot and whistles great, or call a time-out and try to save your smile. We talked with those crack hockey experts at the American Dental Association to determine the best way to deal with a broken or dislodged tooth.

If it's loose: Count yourself lucky that it's still connected, and get off the ice before it gets knocked out. Your dentist should have no problem anchoring that tooth back in place.

If it's knocked out: You may still be able to get it re-implanted, but you need to get to a dentist within the next 30 minutes. After a half-hour, the living tissue in the tooth will start to die, and your chances of re-implantation become pretty slim.

As soon as you scoop that tooth off the ice, gently rinse it in cool water and try to hold it in place in the socket. If that doesn't work, put it in a glass of cool water.

If it's gone: If you're over the age of eight, it ain't coming back. This means you're about to discover the wonders of cosmetic dental repair. Depending on the type of tooth you've lost, you may get a bridge—an artificial tooth cemented to neighboring teeth—or a dental implant, a false tooth that's surgically implanted or screwed into your jawbone. You thought you got checked hard on the ice? Wait until you get hit with the bill for *that*. Don't complain—it's too late to think about the mouth guard you should have been wearing. Just grin and bear it.

need in hockey, especially for shooting," he says. When you play catch with a pal, don't just lob the medicine ball back and forth at one another. In fact, don't stand facing each other; turn to the side. "Then, every time you throw, you have to rotate your trunk and throw. That's what the exercise is meant to emphasize—twisting and throwing, building the torso strength and dynamic stability you'll need when you're shooting and trying to score," says Wharton.

Becoming As Hard As Ice

If hockey puts anything in check, it's the lower body.

"Lower back, hamstrings, hips, groin—we get a lot of groin pulls in hockey," reports Wharton. Because he works with both elite hockey athletes and the average weekend ice warrior, he has seen the broad range of hockey-induced ailments.

"A lot of what I see could be prevented by regular strength and aerobic conditioning. Prep work—that's the key," he says.

This workout program will focus hard on the areas you'll need for hockey—especially your lower body and your flexibility. That said, don't forgo a full-body workout: Use our Core Routine as a basis. Here's what the experts recommend.

Aerobic Exercise

Just because hockey is a sport doesn't mean it's a good aerobic workout.

"Hockey requires a strong aerobic base, but the sport itself does not give you a good aerobic workout," says Connors. As part of your training, then, do at least 30 minutes of aerobic exercise three times a week—four would be better. Run, ride a bike, do some stair-climbing. Build your heart and lungs so you'll have plenty of wind to move you across the ice.

Stretching

Work to keep your lower back, hips and groin especially limber. Back extensions and hip flexions with light weights will help those areas. For the groin, do butterfly stretches. Be sure to do additional stretches as outlined in Flexibility on page 32.

Leg Exercises

Just about every leg exercise you've seen in this book will benefit your leg strength for hockey. Specif-ically, focus on the leg press. "It's one of the best all-around leg exercises you can do," says Connors. Also do hip flexions with heavier weights, dumbbell lunges, dumbbell step-ups and step-downs and standing heel raises for lower-leg stability.

Abdominal Exercises

In addition to being home to your swinging power, your abdominal region helps you meet other essential hockey requirements. "Strong abs will help you with balance. They'll also keep your lower back strong—and it takes a lot of punishment in hockey," says Wharton. Besides the crunches in the Core Routine, do hanging single-knee raises as well as oblique twists and oblique crunches.

Box Jumps

This explosive exercise helps build balance and leg strength at the same time. "We call it bounding. We have our athletes jump laterally over cones or milk cartons. You could use a short box, too," says Wharton. "The idea is to get used to that lateral movement, while building power."

Shoulder Exercises

Because of the endless checking and bouncing off walls, you'll need strong shoulders to survive in hockey. Strong shoulders also come in mighty handy when you need to swing that stick. To protect and strengthen your shoulder joints, do shoulder shrugs as well as one-arm dumbbell rows and alternating front lateral raises, says Connors.

Backcountry Sports

Peak Points

- **Incorporate outdoor equipment such as boots and backpacks into your at-home workouts.**

- **Protect shoulder and knee joints with proper pre-activity training exercises.**

- **Work to increase leg, back and shoulder strength.**

If you're the kind of guy who likes to take it outside, who likes to hike, to fish or hunt, to climb, to get into the woods and mix it up with Mother Nature, you may not do much exercise back home. And that might be your downfall.

"Most people who like the outdoor adventure sports tend to think they're in pretty good shape, and most of them are. But no matter how good a shape you're in, it's foolish to think you can't benefit from a little training back in civilization," says Dave Lillard, president of the American Hiking Society. Here's why: If you're not in peak form for sports like football or baseball, you could, say, sprain your ankle. Not good, but at least someone is there to carry you off the field. But when you're in the backcountry, you're on a playing field that might be days away from the slightest glimmer of civilization. Out there, the same ankle sprain takes on far greater proportions.

"It's a good idea to do some pre-activity training preparation for your outdoor activities," says Byron Crouse, M.D., a physician in Duluth, Minnesota, who studied the health-care needs of hikers on the Appalachian Trail. In that study, Dr. Crouse found that at least 30 percent of hikers suffered some type of muscular injury during the course of a trip, be it a sore spot or muscle strain or tear.

Often as not, those injuries will be in places like the legs, back and shoulders. "After a good hike, my quads are really burning. My knees are pretty creaky, too," says Jim Gorman, senior editor at *Backpacker* magazine. "And no matter how well a pack fits you, hauling that thing around for a few days can do a number on your shoulders and lower back."

Naturally, your off-trail workout should focus on these problem areas, but not to the exclusion of the rest of your body.

"While you want to do exercises that really hit certain areas of your body, those exercises should be part of a broader workout," says Lillard. "When you're out on the trail, your whole body—heart, lungs, muscles, everything—needs to be in shape, not just the parts that are doing the hiking or carrying the pack."

Preparing for the Great Outdoors

Dr. Crouse points out that there are no guarantees out in the wilds; there's always the danger of injuring yourself. But the more you train beforehand, the better your chance of avoiding muscle-based injuries. And that doesn't mean just going to the

First-Class First-Aid

Unless you're completely devoid of common sense, you know you shouldn't venture into the backcountry without a good first-aid kit. But what exactly constitutes "good"? We asked the editors at *Backpacker* magazine, which regularly publishes a "Healthy Hiker" edition of the magazine.

"At the very least, you want something that's going to help you cope with the basic bumps and scrapes that are a fact of life on the trail," says Jim Gorman, senior editor at *Backpacker*. "But if you want to create an ultimate first-aid kit, you can do that, too." Here are a few different options.

The Basic Kit
- Personal prescriptions
- Anti-inflammatory or pain-killing drugs (aspirin, ibuprofen or acetaminophen)
- Antiseptics (alcohol, iodine)
- Adhesive bandages
- Gauze pads
- Medical adhesive tape
- Moleskin or other foot-care products
- Safety pins
- Scissors
- Tweezers
- Sunscreen and lip balm
- Insect repellent
- Water-treatment tablets
- First-aid manual
- Latex surgical gloves
- Medication for diarrhea or stomach upset

The "Peak" Kit
All of the above, plus:
- Irrigation syringe
- Betadine solution (10 percent, diluted)
- Wound-closure strips
- Antibiotic ointment
- Sterile dressings (adherent and non-adherent)
- Elastic bandage
- Lidocaine

gym. We'll discuss exercises in a moment. But first, here are a few simple tips outdoorsmen use to give themselves that extra measure of safety and preparation so necessary for the outdoor life.

Break in your boots. If you've just bought the latest pair of lightweight, weatherproof, indestructible boots, don't make the mistake of breaking them in on the trail. "So many people do that, and it leads to serious problems," says Dr. Crouse. By the end of the first day, you'll be so blister-ridden that you'll be lucky if you can walk. Always spend several weeks breaking in new boots before a trip. And you do that by wearing them everywhere, says Lillard.

Even if you have a pair of old, well-worn boots, wear them for a few days before a hike. "The more you wear them before a trip, the more your sense of balance will adjust to the feel and weight of the boots," says Lillard.

Take the stairs. Whether it's the stair-climber in your gym or the half-dozen flights in your office building, never duck a chance to take the stairs. Because stair-climbing works the knees and leg muscles the same way that hiking does, you'll be building power and strength for your favorite outdoor activities with every step you take. Stair-climbing also helps build better cardiovascular strength, says Lillard.

Walk everywhere. Let's say you have somewhere to go—a friend's house, the store, the post office. If it's within walking distance, then you should walk it. "Too often, people just jump in the car and drive, even if it's only a few blocks," says Lillard.

"That's a missed opportunity for exercise." Remember, in the backcountry, most roads to your favorite mountain peak or fishing hole are open only to two-legged and four-legged vehicles, not four-wheeled ones. The more you walk before a trip, the better and longer you'll walk during a trip.

If you do have to drive somewhere, say, the mall, Lillard suggests parking as far away as possible. "Then walk in. It's good exercise." And you'll eliminate the stress of trying to beat out some other guy for a choice spot close to the entrance.

Wear your pack. As part of your pre-hike routine, start wearing your backpack. "A few weeks before a trip, load it up and start walking around with it," says Mike Hardert, director and senior guide for the International Mountain Climbing School in North Conway, New Hampshire. "The idea is to get your body used to the weight. You'll have better strength and better balance that way." It doesn't matter where you walk—around the block, in the park. One of Lillard's colleagues at the American Hiking Society even goes shopping with his pack, using it in lieu of a shopping cart.

As you get used to the pack, increase the weight until you're hauling a fully loaded pack with ease. Not only does this exercise pre-train your back and shoulders but it will also help you determine what adjustments you need to make to the pack so it will fit you perfectly. "Better to figure that out at home than when you're on the trail," says Hardert.

Carry a pole or two. No matter how much pre-training you do, hiking in the wilds still puts a strain on your shoulders and knees. To help minimize long-term damage to these joints, many serious hikers use trekking poles, says Gorman. They look like ski poles, except they have blunted ends and more shock-absorbing capabilities.

"I think they're the best antidote to shoulder and knee problems on the trail," Gorman says. If you're on steep or rocky terrain, these poles can help absorb the shock that your knees might otherwise bear alone. They also help you maintain your balance on tricky footing. Finally, by getting your arms into the pole-planting swing of things, you'll increase your aerobic workout. A decent pair of trekking poles could run you $60 to $100. Or you could use an old pair of ski poles, which would work almost as well.

Training for the Trail

Rock climbing, hiking, even fishing can be hard on the most rugged of bodies. You already know the trouble spots—the legs, the shoulders, the neck, the back. Focus on these areas, in addition to your core workout, and you'll be able to stay outdoors for as long as you want. Here's your map for true peak performance.

Cross-Training

To improve the cardiovascular power you'll need once you're out on the trail, scaling a cliff-face or wading upstream, make sure you spend your off-trail time doing some other aerobic activity at least once a week. Favorites among outdoor enthusiasts include running, cycling, swimming, snowshoeing and cross-country skiing, says Gorman.

Shoulder Exercises

Hauling a 40- or 50-pound pack through the wilds is a burden you're going to have to learn to shoulder. But you can ease that burden a little bit by strengthening your shoulder joints with lifting exercises. Make shoulder shrugs, lateral raises and upright rows a regular part of your workout, suggests John Graham, director of the Human Performance Center at the Allentown Sports Medicine and Human Performance Center in Pennsylvania.

Back Exercises

Since your back is taking the place of a pack mule, you want to make sure it's going to be ready for hours of hauling your gear. Strengthen the lower-back muscles by performing back extensions. And on the trail, before you cinch up your pack every day, take a few minutes to do a lower-back stretch, suggests Graham. Lie flat on your back and grasp your legs behind your upper thighs. Now pull your knees toward your chest.

Abdominal Exercises

The upper and lower abdominals support your back and, therefore, your pack. They also help you stay on balance when you're on sketchy terrain, such as a boulder-strewn hill or a deep stream.

To strengthen your abs, do crunches. In addition to the traditional crunch, do some raised-leg crunches, says Graham. Finally, to work the oblique muscles on your sides, do crossover crunches.

Thigh Exercises

Flexibility is key in the backcountry. Pounding over rocks, climbing up escarpments—you'll need supple muscles to take the punishment, particularly in your thighs. "Your quads and hamstrings are going to take a beating," says Gorman. Minimize the damage by strengthening your lower-body muscles by performing dumbbell squats with moderately weighted dumbbells, suggests Graham. Leg extensions, leg curls and standing heel raises are also useful.

Grip Strengtheners

You never know when you'll need to get a grip in the great outdoors. The stronger your grip, the easier it'll be to cinch up a pack or land a prize salmon. Grip strength is also essential if you go in for more extreme sports like rock climbing.

"Anything's good—a tennis ball, putty, the old spring-loaded grippers—as long as you work your grip regularly," says Hardert. Keep a grip-strengthener at the office and use it while you work. Hardert uses his grip strengthener eight to ten times a day, but he never grips more than three minutes at a time, and he stops if he feels any soreness. This is for good reason: Overtraining with a grip strengthener can lead to tendinitis in the hands or forearms, Dr. Crouse warns.

Balance Exercises

When you're wading through a fast-moving brook in the backcountry, trying to make your way across an underwater landscape of slippery rocks may give you a workout you never counted on. "It's probably a good idea to do some balancing exercises before you go fishing—it only takes one slip to put you in the water," says Tom Ackerman, director of the L.L. Bean Fly-Fishing School in Freeport, Maine. Here's the simplest one: Close your eyes and stand on one foot for as long as you can—at least 30 seconds. Then switch feet. Keep increasing the length of the balancing act by 15 to 30 seconds until you can balance yourself for as long as you want, says Ackerman.

The Twenties

The twenties guy is the envy of all ages. Youths see him as the realization of manhood; older men see him as the embodiment of youth. Being in your twenties is like surveying the world from the lofty heights of a long, tapering hill: All the declines that take place with age slope gently away from a point still further down your path. But don't let the thin air at the top go to your head.

Two problems arise from the physical confidence and well-being that characterize the twenties. First, it's easy to assume (unless you're recuperating from a crippling mishap or get your sustenance solely from glazed doughnuts) that you have no reason to exercise.

The truth of the matter is that the twenties are a critical time to establish fitness habits, abilities and passions that will stick with you later, when exercise ostensibly matters more. "The problem with sedentary men in their forties is that they have a 20-year history of inactivity," says Bryant Stamford, Ph.D., director of the Health Promotion and Wellness Center at the University of Louisville School of Medicine in Kentucky.

The second problem area for twentysomethings is possessing a lulling sense of invulnerability. This isn't entirely bad, because for those who decide to get with a program of activity, feeling invulnerable allows you to play hard and push yourself to the edge in whatever you do. There's no point in being young if you can't do that. But risk by definition entails real danger. "Intensity tends to be greater with guys in their twenties, especially if they play highly competitive sports that require a lot of agility, like football, basketball or soccer," says Benjamin Gelfand, P.T., supervisor at the Nicholas Institute of Sports Medicine and Athletic Trauma in New York City. "I definitely see more of certain types of injuries at this age, particularly overuse injuries like tendinitis, and knee problems like torn ligaments."

Make the Most of the Moment

Because you're young, your body is more resilient and stronger than it will be in later years, which means you can use (if not abuse) it more heavily and achieve greater results in a shorter period of time. And the gains you make now may have an impact in later decades. To do it all, both effectively and safely, you'll need to follow some tips.

Start lifting weights. Although your body doesn't gradually start to lose muscle mass until you're in your thirties, it's important to bulk up now, says Gary Hunter, Ph.D., director of the exercise physiology lab and associate professor of health and physical education at the University of Alabama at Birmingham. Think of your body as a retirement investment: If you build up and maintain resources early, you'll have that much more to draw from when you start to cash out later. And as with finances, an early contribution may produce bigger yields: At this age, your body is still pumping out ample amounts of growth hormone. This chemical keeps muscles strong, but its production will taper off as you age.

Beyond muscle, weight lifting also builds bone. Men don't lose bone as early or as dramatically as women, but it will still be a problem when you reach your late forties or early fifties. Building bone now won't prevent loss from occurring later, but "if you increase bone density up until age 25 to 30 and maintain it, you'll lose bone more slowly," says Dr. Hunter.

Make intensity work for you. In the pre-marriage and pre-kids years, you have more time (not to mention inclination) to participate aggressively in lots of different activities, from pickup basketball to mountain biking to snowboarding. Because you're engaged in multiple pursuits, you need to keep your body well-conditioned to meet different kinds of physical demands. This means that in addition to keeping your body strong, you need to keep it in prime aerobic condition. You may be getting a lot of the conditioning you need from your activities themselves, but adding an aerobic component to your regular workout schedule doesn't need to take a lot of time, says Carol Espel, program director for The Sports Center at Chelsea Piers in New York City.

If you're already in decent shape, Espel suggests cramming all your aerobic requirements into a short, highly intense bout in which you work at 80 to 85 percent (as opposed to the more customary 60 to 70 percent) of your target heart rate—something that's not recommended for older or (even if you're young) out-of-shape men. At that intensity, you'll get a superior aerobic workout in about 20 to 25 minutes. "It's

Dividing Your Time

You can accomplish your objectives in workouts of no longer than 45 minutes to an hour by following this schedule, says Benjamin Gelfand, P.T., supervisor at the Nicholas Institute of Sports Medicine and Athletic Trauma in New York City.

Monday, Wednesday and Friday
• 30 minutes of strength training using the Core Routine on page 121, aiming for three sets at each station. If you're short on time, omit the alternating press with dumbbells.
• 15 to 20 minutes of aerobic exercise paced at 80 to 85 percent of your maximal heart rate.

Tuesday and Thursday
• Do the extra exercises recommended in this chapter as a separate, easy workout.

tough to sustain that kind of effort much longer than that," Espel says.

Protect knees and shoulders. Being in great overall shape goes a long way toward warding off injury, but you need to pay special attention to areas of the body that are prone to damage during intense exercise, especially competitive sports, Gelfand says. Specifically, he recommends you shore up your knees and shoulders through extra exercises that will bolster the muscles and ligaments supporting these crucial joints. You don't have to add more to your gym routine; just do a few extra moves using little or no equipment at home when you're watching TV or listening to music. Here's what he says to do.

Hamstring Curls ►
Put a weight on one ankle for this simple exercise, which works the muscles at the back of the upper leg.

Lie on your stomach with both legs extended. Slowly bend the knee of the weighted leg, moving your foot through an arc until the heel is almost touching your butt, then slowly lower it to the floor again. Do two sets of 15 raises, resting ten seconds in between, then repeat with the other leg.

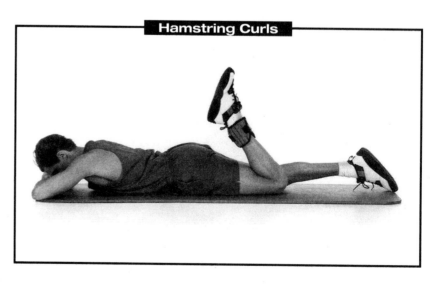

Hamstring Curls

Straight-Leg Raises

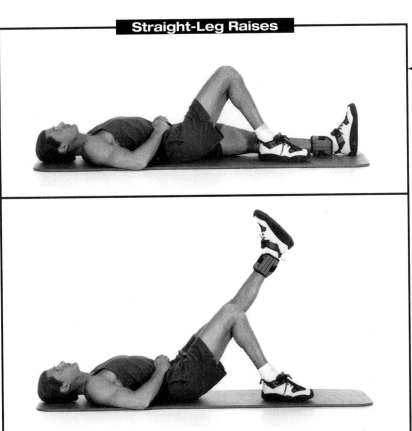

◄ Straight-Leg Raises

This exercise keeps the knee neutral but strengthens muscles and ligaments of the hips and quadriceps, which support, stabilize and protect the knee.

Lie on your back with one leg extended and one leg bent. Your foot should be flat on the floor with the heel about 12 inches from your butt.

Slowly raise the extended leg, toes toward the ceiling, until it reaches the height of your bent knee, then gradually bring it back down. Do two sets of 15 raises, resting ten seconds in between, then repeat with the other leg. For added resistance, put an ankle weight on the extended leg, but don't make it any heavier than 10 to 15 percent of your body weight.

Wall Sits

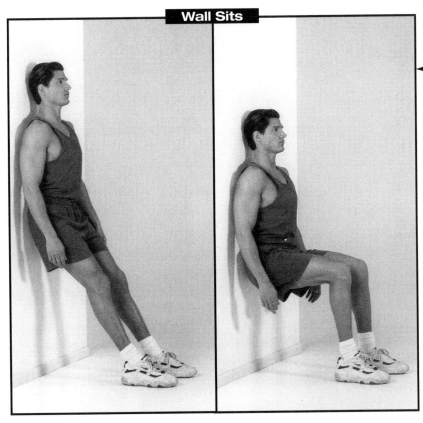

◄ Wall Sits

Here's a deceptively easy-looking exercise that's a terrific, low-stress substitute for lunges if your knees are prone to problems.

Stand with your back flat against a wall with your heels about two feet from the baseboard and each foot about six inches from the other.

Slowly slide your back down the wall, bending your knees as you go until your thighs are almost parallel to the floor. Hold the position. You should feel your muscles begin to burn by about 20 seconds, but shoot for holding for a full minute before standing up straight again. Do a total of five sits, resting 30 seconds between each one.

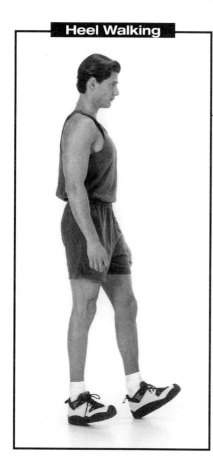

Heel Walking

◄ Heel Walking

To strengthen the front of the lower leg, revisit a move you probably last did when you were a kid.

Lift your toes so that your weight rests on your heels. Now walk 20 to 30 steps, using the muscles at the front of your lower leg to maintain your position and balance. Rest 30 seconds, then repeat.

Heel Drops

The knee isn't the only leg joint vulnerable to injury during vigorous activity. The ankle, too, can use all the support it can get in the form of strong muscles in the calf and front of the leg.

To strengthen the calf, stand on a platform, weight or block, with your heel sticking past its edge. With a smooth motion, let your heel drop past the level of the platform, then raise it back up again. (There are variations on this; see page 260 for another technique.)

Outside Shoulder Rotations ►

A major shoulder problem for men in their twenties is rotator cuff impingement, an overuse injury of the shoulder, Gelfand says. Strengthening the rotator cuff requires exercises that hit the area from two angles. For the first exercise, you'll lift a dumbbell toward the outside of your body.

Lie on your left side with a dumbbell on the floor in front of you, close to your stomach. Keeping the upper part of your right arm parallel to your torso, with your elbow close to your body, bend your right arm at 90 degrees so you can grasp the dumbbell with your right hand.

Lift the dumbbell from the floor, raising it from your stomach toward the ceiling and your right torso, keeping your elbow close to your body. Then lower the dumbbell back to the floor. Do two sets of 15, then repeat on the other side.

Outside Shoulder Rotations

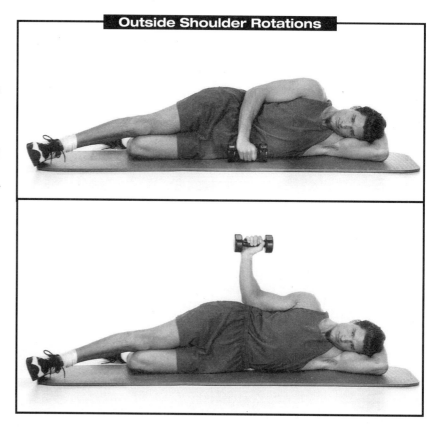

Inside Shoulder Rotations

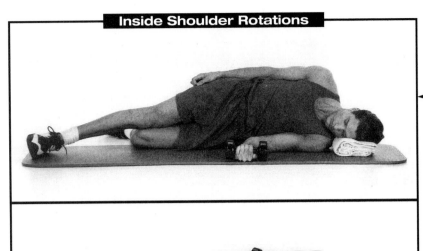

◄ Inside Shoulder Rotations

To strengthen your shoulder from a second angle, lie on your left side again, with a dumbbell on the floor in front of you. This time, grasp the dumbbell with your left hand, with your upper left arm parallel to your body and your elbow close to your torso, bent at 90 degrees.

Lift the dumbbell from the floor up to your right side, keeping your elbow close to your body. Again, do two sets of 15, then repeat on the other side.

The Thirties

Life fills the thirties with transitions. It's a time of incremental changes that, when the decade is over, you realize amount to an epic journey from carefree youth to high-stress adulthood. Girlfriends become wives, marriages produce children, jobs turn into careers, promotions deliver power. There hasn't been much time to think about your body, but what the heck: Your twenties were just a few years back.

And that's the dilemma of the thirtysomething man, this tendency (physically speaking) to look back, not ahead. Once you reach the middle years of this decade, however, there's no escaping the fact that you have just as much in common with a 40-year-old as a 29-year-old.

Granted, there's not much reason to start thinking like a 40-year-old at first. For much of your thirties, your body is not significantly different than it was in your twenties. But the imperceptible declines that occur with age start kicking in during this decade: Muscle mass, strength, aerobic capacity and metabolism (the rate at which the body burns fuel) all begin a shallow downward glide at about the same time. From here on, your overall physiologic function dips by about 1 percent a year.

The critical caveat to all this, however, is that declines are influenced to a huge extent by your level of activity. Look at the "Exercise and Age" chart. The top line shows how slowly the aerobic capacity of a fit man falls off over the years. The lower two lines, in contrast, show how fast the aerobic health of a less-active and a sedentary man decline with time.

With activity, "you're still declining at 1 percent a year, but you're at a much higher level," says Gary Hunter, Ph.D., director of the exercise physiology lab and associate professor of health and physical education at the University of Alabama at Birmingham. Follow the top line down to the 100 percent mark and you'll see that if you stay active, you won't drop to the fitness level of the average 30-year-old for another 30 years.

Acting Your Age

The main challenges of the thirties, then, are a paradox. You want to (and can) maintain the physique of a college boy, but at the same time, you want to (and must) start adjusting to some limitations and liabilities. There are a few points to remember.

Reduce high-impact activity. "Back off just a bit," says Carol Espel, program director for The Sports Center at Chelsea Piers in New York City. "You're still in good shape and shouldn't stop doing high-impact exercise, but if you run three days a week, consider skipping it one day and replacing it with biking, swimming or stair-climbing." Think twice about participating in aggressive contact sports like football and soccer, unless you are already participating in them on a regular basis.

Exercise and Age

The following chart shows how aerobic power declines for men with differing levels of fitness and body fat. Aerobic power is given here as "VO_2 peak," a measure of the maximum amount of oxygen your lungs and heart can transport. The following criteria was used to distinguish between lean, moderate and sedentary men.

- Lean (15% body fat), men who habitually do three hours of heavy aerobic exercise weekly
- Moderate (20% body fat), men who do 30 to 60 minutes of aerobic exercise per week
- Sedentary (30% body fat)

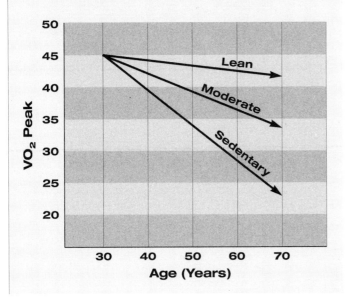

Be prepared. With all the responsibilities in your life, it's common for your exercise plans to get derailed. As long as you later get back on track, that's not a big problem—unless. Being young at heart, there's a tendency to assume you can launch yourself at full throttle into any activity, even if your body isn't up to speed. "I often see men who decide out of the blue to play an intense game of tennis," says Benjamin Gelfand, P.T., supervisor at the Nicholas Institute of Sports Medicine and Athletic Trauma in New York City. "If they're not prepared for it and make a sudden cut to the sideline, they can tear a muscle and tendon."

Nobody's saying you can't play anything without training first; just don't let your competitive urges propel you beyond your capabilities.

Pay attention to your body. When gauging your capabilities, how do you know where the line is? Your body will tell you. Pain, stiffness, soreness, a sense of holding back—these are the body's dashboard lights. But the best early warning system won't help if you ignore its signals. If ever you find yourself saying, "I'm not going to let that stop me," stopping may be exactly what you should be doing.

Make flexibility a priority. "Stiffness is one of the first signs of aging that you'll notice," says Gelfand. That's not surprising, since loss of flexibility starts earlier in life than other signs of aging—as early as your teens. Beyond that, Espel observes that stretching is the most often overlooked part of a man's workout. Yet flexibility is crucial not only for preventing injury but also, because muscles build strength and endurance only in the range through which they move, for achieving all forms of fitness goals. Flexibility also becomes an issue in the thirties because you're likely to be spending less time moving your body and more time chained to a desk. "That's especially important when it comes to the back," Gelfand says, "because the forces on your back are greatest when you're sitting."

The thing about flexibility is that you achieve it one joint at a time. "Your hamstrings can be flexible, but the rest of your body could still be tight," says Espel. In other words, you'll need to devote more time to stretching. Here are some stretches to supplement those described in Flexibility on page 32.

Dividing Your Time

The thirties workout differs from the twenties workout in that you're easing off ultra-high-intensity aerobic exercise, which means your aerobic exercise will require slightly more time. To make up for lost minutes and make room for stretches, you're doing only two sets in the weight workout instead of three (consider compensating by completing more reps in the sets you do), says Carol Espel, program director for The Sports Center at Chelsea Piers in New York City. You should still be able to keep your workouts to 60 minutes or less with this schedule.

Monday, Wednesday and Friday
- 30 minutes of aerobic exercise at 70 percent of your maximal heart rate
- 20 minutes of strength training using the Core Routine (two sets) on page 121
- 5 to 10 minutes of stretches

Tuesday and Thursday
- An easy workout of either the extra exercises described in the workout in the Twenties chapter or the stretches described in this chapter

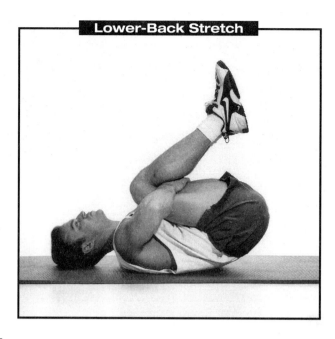

Lower-Back Stretch ➤

We torture the lower back all day, slouching in office chairs and hunkering over computers. Waking up lower-back muscles is a simple matter of assuming a position to which the spine is unaccustomed. Here's one move you can do right in your office without looking like you're rehearsing a bit from your secret life as a contortionist.

Lie on your back, bend your legs and tuck them in toward your chest. As you do this, place your hands on the backs of your upper thighs and gently pull them closer to your chest. Hold for 30 seconds. Remember to keep breathing throughout the stretch.

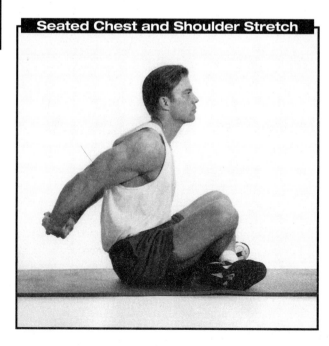

◄ **Seated Upper-Back Stretch**

Sit cross-legged on the floor and interlock your fingers in front of you, palms facing away from your body. Straighten your arms, keeping your fingers locked, and roll back onto your hips while extending your arms forward, so that your back makes a C shape. Hold for 30 seconds; don't hold your breath.

Seated Chest and Shoulder Stretch ➤

Remain sitting, this time placing your hands behind your back. Interlock your fingers with your palms facing your back and slowly raise your arms toward the ceiling, back and away from the body as far as is comfortable. Keep your back straight. Hold for 30 seconds; again, keep breathing throughout the exercise.

Forward Neck Stretch

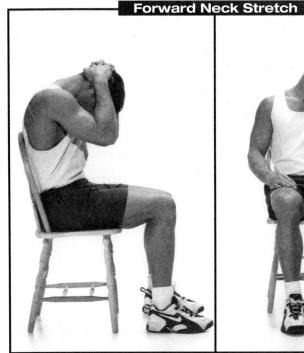
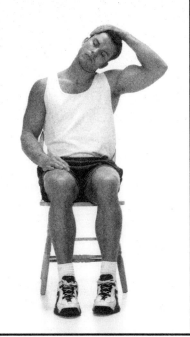

◄ Forward Neck Stretch

The neck is overworked and underappreciated. "Some men's necks are so tight, they're like rocks," Espel says. If that doesn't strike you as a factor in physical performance, ask yourself if having a headache is: Stiffness in the neck is a leading cause of headache pain.

Sit upright in a chair and interlock your fingers behind your head. Gently press your head forward with your hands so that your chin moves toward your chest. Keep your arms relaxed. Stop when you feel a tug along your neck, and hold 30 seconds.

Now hold your head up straight again. Slowly let your head fall to the left side, with your left ear dropping toward your left shoulder, using your left hand to pull your head downward—but not too far. Relax the opposite shoulder. Don't shrug. Hold 30 seconds, breathing throughout the exercise. Repeat on the other side.

Lying Hamstring Stretch

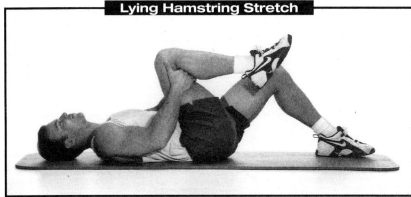
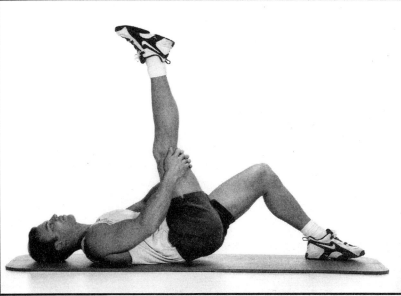

◄ Lying Hamstring Stretch

To stretch the muscles at the back of the upper leg without putting stress on the lower back (which many hamstring stretches do):

Lie on your back with your knees bent and both feet flat on the floor; then bring your right knee to your chest. Remember to breathe. You can hold this position for 30 seconds for a stretch of the hamstrings and lower back, or proceed to the next step.

Extend your right leg straight up toward the ceiling. For an extra stretch, you can use your hands to pull your extended leg back so that your raised foot is directly above your chest. If you can't comfortably reach the extended leg, use a towel around your ankle. Hold both ends as you gently bring the extended leg toward your chest. Remember to keep your extended leg straight, but don't lock your knee. Repeat with your other leg.

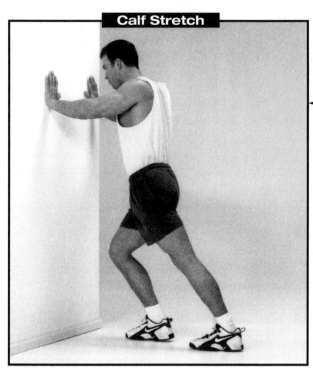

Calf Stretch

◄ Calf Stretch

If you don't have a step handy for the heel-drop calf stretch described in the Flexibility chapter, stand about three feet from a wall, with your toes pointed toward the baseboard. Step forward with your right foot, bending your right leg. Keep your left leg straight, with your left foot planted at its starting position. Placing your hands on the wall for support, lean forward as far as is comfortable. Be sure to keep your left heel on the floor. You should feel this stretch in your left calf. Hold for 30 seconds, then repeat with the other leg. As you become more flexible, try standing farther away from the wall.

Seated Torso Twists ►

Sit on the floor with your left leg extended straight in front of you and your right leg bent, with your right foot positioned on the outside of your left knee. Keeping your back straight, place your right arm on the outside of your right knee. Twist your torso until you can touch the floor on the left side with your left fingertips. Turn your head so you are looking over your left shoulder and behind. Hold for 30 seconds, breathing the entire time, then repeat on the other side.

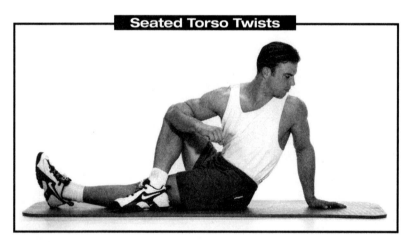

Seated Torso Twists

Modified Raised-Leg Crunches

◄ Modified Raised-Leg Crunches

In the Abs chapter we explained raised-leg crunches, in which you "crunch" while lying on your back with your legs propped up on a bench or chair.

As your abdominals become firmer, stronger and able to take on greater challenges, add difficulty to the raised-leg crunch by making the usual 90-degree angle of your extended legs shallower—to 80, 70 or even 60 degrees. "The lower the angle and the closer your feet move toward the floor, the harder it is," Espel says. To be sure you're isolating your abdominals, however, keep the small of your back pressed to the floor at all times.

The Forties

Peak Points

- **Devote more time to aerobic exercise to improve cardiovascular health and keep fat from padding your midsection.**

- **Pay stricter attention to a properly balanced diet to avoid undermining exercise.**

- **Continue working out with weights, but schedule at least one day of circuit training into your program.**

- **Do more abdominal exercises to keep your belly looking lean.**

In some ways, being in your forties is as much a state of mind as a state of body. Decade boundaries are like borders on a map: Just as land and water don't care where the lines are drawn, your body doesn't care that you've crossed an arbitrary demarcation into your fifth decade. For a while at least, it's just the thirties, continued, and the same concerns remain pertinent: keeping active to stave off aging, approaching activity with prudent caution so as not to exceed your body's abilities, and religiously maintaining flexibility even at times when the rest of your formal exercise plan falls temporarily by the wayside (a basic stretching regimen takes only five minutes, after all).

But the declines that shave 1 percent off your physical function per year have now had some time to aggregate. Age is sneaking up on you, incrementally. The idea of physical decline, which was largely abstract and theoretical in your thirties, gradually is becoming a tangible reality. This means that contributing to your fitness reserve is no longer a luxury with deferred benefits; it's a necessary investment you will increasingly depend upon to maintain your quality of life.

The Injustices of Middle Age

The tangible effects of aging in your forties fall into two broad areas, the first of which is the toll that genetics and a less-than-optimal lifestyle can take on cardiovascular performance. It's time to start paying attention (if you haven't already) to heart-related factoids—for example, that 88 percent of heart attacks in men occur after age 44.

But let's not be alarmist. "A lot of men worry about heart disease more than they need to," says Paul D. Thompson, M.D., director of the Cardiovascular Disease Prevention Center at the University of Pittsburgh Medical Center. He describes how men often visit his office after they turn 40, assuming heart disease is automatically an issue for them. It's not. The likelihood of heart disease being a problem depends on a number of risk factors, one of which is your fitness level. The men Dr. Thompson worries about are the ones who don't worry about heart disease enough.

You probably won't fall into that category if you've been active up to this point. But if you haven't, or if your exercise rou-

Reference Points

Dividing Your Time

While many of the general recommendations for the forties workout are similar to those of the thirties workout, your individual needs and abilities are becoming more of an issue. Be sure to get a checkup with your doctor, especially if you've laid off exercise for an extended period of time, says Carol Espel, program director for The Sports Center at Chelsea Piers in New York City. If you feel pain, or if old injuries begin to act up, lay off activities that cause discomfort, substituting or rotating less stressful alternatives. For example, if running makes your ankles hurt, walk more. If the sheer off-the-saddle physicality of mountain biking bothers your knees, ride more level grades or take to a road bike. With that in mind, consider the following guidelines, says Espel.

Monday and Friday
- 25 minutes of aerobic exercise at a comfortable pace of 60 to 70 percent of your maximal heart rate
- 20 minutes of strength training using the Core Routine (two sets) on page 121
- 5 to 10 minutes of stretches

Wednesday
- 45 minutes of circuit training using the stations of the Core Routine. Do three sets. If you have time left over, do an aerobic exercise like rowing or stationary cycling, using the last five minutes for an easy-paced cooldown.

Tuesday and Thursday
- Light activity such as stretches and/or 30 minutes of brisk walking

---

tine has focused primarily on weight training, now's the time to work more aerobic exercise into your life, according to Dr. Thompson. As we pointed out in Aerobic Exercise on page 27, aerobically active men between the ages of 35 and 74 have a 64 percent lower risk of suffering a first heart attack than their more sedentary peers. Aerobic exercise defends against heart problems across a wide front, reducing risks from (among other things) blood pressure and cholesterol. Exercise may also play a role in fending off diabetes and cancer.

The other major way age now makes itself obvious is the birth of middle girth. You find yourself standing before the mirror, gathering and tugging the folds of flab just above your belt line and wondering, "Where is this coming from?" The problem, however, isn't about coming, it's about lack of going. What's happening is that your body is losing fat-burning

efficiency, says Dr. Thompson. The jets of your fuel-burning metabolism—one of those declining physical functions we've talked about—have been turned down a notch or two. You've also lost a certain amount of lean muscle mass, which means your body needs fewer calories, yet you're probably eating the same amount of food. And your diet (despite your best intentions) is probably too high in fat, which in men gets stored primarily in the bulkhead of the belly.

If you feel all of this is patently unfair because you're not doing anything differently than you ever did, you're right. But not doing anything differently has now become part of the problem. You have to make some changes. Fortunately, both primary problems of the fortysomething man can be confronted with the same countermeasures and the same workout plan. "Weight control and cardiovascular health go together," says Benjamin Gelfand, P.T., supervisor at the Nicholas Institute of Sports Medicine and Athletic Trauma in New York City. "If you address one, you address the other." Before getting the workout specifics, take to heart the following points of action.

Get a checkup. Doctors and trainers alike start getting nervous when men over age forty exercise without having had a physical. Sure, there's nothing to worry about, but it's a peace-of-mind thing. Get the checkup, says Dr. Thompson. Find out your blood pressure and cholesterol levels. You're a winner no matter what the outcome: If there's some unforeseen problem you should be cautious about, you'll be glad for being wiser. And if the doctor pronounces you a fine specimen—well, there's no better news than that.

Be diligent about diet. Now, more than ever, what you eat makes a difference. "All the data says that you need both exercise and diet to keep weight off," says Dr. Thompson. Stick to the classic proportions you've already learned: 60 percent carbohydrate (beans, cereals, breads, pasta, corn, potatoes), 10 to 15 percent protein (lean meat, fish, dairy products) and 25 to 30 percent fat.

Don't abandon your weight workout. Aerobic exercise is crucial, but it's not the whole story. Keeping muscles strong and firm elevates the body's calorie requirements and helps protect against injury, says Carol Espel, program director for The Sports Center at Chelsea Piers in New York City.

Include circuit training. Typically, weight training doesn't burn many calories while you do it—unless you modify the typical program. With circuit training, you lighten the resistance for each exercise and increase the repetitions, usually to 15 to 20. Instead of doing multiple sets, you proceed immediately to the next station, resting only about 15 seconds in between exercises. In one study, circuit training boosted heart rates to aerobic territory—

The Heart Disease Risk Checklist

The reason exercise and nutrition make a difference in heart disease is that both can influence a wide range of risk factors—or offset risk factors that can't be controlled. Here are the primary markers of potential cardio-problems.

• Family history. A lot of factors leading to heart disease run in families, but when counting the heart attacks among parents, take age into account. Research suggests that if neither of your parents had a heart attack by age 70, your own chances of having one by that age are cut in half. If either parent had a heart attack before age 70, look first at controllable circumstances that may have played a role, such as some of the factors that follow.

• Smoking. Habitual smoking narrows blood vessels and makes blood more prone to clotting. If you don't smoke, you've cut your chances of a fatal heart attack by at least 50 percent.

• Obesity. Having a potbelly is a risk factor all its own. If you measure your waist between your ribs and your hip bone, and your hips at their widest point, then divide the waist size by the hip size, you get your waist-to-hip ratio. If it's .95 or less, you can cross this risk factor off your list of worries.

• Cholesterol. The blood test you get during your physical will provide two numbers: your total cholesterol and your HDL cholesterol. Divide the total by the HDL. If the number you get is under three, you probably don't have to worry about this risk factor.

• Blood pressure. Having hypertension makes you six times more likely to have a heart attack. Don't believe the first number you hear, though: It's best to take two readings and average the results. Numbers of 120/80 or lower put you in good shape. Risk increases as the numbers rise, but you don't need to worry until you cross the borderline hypertension line, which is 140/90.

• Diabetes. Chances are you don't have it, but if you do, your heart disease risk increases two to four times. Be alert for symptoms like slow-healing bruises, recurrent infections and tingling or numbness in your hands or feet.

• Too much alcohol. A nip here and there won't hurt and may even help. But try to keep it to one drink a day: A 12-year study of 1,455 men found that blood pressure readings began rising steadily if they drank more than six beers a week.

• Social support. Men without close friends or confidants are more susceptible to heart disease than men with no social web. But you don't have to wear a funny hat and learn secret handshakes to be social: Just having one good friend—your wife counts—makes a big difference.

---

72 percent of maximal heart rate for men, on average. That's the equivalent of slow jogging, playing basketball or fitness hiking in hilly terrain.

Firm up your abdomen. It's an old guys' tale that doing sit-ups and crunches will burn fat from the belly. Burning fat is a whole-body metabolic deal that can't be done on a spot-specific basis. Still, crunches really can make you look better because they firm up the muscles underneath whatever fat is girding your gut. "Think of what you do if you want to instantly look better in a swimsuit," says Espel. "You suck in your stomach." If the muscles there are firmly toned, it's like a permanent gut-suck effect. Except you're not faking it. "Good abs account for half of good posture," Espel adds.

The Forties Workout

The exercises you should do in your forties are not substantially different from those of your thirties or twenties. Follow the Core Routine on page 121: Even when you're doing circuit training, the stations you use are the same as for standard strength training. Continue with the regular stretches from the Flexibility chapter on page 32 or the workout in The Thirties chapter on page 244. The major addition is a battery of abdominal exercises. If you can, do each of the following exercises ten times, proceeding to the next one after resting no more than 15 seconds, says Espel. If your abdominals fatigue before you can finish them all, just take them in order and work toward doing more.

Reverse Curls

In this version of the curl, you start with your thighs raised perpendicular to the floor and your feet off the ground, hanging loosely by your butt. Lift your shoulders as you would in an ordinary crunch, but also bring your knees toward your chest. "This is my favorite abdominal exercise, especially if you only have a few minutes. It engages the abdominal wall in a very intense way," says Espel. If you can only do one ab exercise, this is it, she says.

Crossed-Ankle Reverse Curls ➤

Do another set of reverse curls, but add a level of difficulty by making one change: Cross your ankles so that your knees are one to two feet apart.

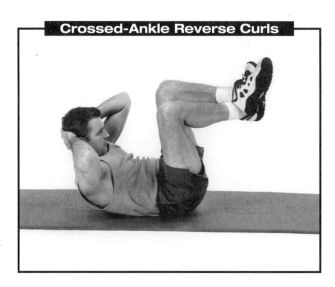
Crossed-Ankle Reverse Curls

Crossed-Ankle Oblique Curls ➤

For an advanced, difficult variation on the curl that also works the important oblique muscles at the sides of the torso, assume the crossed-ankle starting position of the crossed-ankle reverse curl. But instead of raising your chest and knees toward each other, perform the following move.

With your hands kept behind your head, elbows pointing out to the sides and knees in a fixed position, raise your left shoulder (not elbow—that would put stress on your neck) toward your right knee.

Lower your torso to the starting position, then raise your right shoulder toward your left knee.

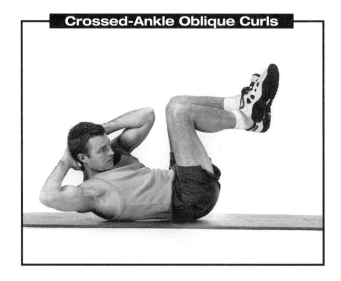
Crossed-Ankle Oblique Curls

Over 50

Peak Points

- **Don't compare yourself to any other man of any age: More than ever, you're working within your own personal parameters.**

- **Maintain vitality indefinitely by keeping up a regular schedule of vigorous workouts.**

- **To offset changes with age, eat more nutrient-dense foods, do more weight-bearing exercise such as walking, and modify exercises to avoid potential injury.**

There's an unfortunate tendency for people younger than age 50 to lump everybody over the half-century mark into one group labeled "older." This presupposes that a man who's 51 will identify with—and more or less be the same as—a man who's 71. No doubt you've noticed by this chapter's heading that we're guilty of such unfair categorizing ourselves.

There's justification for this, however, and it's as follows: A 71-year-old man actually may be similar to a 51-year-old man in terms of fitness. The fact is, the older you get, the more difficult it is to generalize about what's typical, because your individual limitations and problems, your individual habits and your individual fitness history—all increasingly important—could make you vastly different than another man your age.

Take, for example, Hank Kiesel, who's in his late sixties, of St. Louis, Missouri. Kiesel runs five to seven miles three or four times a week and exercises as often as twice a week on a rowing machine. Periodic measurements show that his heart and lungs work as efficiently as they did in 1988, when he started exercising regularly shortly after retirement.

"The latest tests showed a slight increase in my VO_2 max," Kiesel says. (VO_2 *max* is a measure of how much oxygen your body can consume during extreme exertion; it is considered one of the best ways to read your aerobic capacity.) With age, "you don't necessarily start dropping off." A researcher who's following Kiesel and other older adults as part of a study, Robert Spina, Ph.D., of the Division of Geriatrics and Gerontol-

ogy at Washington University School of Medicine in St. Louis, Missouri, has found that between ages 60 and 72, cardiovascular performance can improve by about 25 percent in nine months of endurance training. Every year, Kiesel puts himself to the test in a major rowing-machine competition held in St. Louis. In 1996, he rowed the equivalent of 2,000 meters in 7 minutes, 56.3 seconds, besting men 17 years his junior who were competing in a younger age group.

All of which goes to show that the real crime of perception isn't when younger people think of you as older, but when *you* think of yourself as older, assuming—as many men do—that physical activity won't make much difference anymore. Doctors note that physical activity tends to decline with age. Men start exercising less frequently and less vigorously. It's easy to understand why: The body isn't all it used to be, and trying to keep up the energy and power of younger years—or even to match the efforts of spectacular specimens like Kiesel—can be discouraging.

But the fact is, all that's required is that exercise be challenging for you as you exist *now*. No, your aerobic capacity isn't what it was when you were 30. But that doesn't matter: The goal isn't to regain past fitness levels, but to sustain and improve upon your current condition. There's an elegance of design at work here in which your body's needs are paralleled by your body's abilities.

Maintenance is the operative word here. "After age 50, that's the primary goal," says Carol Espel, program director for The Sports Center at Chelsea Piers in New York City. "Strength and endurance are still important, but the gains you make won't be as great." As you become older, holding firm and steady, as Kiesel has done, becomes a form of progress. If working hard to stay in one place strikes you as futile, just ask Kiesel how he feels about it. "I hardly ever sit down," he says. "Through the whole day, I feel good. And it's fantastic mentally to know that I can still do things like maintain the house and cut the grass with a hand mower."

Issues of Aging

The concerns we've discussed in other age groups—flexibility, cardiovascular health, healthful weight—are still important, of course. But there are a number of other issues to pay close attention to as you get into your older years.

• Preventing bone loss. As we've noted, the body starts losing bone earlier in life. But as you age, loss begins to accelerate for a number of reasons. The body becomes less able to absorb nutrients such as calcium and vitamin D, both of which are important in bone synthesis. Intake of these nutrients also tends to decline. Add these factors to a more sedentary existence, and you have extra-bad news for bones.

From a fitness viewpoint, it's increasingly important to do weight-bearing exercises. That doesn't mean you should lift more weights; it means you should be on your feet as much as possible so that both bones and muscles are called upon to support your body and whatever loads it carries. "The important thing is that the feet are making contact with the ground," says Benjamin Gelfand, P.T., supervisor at the Nicholas Institute of Sports Medicine and Athletic Trauma in New York City. Walking is an excellent bone protector, as is running or even dancing—any activity that keeps you on your toes counts.

• Changing nutritional needs. Declining calcium and vitamin D synthesis aren't the only nutritional changes that occur with age. As metabolism slows, the body also starts needing fewer calories—something you knew from your forties. But here, too, the trend accelerates with age: According to the World Health Organization, the body needs 5 percent less energy per decade between ages 39 and 59, but needs 10 percent less from age 60 to 69 and 10 percent less over age 70. That would seem to argue in favor of eating less, but paradoxically, studies also

Dividing Your Time

You can see by comparing this workout to the one from the forties that being over 50 (or even over 60) is no reason to significantly curtail the amount or intensity of your exercise. Here's what to do, according to Carol Espel, program director for The Sports Center at Chelsea Piers in New York City.

Monday and Friday
• 20 minutes of aerobic exercise at a comfortable pace of 60 to 70 percent of your maximal heart rate
• 20 minutes of strength training using the modified Core Routine in this chapter
• 5 to 10 minutes of stretches

Wednesday
• 45 minutes of circuit training, doing three sets of the exercises in the modified Core Routine. If you finish three sets before 45 minutes are up, cool down with walking.

Tuesday and Thursday
• 30 minutes of brisk walking, followed by 5 minutes of stretching

find that older people tend to take in too little of the nutrients they need. What this suggests is that it's increasingly important for the foods you eat to be low in calories but nutrient-dense. That's why it is important to cut back further on fat, sugar, alcohol and other "empty" calories in favor of fruits, vegetables and grains.

• Side effects from medications. Drugs you might start taking at this point in your life can have an effect on things like appetite and nutrient absorption. Just one cholesterol medication, for example, interferes with the body's use of vitamins A, D, E and K and can cause folate deficiencies. Each drug has its own set of side effects, but this is why you should consult a doctor: He will tell you how the medications you take can affect your ability to exercise or fuel your body.

• Increased vulnerability to injury. By now, you've heard us talk about taking it easy so many times, we're not going to bore you with reminders. In fact, we're not the ones whose word you should take on what you can or can't do, anyway. As a rule, we wouldn't recommend that you run three times a week, but Hank Kiesel manages to do it without any problems, and every major marathon has its contingent of men well over 50. Instead, this is something you need to work out with your doctor, says Dr. Spina.

The Fifties Workout

The basic outline of the fifties workout is the same as the forties workout—a mix of strength and aerobic exercise, with one day of circuit training for combined cardiovascular and muscular fitness. One specific suggestion, however, is to be less cavalier about regular walking, which is both aerobic and weight-bearing: Try to walk for 30 minutes at least three times a week. In addition, it's a good idea to modify some of the exercises of the Core Routine on page 121 to ensure you don't put undue stress on joints or muscles. Here's your Core Routine, with slight safety-minded alterations to a number of free-weight exercises, says Espel.

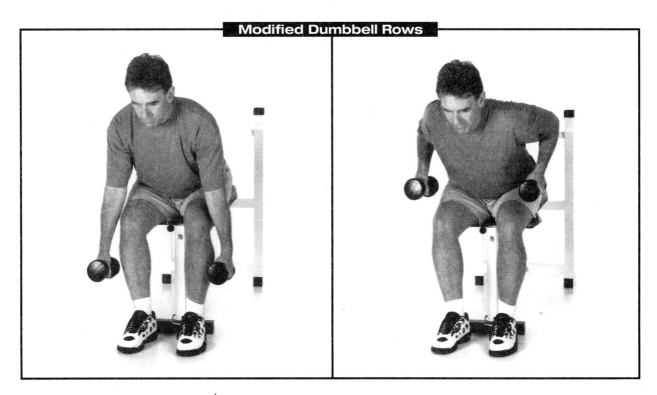

Modified Dumbbell Rows

Modified Dumbbell Rows ▲

The one-arm dumbbell row in the Core Routine is a safe exercise, but if you want to save a little time in order to make room for aerobic exercise or stretching, try this variation, which uses both arms at the same time, yet is easy on the back.

Sit on the edge of a bench with your feet flat on the floor and dumbbells positioned on the floor to either side.

Keeping your back straight, lean forward and grab the dumbbells, holding them with your arms extended. This is your starting position.

Lift both dumbbells by pulling both arms back in a rowing motion. Try to squeeze your shoulder blades together as you lift. Return to the starting position and repeat.

Modified Bench Press ▶

Perform the bench press as described in the Core Routine, but with one difference: To avoid stressing the anterior deltoid area at the front of your shoulder and possibly tearing a tendon or damaging the joint, bring your elbows out to the side, no lower than shoulder level during the down phase of the movement. Said another way: When your elbows become parallel to the floor, halt your downward movement and begin raising the bar back up. Make sure the small of your back is pressed into the bench.

Wall Sits

"Stay away from squats, which hit many areas of muscle but put tremendous stress on the knees," Espel says. This is a concern for much younger men as well. For a safer alternative, see the wall sits exercise described in The Twenties on page 241.

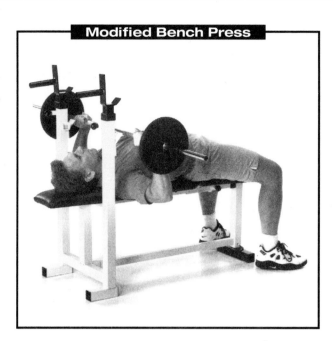

Modified Bench Press

Alternating Press with Dumbbells

Perform as described in the Core Routine.

Concentration Curls

Perform as described in the Core Routine.

Seated Triceps Press

The Core Routine calls for you to do overhead extensions to work out your triceps. We're going to make a substitution, however: Do the seated triceps press (described in Arms on page 51). The basic move with this exercise is the same as in the overhead triceps extension, but with two important differences: You're using a dumbbell instead of a barbell, and you're sitting instead of standing. "Dumbbells are easier to control than barbells, and you can use a lighter weight to get the same effect," says Espel.

Crunches

Perform as described in the Core Routine.

City Living

They say there are nine million stories in the naked city, but where exercise is concerned, it's more like nine million excuses. Joining a gym is too expensive. Or if you do belong to one, it's always too crowded. Or you can't go running because you might get mugged. Or your commute takes so long, you never have time to work out.

If you've ever lived in a big city, you already know that it's strenuous enough just making your way amidst the teeming humanity—the crowds, the traffic, the stress, the endless demands on your time, your energy, your money. Add a workout on top of that? Not in a New York minute.

Think again, says Bob Arnot, M.D., CBS News medical correspondent and author of *Dr. Bob Arnot's Guide to Turning Back the Clock.* "I live in New York City and have a job that keeps me pretty busy. But I discovered there are plenty of ways to exercise in the city and make it part of your routine," he says.

Exercising in the Big City

Working out in the city requires two things: some small sense of time management and a willingness to explore new venues for old-fashioned exercise.

"Finding a time and a place for exercise is a little like making your way around on the subway. The first couple of times you do it, you'll probably miss a stop or lose your way. But the more you do it, the easier and more instinctive it becomes. Pretty soon you'll know the whole system," says Charles Kuntzleman, Ed.D., adjunct associate professor of kinesiology at the University of Michigan in Ann Arbor. Consider this chapter your pocket guide to a city fitness system. Here are a few pointers to get you headed in the right direction.

Be a power-commuter. The time you spend commuting is time you could spend exercising. For example, Dr. Arnot gets up early and commutes to work every day by bike or in-line skates, then showers and changes when he gets to work. "If you can bike to work, it's certainly a great idea," says Dr. Kuntzleman. "You can either pack your work clothes and take them with you, or leave a change of clothes at the job."

Take the road less traveled. If you decide to follow in Dr. Arnot's tire tracks and commute to work by bike or skate, try to stay off busy streets. Instead, develop a network of parallel side streets that will get

Rules of the Road

As philosophical questions go, it's not as pressing as, say, the meaning of life or the existence of God, but it's one you need to ask yourself if you're planning to commute in the city on a bike: Are you a vehicle or a pedestrian?

The answer, of course, is both. Any time you want, you can always jump off a bike and walk it, so boom, you're a pedestrian. "But if you're on a bike, on the road, then you should consider yourself a moving vehicle," says Sandra Woods, past bicycling coordinator for the engineering department of the city of Seattle, which has one of the best city-bicycling programs in the United States.

As a vehicle, you need to follow basic rules of the road to keep motorists aware of your actions and, more important, to keep you from becoming street pizza. Here are a few tips she mentioned.

• Obey all traffic signs and signals, just as if you were in your car.

• Use hand signals to indicate what you're doing next. Left arm extended horizontally means left turn; left elbow bent, hand extending upward means right turn; left hand extending downward means slow down or stop.

• Keep to the right as far as possible. In general, you want to be just outside the actual flow of traffic. If you have to make a left turn, signal your intentions. If it's a turn-only lane, ride to the right in the turn lane. Once you make the turn, get back over to the right.

• Stay off the sidewalk unless absolutely necessary. Woods warns that some city police departments are authorized to ticket cyclists on the sidewalk, especially if they ride in an unsafe manner. Whether local ordinances mandate it or not, it's a good idea to stay in the street. It is difficult to predict what a pedestrian is going to do.

• Watch out for car doors or people in parked vehicles. If the road is wide enough, try to ride at least a car door's length from all parked cars.

• Make yourself conspicuous by wearing bright colors and using reflectors or bike lights in dim light. The more obvious you are to motorists and pedestrians, the more likely you'll all be able to go your own way without incident.

• Assume you are invisible to drivers and pedestrians. Never assume that a turning motorist will see you. Always be as cautious as you can.

---

you to your office. Less crowded streets mean less danger to you, less stopping and starting and less exposure to exhaust and other harmful pollutants you could inhale.

Stop and walk. If you don't have a bike, or don't have a shower where you work, you can still get in some exercise. Let's say you take a train or bus to work. "I'd suggest that you pack some sneakers, get off one stop early and walk the rest of the way to work," says exercise physiologist John Amberge, director of corporate programs for the Sports Training Institute in New York City. Do the same thing on the way home. "With the way traffic is in the city, you may find you can get where you're going faster on foot," Dr. Kuntzleman adds.

Grab a partner. Early morning or evening is often the only time city dwellers can conceivably work in a workout. But one of the realities of city life is crime, and many of us are understandably reluctant to go out alone in the dark, lonely hours.

"If you have an exercise partner—a neighbor, a co-worker, someone who can exercise with you—you are more likely to be consistent with your exercise routine, which will result in greater improvement in your fitness levels," says Amberge. First of all, if there are two or more of you, you'll be a less appealing target for a mugger. Second, because of that tacit

commitment to another person, buddying up tends to make you more likely to roll out of bed for that morning run than to blow it off. After all, you don't want to let a friend down.

Do an all-building workout. If you live in an apartment building or complex, you can use the whole building as your own personal exercise facility. "From an aerobic standpoint, you can use your apartment building stairwell for stair-climbing, or you could do laps in the hallways," says Dr. Kuntzleman. Plus, Dr. Kuntzleman points out that the confines of where you live may be safer than exercising on the street or in the local park.

Seek alternative workouts. One of the great things about city life is that there's always a broad range of choices. That applies to restaurants, theaters and places to work out.

"Never mind that, the bigger the city, the more health clubs there are. If those clubs are always crowded, look to other options for exercise, places where you'll get a good workout and maybe even learn a new sport at the same time," recommends Dr. Kuntzleman. Racquet clubs and martial arts studios are some obvious choices. Other options you might want to try include indoor climbing walls or boxing gyms.

Join an alternative club. While that fashionable

Urban Exercise Essentials

If you plan to exercise out on those wild city streets, exercise physiologist John Amberge, director of corporate programs for the Sports Training Institute in New York City, suggests that you don't go out without the following items.

• Spare key. Don't take a whole ring of keys—they'll just weigh you down. Instead, take one key, something you can put on an elastic band and slip around your wrist.

• ID. Slip your license in your sock or put it in a zippered pocket.

• Medical alert necklace or bracelet. If you're out cold in the middle of the street, this little trinket may just save your life.

• 20 bucks. Long-time veterans of city life are well aware of the principle of mugger money. If you get accosted, give it up. This strategy may actually be safer than carrying no money. If you're penniless, your would-be robber may get a little testy and take his frustrations out on you.

• Exercise partner—or partners. There's strength in numbers. If you can get some co-workers, neighbors or pals to exercise with you, you'll be far less vulnerable than if you went out all by your lonesome.

health club in your neighborhood may be too much for your budget, there are other fitness clubs that will be a lot easier on your wallet to join.

"The YMCA is an obvious choice. Membership is usually much cheaper than most health clubs. And the Ys in bigger cities have comparable facilities," says Dr. Kuntzleman. Also, most large cities subsidize an athletic or social club that sponsors intramural team sports or lessons in various sports, from swimming to in-line skating. To see if your city has one, check your local government telephone listing. "You may have to pay a nominal fee to join or take lessons, but once again, these options are likely to be far less expensive than a health club," points out Dr. Kuntzleman.

Urban Workouts

City life doesn't require muscle so much as flexibility and cardiovascular strength. You need a good set of heart and lungs if you want to catch the bus before it heads downtown. And it helps to be supple if you need to slide between the train doors, just before they close.

We had our experts recommend a few stretches and cardiovascular exercises that will help keep a good level of aerobic fitness and flexibility. The best

thing about them is that you can do them anywhere in the city.

"You don't want this to be your only workout, of course," says Dr. Kuntzleman. But these exercises make a nice addition to a basic routine. Some of them even help you turn some basic elements of city life into effective workout tools.

Shoulder Exercises

Your shoulder joints have it hard in the city. Whether you're shouldering your way through a crowd or trying to force a temperamental subway door open, you'll want to protect your shoulders. Do plenty of shrugs as part of your regular workout. Lateral raises will also help increase shoulder strength.

Abdominal Exercises

Even in the most cramped apartment, you ought to have room to do crunches. And you should do them—every day. Besides improving your maneuverability, your abdominals also help shore up your lower back, which gets sore when you sit on public conveyances for hours at a time, and absorbs a lot of impact when you walk on hard, city pavement. Do crunches, including oblique crunches and oblique twists.

Arm Exercises

Whether you're hauling shopping bags across town or trying to hold on while the bus is swaying wildly through rush-hour traffic, you'll need arm strength aplenty. Keep a couple of dumbbells handy in your apartment so you can do biceps curls and standing kickbacks on a regular basis. Push-ups are also another handy exercise you can do in your apartment—and they work the chest muscles to boot.

Stair-Climbing

Every day at work, every night at home, avoid that elevator. Stair-climbing delivers an important aerobic benefit most urban dwellers overlook, says Dr. Kuntzleman. "When you're commuting every day, on the train, the bus or by car, you're probably not getting much of an aerobic workout as it is. This gives you a little extra workout. And it's something you can do every day."

To give the exercise a little extra kick, vary your stair-stepping. "For example, on the way down, take the steps two at a time. On the way up, with each step you take, rise up briefly on the toes of your stepping foot, then take another step, rise up on your toes, and continue down the stairs that way. It looks funny, but it's a great calf exercise," says Dr. Kuntzleman.

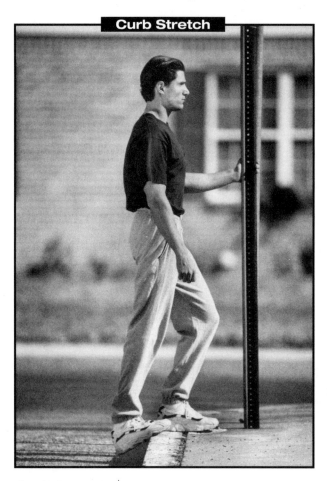

Curb Stretch

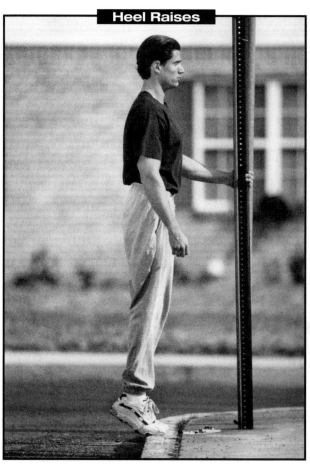

Heel Raises

Curb Stretch ⋀

To stretch your Achilles tendon and ankle before a run, or while you're waiting for the bus, stand with the ball of your right foot on the edge of a curb—the rest of your foot should be hanging off the edge. Your left foot should be fully on the curb.

Now slowly lower your right heel below the level of the curb. If you need to, place one hand on a sign or parking meter for balance. Your right leg should remain straight as you stretch the ankle. Hold for 20 seconds, then switch your legs.

Heel Raises ⋀

To exercise your calf muscles, stand with your feet hip-width apart. Your toes should be resting up on the edge of the curb; your heels should be hanging over the edge. Hold your arms loosely at your sides (if you have hand weights or dumbbells, hold them in each hand, palms facing in). You should be leaning forward slightly.

Now rise all the way up on your toes. Feel the contraction in your calves, and pause briefly at the top. Your arms should remain in position, though your body will probably be more upright. Lower, repeat.

Chain-Link Fence Chest Stretch ➤

You can use this handy shoulder and chest stretcher on any doorway or chain-link fence.

Stand with your back to the fence. Hold your arms behind you at shoulder level and grab the fence. Your palms should be facing away from you.

Now lean slightly forward, feeling the stretch across your chest and shoulders. Hold your chest up and tuck your chin slightly in toward your chest.

Note: You can also modify this stretch for your daily commute. Instead of a doorway or fence, use the support poles found on either side of the aisle in most trains or buses.

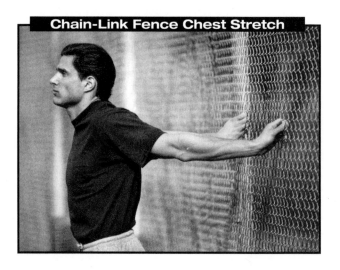

Chain-Link Fence Chest Stretch

Country Living

Peak Points

- **It takes stamina to live in the country. You need a year-round aerobic fitness program.**

- **Strengthen your arms, shoulders and back. Country living is tough on your upper body.**

- **Use the hills and fields around you as exercise tools.**

For some men, it all comes down to a single choice: city living or *real* living—in the mountains, or desert, or forest, or rolling countryside. Days spent in the great outdoors, away from the cacophony and mass of urban dwelling.

Of course, you can spend time outdoors each day in cities and towns. You can walk in a park. You can get an outdoor job steaming bubble gum off sidewalks. But that just doesn't compare with true country life. Certainly it's more beautiful, perhaps even spiritual, to live in the country or mountains. But it's also much harder: longer drives, harder chores, physical isolation. It's a different day-to-day life, to be sure.

This being a book on conditioning, we'll focus on just one aspect of the country life: The man living in rural and mountain environs faces fitness opportunities—and challenges—the urban and suburban man does not.

For instance, he probably doesn't have access to a gym.

He may have a long daily commute to and from work in an urban area, meaning he spends even more time sitting than his urban counterpart and has even less free time available for working out.

He probably doesn't have a patch of grass he can mow in 20 minutes like his suburban brothers, but rather a gangly field-size lawn that takes all Saturday afternoon to tame. Good exercise, by the way, if you use a push-mower, says Jonathan Robison, Ph.D., an exercise physiologist, nutritionist and executive co-director of the Michigan Center for Preventive Medicine in Lansing.

He's more likely to have a quarter-mile-long driveway in constant need of maintenance—snow shoveling in the winter, pothole and rut smoothing in the spring and summer. Good exercise, by the way, if you're physically up to it, says John Emmett, Ph.D., exercise physiologist and associate professor of physical education at Eastern Illinois University in Charleston.

He's more likely to have animals that need to be fed and watered, stalls that need to be cleaned, fences that need to be maintained. All fine physical labor.

The mechanical equipment required to maintain a rural spread is heavy and bulky. Just hooking up a plow to a tractor is a major, albeit short, weight-lifting routine.

The lifestyle may require and encourage substantial physical activity. And the environment and terrain offer opportunities aplenty for recreational fitness activities.

We'll help you work on the strength and conditioning needed to live the outdoors life in style. Then we'll suggest ways to enjoy the unique environment. Finally, we'll show you the right way to do that most common of chores: splitting logs.

The Strength You Need

The air in most rural areas is cleaner than in cities, notes Dr. Emmett. And that's good, because he wants you huffing and puffing.

Often the demands of rural living are sudden or seasonal, he notes. Like a mountain of snow to shovel. Or a mountain of logs to split. You may have bulging biceps, but your heart may not be up to the task, he says.

So Dr. Emmett's first prescription for rural and mountain dwellers is aerobic training. Build up your stamina so you can put in long, hard days and still have energy remaining for short blasts of hard effort.

The base-level cardiovascular routine would be to get your heart pumping hard for stretches of 20 minutes or more, at least three times a week, Dr. Emmett says. You don't want your heart beating *too* hard—just enough so you work up a sweat. You can do this gardening—hoeing, for instance—or pitching hay, or posthole digging, or recreationally—biking, running, playing basketball.

It's important that you find a way to get an aerobic workout indoors, as well, advise Dr. Emmett and Charles Swencionis, Ph.D., head of the health psychology program at Yeshiva University in New York City and co-author of *The Lazy Person's Guide to Fitness*. You need to keep your heart and lungs in shape year-round—even when you can't get outdoors comfortably. Snow is no excuse for falling out of shape.

Second, Dr. Emmett says, work on upper-body strength.

So many physical demands of rural life involve the upper-body muscles—arms, back, shoulders—he points out. Actually, Dr. Emmett recommends a regular, full-body strength-training program, like that found in the Core Routine on page 121. But, he says, pay particular attention to upper-body conditioning. "If your upper body is weak and you're engaged in activities requiring upper-body strength, you're putting an even greater strain on your heart," he says.

Next priority in terms of muscles is to strengthen your back and abdominals, Dr. Emmett says. All that lifting, carrying, chopping and shoveling puts a mighty large strain on your back; conditioning can keep you from aching or getting laid up.

Particular exercises Dr. Emmett recommends:

- Bench press for chest and shoulder strength
- Biceps curls for lifting power
- Overhead triceps extensions for chopping power
- Crunches for back support
- Back extensions for lifting support
- A stretching routine to guarantee you have a full range of motion

The third aspect of health and fitness for the outdoor worker, says Dr. Emmett, is hydration. Carry a water bottle, cooler or thermos with you. Think of yourself as an athlete, whether you're working in the garden or digging postholes. You need about eight ounces of fluid every 20 minutes during heavy physical activity, he says.

The Wilderness Gym

The rural outdoors lend themselves to myriad fitness possibilities. Among them:

- **Incline work.** "Literally use the hills as resistive equipment," says exercise physiologist John Amberge, director of corporate programs for the Sports Training Institute in New York City. "When you're walking, hiking or biking on an uphill elevation, you don't have to go at the same pace as on flat terrain to get a great workout."

- **Running.** Try cross-country running, says Dr. Emmett. "Instead of following a specific road or track or being on a particular piece of equipment all the time, get outdoors and run up hills, down hills, on gravel, on grass. The different surfaces and terrains offer great cross-training. Work different muscles. You get in a little endurance work, a little speed work, just by virtue of the changing terrain."

- **Cycling.** You could do both on and off-road cycling. Rural and mountain areas often offer quiet, safe trails and roads to ride. While not a total-body fitness activity, bicycling does build lower-body strength and, if done at a level that gets the heart into training range and holds it there for 20 minutes or so, is a good cardiovascular workout. "Get a training stand for your bike and bring it indoors and use it as a stationary cycle during the winter months," advises Dr. Swencionis.

- **Advanced mountain biking.** "Take advantage of beautiful nature and get a real workout on rugged trails," advises Amberge. Serious mountain biking, he says, combines muscular and aerobic work.

- **Rock climbing.** "Most of us probably wouldn't climb at a pace and pattern for a long enough period to qualify this as a cardiovascular exercise, but it's a great muscular strength and endurance activity," says Amberge.

- **Chores.** "Gardening, wood chopping, these sorts of activities are rarely done continuously in fitness training range—which would really be quite a workout—but the activities themselves have a caloric expenditure value and build muscular strength," says Amberge. "When they're added to your weekly volume of activities, you see a beneficial lifestyle pattern."

Study the exercises in the Core Routine on page 121 and you'll see ways to incorporate their moves into your daily chores, Amberge adds. For instance, you can do curls or squats or lunges gripping buckets of feed corn in each hand, or with logs at the log pile. You don't have to have specialized equipment.

• Skiing and skating. "Cross-country skiing and ice-skating both offer muscular strength and endurance benefits," points out Amberge. When sustained for continuous bouts of 15 to 20 minutes or more, these activities will improve aerobic capacity, he adds.

Proper Log-Splitting Technique

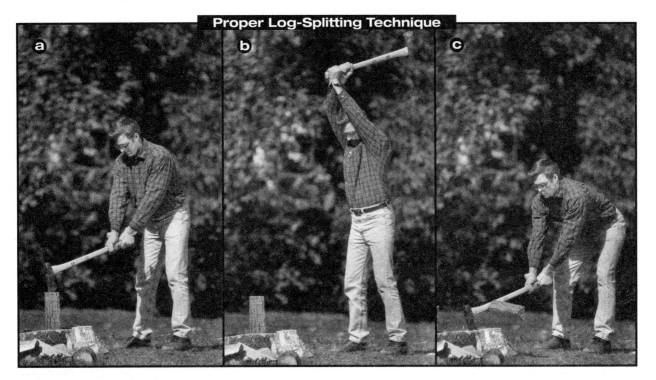

Sharpening a Skill ▲

We may split hairs over technique, but we all think we know how to split a log.

But 18,000 would-be Paul Bunyans injure themselves with an ax or hatchet every year. So, really, we don't want to chop you off at the knees, Bud, but what's the harm in reviewing a little technique?

● Start by getting your ax together. A maul is the preferred variety. A maul has a head like a wedge, with some weight on it. Make sure the head is on tight and the blade is sharp. Save the hatchets and handheld tools for kindling. For log-splitting, you want the big guy.

● Get your gear on. Veteran log whacker Bob Billings of Maine recommends heavy-weight high-topped boots and safety goggles.

● Use a hardwood chopping block. It should be at least 16 inches in diameter.

● Stand your log upright on the block. You'll cut with the grain. Spread your feet wide, plant them firmly and grasp the maul. Hold the handle with your hands close together, about two inches from the end.

ⓐ Get in position. Rest the blade on the center of the log in front of you and keep your eye there.

ⓑ Raise the maul. Now gently, smoothly, swing it straight up over your head.

ⓒ And let it drop. The maul should fall directly on the target, using your hands to guide it. Let the maul do the work. That's what you bought it for.

Some don'ts:

● Don't split unseasoned wood. It will fight you and, besides, it won't burn right and will soot up your chimney. You'll know dry wood by its weight and its cracks and splits. A log gets lighter as it sheds its moisture.

● Don't use an ax as a wedge, pounding it into a log with a sledgehammer. You'll hurt the ax—mess with its head, so to speak.

● Don't use the back side of an ax head as a hammer to drive a wedge. Why? Well, when you raise the ax, you have the blade pointing at you. Enough said? If using a wedge, pound it with a sledgehammer.

Oceanfront Living

You don't have to wax your chest, hoist dumbbells and pose on Muscle Beach to get fit at the ocean.

If you're fortunate enough to live in a coastal area, then you must know the enlivening effect of salt air, sunshine, glistening water and offshore breezes. The combination simply lends itself to fitness.

Listen to San Diego–area lifeguard supervisor Leonard Ortiz.

"When it comes to exercise, most people find it hard to get motivated about going to a weight room or getting on a machine just to do an aerobic thing. But when you come down to the coast, even if it's just for a brisk walk or a job like mine, or you're slipping the roller blades on, there's something in the air. It's a lot more enjoyable. You have the ocean to look at, a nice breeze; it's energizing. Hey, I'm here every day. I know. I'm in paradise."

Ortiz gives talks on beach fitness activities for the California State Department of Parks and Recreation; he's particularly an expert on surfing.

We asked him and others for guidance on how to use the beach as an exercise tool. There are endless alternatives. Here are just a few.

When Ortiz sits in his elevated lifeguard station, as far as his eye can see, people are engaged in myriad fitness activities. Here are a few he recommends.

Running

Choose your terrain, choose your level of workout. Lifeguards know all about running. After passing a test requiring them to swim 1,000 yards in the ocean under 20 minutes, they must then complete the "Run-Swim-Run." "You must run 200 yards, swim 400 yards and then run 200 yards in 8 to 10 minutes—depending upon ocean conditions. It's not very easy," says Ortiz.

Lesson one: Running in soft sand is an entirely different workout than running on solid ground. What you run in soft sand, "the range of motion and the quantity of muscles incorporated in the running movement increase. It takes a lot more power and stresses the joints and muscles in ways in which they are not stressed on a flat surface," explains Ken Sprague, coach and strength trainer, owner and operator of the original Gold's Gym and author of *Sports Strength*.

"Running in the soft-pack—the soft sand—is good if you're working on strengthening your muscles for more push, more lift," Ortiz adds.

To avoid serious soreness the next day, Sprague recommends that you start slowly and don't overdo soft-sand running.

Lesson two: If you want to do distance running along the ocean, you'll need to be a student of the tides. Literally. "Look at a tide book and run at lower tide down close to the water where the water has already packed the sand," says Ortiz. "You can even run barefoot, provided it's not rocky."

But know your beach before heading out without shoes, he advises. Some beaches have a lot of broken shells; some have boulders and cliffs or other rugged terrain.

If running in the sand is a bit too hard on your joints or calves, slow it down. "Walking is excellent conditioning if you walk on the soft-pack," says Ortiz. Or walk vigorously along beachfront walkways. There are usually a lot of good walking trails in beach areas.

Swimming

"Swimming in the ocean is a lot different from swimming in a pool," notes Ortiz. You deal with currents and rip currents and waves and swells. You have a wide-open expanse of water, so it's easy to lose direction. And you have more buoyancy. Ortiz considers that a benefit.

"I'm a very strong pull-swimmer, but I have heavy leg drag—very little flutter kick," says Ortiz. "In a pool my legs sink. But in the salt water, I float better. I can outswim guys in the ocean who swim circles around me in a pool."

Dealing with Currents

"Pay attention to what the ocean is doing, what the currents are, what the rip currents are doing," says Ortiz. You can ask surfers and lifeguards or watch the TV weather. Coastal TV stations all give water-condition reports, he says.

"If there is a longshore current, and you're going to swim parallel to the shore, you need to swim with the longshore current, not against it."

Longshore current?

"Along the California coast in the summer, we get south swells from storms off the Baja in Mexico. The weatherman will talk about 'south swells.' Well, south swells bring a north longshore current. So in the summer, along the Southern California coast, plan to swim north so you aren't fighting the current."

The theory, he says, holds for "the East Coast, any ocean, anywhere. There are different variables, and you need to check the local information, but you're going to have rip currents and longshore currents. In some places it'll be more dramatic than in others. So be aware of them."

Dealing with Direction

The current is going to mess with you as you try to swim from Point A to Point B, notes Ortiz. If you're fitness swimming to and from a distant buoy, "you need to know how the current is pulling so you end up close to the buoy, while swimming in as straight a line as you can," he says. This is sort of like how a skeet shooter must take into account his moving target and shoot a bit ahead of it.

And swimming in a straight line in the ocean is no easy feat. "Periodically, lift your head up and set

---

Coping with Rip Currents

Rip currents (also known as riptides) are narrow currents that move water along the shore's edge back toward the ocean. They are usually between 50 and 150 feet wide and can flow hundreds of yards behind the surfline. They sometimes flow out of large holes not too far offshore. Rip currents can drag swimmers away from shore.

The best strategy, if you find yourself suddenly caught in one, is to start swimming parallel to the shore until you are out of the rip current. Most serious riptides are only a few hundred yards across at best, and by swimming parallel to the shore, you'll swim out of it. Once you are out of it, you can swim toward shore. If you try to swim toward shore while you are still in a rip current, you'll wear yourself out fighting it and trying to stay afloat. The other strategy is to just call or wave for help. Rip currents can be dangerous—don't take them as a personal challenge or a test of manhood. If someone can help you get out of one, by all means, take advantage of it.

Better yet, avoid them when you can. You can spot a rip current by its choppy, foamy surface and by the dirty brown color of the water, which is caused by the sand it churns up.

---

your bearings. Every three or four strokes or so," says Ortiz. "There's no pool wall or lane lines to keep you moving straight. And most swimmers don't have equal arm pull. One arm is stronger, pulls harder than the other. And if you aren't paying attention in the ocean, you'll find yourself swimming in circles or at least a pretty crooked line."

Ortiz's secret: "It helps if you pick a land mass or some fixed object (like a fishing boat or a buoy) even before you get in the water that you'll use as your setting."

Surfing

Surfing is probably the most popular ocean activity in Southern California, notes Ortiz. It takes a lot of skill and involves delicate balance, lots of quick, lithe movements and a fair amount of vigorous swimming, so it is a fitness activity, he says.

One rarely sees a surfer dancing atop a board who looks out of shape or significantly overweight. A more robust build lends itself better to bodysurfing.

"There are many forms of surfing," Ortiz says. "The purest form is bodysurfing, the guy with a pair of fins; then boogie boards; regular surfboards; then long boards. And now there are guys out there kayaking in the surf, and people surf-skiing."

A Beginner's Guide to Bodysurfing

No boards, no gizmos, just you and the water. Bodysurfing—when you ride the top of a wave on your chest and stomach—is a pure thrill. And it can be quite a fitness activity. Here are the basics so you can try bodysurfing.

• Walk or swim out to just beyond where the big waves seem to be breaking, and feel and watch the swells. Pretty soon you'll have some idea which ones are likely to break soon after they pass you.

• Pick a good-candidate swell and swim furiously forward atop it—your body pointed toward the shore.

• As the wave breaks, fight to get your chest just ahead of the curl of the wave, hold your body rigid and let the wave's power propel you forward.

When perfect, your body rides the wave like a surfboard. It's a charge. When less than perfect, you flail your arms and kick like mad, and the wave gets away from you. Or doesn't break when you expected it to. Or breaks suddenly and splats you in the sand.

Seasoned bodysurfers wear swim fins, which give them more kick-power and better control. Some wear high-tech wetsuits so they can stay in the water for hours almost year-round. More recently, bodysurfers have taken to boogie boards for faster, easier, longer wave riding.

Bodysurfing is a workout because no one catches every wave. You do get better at it with practice. Better at timing. Better at positioning. Better at form and technique. But still, you do a lot of swimming between great rides. And for every good ride, you have a long walk and swim against the swells to get back out to the wavebreak.

Other Activities

The possibilities for fitness fun on the beach don't have to involve the water. Here are some other activities Ortiz recommends.

• Beach volleyball. "Anywhere where there's a nice sandy beach, you find people putting their poles and nets up for volleyball," he says. If you want a game right now, bring your own poles, net and group, he says. Most existing groups are pretty experienced and have established rotations; you don't just join a game in progress.

• Skating. "Anywhere there's a sidewalk or parking lot, you'll find people roller-blading and skateboarding," Ortiz says. Both, he says, are good aerobic, lower-body muscle-builders.

• Bicycling. "People don't ride their bikes in the sand, of course, because that's bad for the bikes. But in the West, the Pacific Coast Highway runs along the beach, and in many areas there are bike trails right along the water, and people ride their bikes in packs of 100 and more. Bicycling is big."

Beyond that, there's Frisbee throwing, kite flying (the new high-tech kites that fly circles and dive involve several pull lines and might give you a bit of an upper-body workout), surf fishing and even metal detecting—folks walking along the beach waving their metal detectors and locating coins, pop-tops and what-have-you—nature walks and birder's hikes, and. . . . Gotta go. Someone just yelled, "Surf's up!"

Cold Weather

Peak Points

- **Think of the cold as an exercise tool, not an exercise excuse.**

- **Dress appropriately to conserve heat and keep your body dry.**

- **Use common sense—learn to recognize when it's too cold to exercise outside.**

When the temperature starts to drop, so does our interest in working out. It's cold. It's icy. We might slip. We might fall. And even if we're exercising indoors, it just seems like too much effort to get from the car to the gym, change, work out, shower, and drive home in a cold car with wet hair. Plus, the days seem shorter—it's dark when we get out of work. We don't want to waste any time exercising; we just want to get home and hibernate until spring.

If you live in a place where cold weather strikes, you're probably all too familiar with this litany of excuses. What you may not know is this: You get a better workout in cold weather than in hot. It's true. You don't lose as much water and you don't overheat as quickly, so you can work out longer and possibly harder. Also, there's some evidence that cold weather actually causes your body to work harder—your heart has to contend with pumping blood faster not only to keep up with your exercise but also to keep you warm.

"There's plenty of anecdotal evidence to show that people respond better to exercising in the cold," says Al Paolone, Ed.D., professor of exercise physiology in the physical education department at Temple University in Philadelphia. "They tend to feel more invigorated after a chilly morning run than after a jog through sweltering heat."

Frigid Fitness Factors

That's not to say you shouldn't be a little more careful when you exercise in the ice and snow. A cold-weather workout—for our purposes, that's any exercise you do outside in temperatures in the low 40s or colder—can be hard on your body. We're talking frostbite, injuring yourself from a slip on the ice, throwing your back out from snow-shoveling—you get the idea.

And if you have a history of heart or lung trouble, a cold-weather workout could be dangerous. "You definitely want a doctor's okay before you work out a lot in cold weather," cautions David Spodick, M.D., professor of medicine at the University of Massachusetts Medical School and director of the cardiac fellowship program at St. Vincent Hospital, both in Worcester. "Winter exercise puts more strain on your cardiovascular system, both from the cold itself and from whatever exercise you're engaged in. It requires that you have a little common sense and the presence of mind to prepare for the cold," he says.

Making a Cold Start

How then do you prepare for a cold-weather workout? Follow these tips and you may just earn the best, safest—and certainly the coolest—workout of your life.

Warm up first. You'll be able to exercise more efficiently in cold weather if you take a few minutes to warm up indoors first. "Something as simple as jogging in place for a few minutes before going outside will limber up your muscles and get your heart and lungs working. Then when you go outside, you'll find that the cold isn't so bad," says Dr. Paolone.

Reference Points

Windchill Chart

Wind Speed (MPH)	Thermometer Reading							
	50	40	30	20	10	0	-10	-20
Calm	50	40	30	20	10	0	-10	-20
5	48	37	27	16	6	-5	-15	-26
10	40	28	16	4	-9	-24	-33	-46
15	36	22	9	-5	-18	-32	-45	-58
20	32	18	4	-10	-25	-39	-52	-67
25	30	16	0	-15	-29	-44	-59	-74
30	28	13	-2	-18	-33	-48	-63	-79
35	27	11	-4	-20	-35	-51	-67	-82
40	26	10	-6	-21	-37	-53	-69	-85

Little Danger   **Increasing Danger**   **Great Danger**

Watch the weather. Before you go out for a wintertime run, be sure you know what the temperature is out there and, more important, the windchill factor. "That's your best indicator of how cold it really is outside," says Dr. Paolone. "And if you know that, you'll know how much to bundle up—or whether you should stay indoors." We've included a handy windchill chart to help you prepare for the cold.

Cover your mouth. Mouth and nose feeling raspy from breathing in all that cold air? Don't let it slow you down.

"When you're doing moderate exercise, wear a scarf or some kind of covering over your mouth," says Henry Gong, M.D., chief of the environmental health service at Ranchos Los Amigos Medical Center in Downey, California. This will slightly warm up the air before it gets into your airways, thus making breathing easier. "It's especially good for people with a history of respiratory problems, such as exercise-induced asthma. Cold air really agitates these problems," says Dr. Gong.

Live in layers. Layering is your best weapon against cold weather. "By wearing several layers of clothes, you create cushions of warm air between the cold and your skin. That will keep you warmer and prevent loss of body heat and possible hypothermia," says Dr. Paolone. If you're seriously exercising outdoors, you'll want to wear three layers.

• Under layer. That sounds like "underwear," and for good reason; this is the layer closest to your skin. Ideally, you'll want a set of long johns made of a synthetic material like polypropylene or Capilene—these are designed to wick sweat and moisture away from your body, thus keeping you dry and warm. Avoid cotton, which soaks up moisture, leaving you wet and cold.

• Insulating layer. This layer helps trap body heat. You'll want some insulating bulk, but nothing so thick that you can't fit the last layer over it. Wool pants or shirts are okay, but because they soak up a lot of moisture and are bulky, think about investing in lightweight synthetics like Hollofil, Thinsulate or polyester fleece.

• Outer layer. This is also known as your shell layer. Your main concern here isn't how thick it is, says Dr. Paolone, but how waterproof and breathable it is. Coated nylon or materials like Gore-Tex help move moisture out, but also keep it from getting in.

Wear a hat. You can lose as much as 40 percent of your body heat through the top of your head. You'll be able to work out longer and better by wearing a hat. So wear one—and we mean a hat, not just ear warmers or a headband. Preferably, the hat should be made of an insulating material like wool and should cover the top of your head and most of your ears, says Dr. Paolone. That rules out baseball caps.

Protect your fingers. Don't overlook your fingers in cold weather. They are susceptible to frostbite. The best way to prevent that is to cover your fingers. Mittens are better than gloves, says Dr. Paolone, because they trap warm air around your fingers.

Wear sunglasses. You have to worry about ultraviolet rays even in winter. If you are out skiing down a snowy mountain on a sunny day, you'll need sunglasses to protect your eyes from damage. Buy a brand with ultraviolet blocking on the lenses, says Merrill Allen, O.D., Ph.D., professor emeritus of optometry at Indiana University in Bloomington.

Warming to a Winter Workout

Now that you know what to do before you go out in the cold, you'll want to make the most of the actual workout. Whether you're running, cycling or shoveling snow, there are ways to stay as warm and safe as possible, even when the mercury is dropping faster than a crashing stock market. Try these.

Use the buddy system. Indoors or out, if you want to work out when it's cold, drag a friend along with you. "If you're having trouble motivating yourself to get to the gym, having a friend to work out with makes you less likely to blow off exercise. You'll feel obligated to one another to work out, and that's good," says Dr. Paolone.

Outdoors, the buddy system takes on even greater significance for your general well-being. "If

Cool Sports

There's a whole cluster of exercises and sports you can enjoy in the winter that you'll never be able to do when it's warmer. Here's a list of some old favorites, along with ones you may never have tried.

• Snowshoeing: With this hybrid of running and cross-country skiing, you can burn about 735 calories in just an hour of tramping across the snow-steeped landscapes. Beginners may notice pains in their upper legs and lower torso. Snow shoes make a lot of people feel like they have to walk in a wider stance—that wide step is going to put an extra strain on hip and groin muscles. Stretching before you step out in the snow is key. Meanwhile, check out newer-design snowshoes—they're smaller and faster, making you feel less like you have tennis racquets strapped to your feet.

• Snow hiking: Snowshoeing is a good cardiovascular sport, but if you don't have the money or the inclination to buy snowshoes, walking around in snow, especially deep snow, can be great exercise, too. "It's certainly harder on the legs and heart than just walking around," says Al Paolone, Ed.D., professor of exercise physiology in the physical education department at Temple University in Philadelphia.

Note: Wear good, insulated boots for this exercise; otherwise, your feet will get too cold too fast.

• Sledding: As a kid, you'd never have known what a grueling form of exercise this could be. Now that you're an adult sledding with your kids, the rules have changed dramatically, and your body is lodging a formal protest. That's because sledding does offer some good exercise, a fact you'll realize by your third trip to the top of the hill with your trusty old Flexible Flyer in hand. A good hour of sledding can burn about 420 calories off your less-than-aerodynamic frame.

But sledding can also cause muscle pulls in older guys—the result of scrunching middle-aged bodies onto sleds designed for 12-year-olds. Plus, sliding pell-mell down an icy slope may make you a little more tense than you were in your youth and—hey, what's that giant oak doing in the middle of the hill?

To avoid serious muscle pain later on, stretch before you slide. And don't use your kid's sled; buy yourself a nice, roomy, adult-size, five-foot-long toboggan. Finally, don't slide on your stomach or lean too far forward when you're sledding (especially on a toboggan—you'll hit your chin on the curved front). These positions will force you to arch and bend your back unnaturally.

• Ice climbing: This extreme sport is fundamentally like mountain climbing, only really slippery. Ice climbing requires strong arms and legs to hoist your body up a slippery slope. But that's just one aspect of the sport. "We emphasize intelligence and technique rather than brute strength when ice climbing," says Mike Hardert, director and senior guide for the International Mountain Climbing School in North Conway, New Hampshire. "And it helps to have really good balance." Learning this cold and dangerous sport might leave your wallet muscle sore, too: Lessons can run you $175 a day.

• Playing in the snow: We don't have exact figures for how many calories you burn during a snowball fight or while you're building a snowman, but you'll get a workout, trust us. Just be careful when you're throwing. You're probably on a slippery surface as it is. Hurling a snowball with all your might could knock you over or cause you to twist something. And when you're rolling Frosty's head over to the rest of his body, be careful picking it up. Remember that a giant ball of wet snow is pretty heavy. So lift with your legs, not your back.

one of you gets injured or pulls a muscle, the other can go for help," says Dr. Paolone. Once you're sitting still in the cold, nursing that sprain, you become a ready victim for hypothermia, a drastic loss of body heat caused by cold exposure.

Stay in the sun. Despite what the mercury tells you, some places outdoors are colder than others.

"You can modify your workouts so that you're exercising in the warmest possible places," says Dr. Paolone. For example, try to work out when and where you can see sunlight. "Even though it's cold, you'll get some radiant heat from the sun—far more than if you're exercising in the shadows," he says.

Do a dry run. Streets, sidewalks and parks that have been cleared of snow are going to be much warmer running tracks for you than surfaces with even a light dusting of snow or ice. "Besides being less slippery, dry surfaces like cement or tar, instead of snow and ice, will keep your feet warmer," says Dr. Paolone.

Seek sheltered areas. Because of the danger—and the real bone-numbing cold—of icy winds, try to exercise in places where there are plenty of natural and manmade barriers to block the wind. In general, says Dr. Paolone, tree-lined streets are much warmer than a wide-open road or trail where the wind can build up and freeze your butt off.

Put your back to it. You can't always avoid a

stiff winter wind. When you're out running or biking and there's nothing between you and that blustery breeze, turn around and let it blow you the other way. You won't feel as cold with the wind at your back, says Dr. Paolone. If you have to exercise against the wind, do it on your outward trip. Even in winter, you'll be sweating on the return trip. That's why it's better to take the wind on your back coming home. If the wind hits exposed sweaty skin such as your face, you'll rapidly lose body heat through evaporation.

Shovel Smartly

Every winter the number of men dying from heart attacks suddenly doubles or triples. Why? "Some of them are killing themselves by shoveling snow," says Dr. Spodick.

Here's why snow-shoveling is so hard on the heart. First, in cold weather, your ticker has to cope with the stress of pumping more blood to keep you warm; now your blood pressure is elevated. On top of that, when you shovel snow, you're mixing two very different kinds of exercise. "First you're lifting a static weight, then you're throwing it. And you're doing the two in quick succession," says Dr. Spodick. Each action is tough on the heart by itself; taken together, they're a brutal combination.

And yet, if you don't have a history of heart trouble and you've been working out regularly, snow-shoveling can be one heck of a cold-weather exercise. Here's how to do it right, according to John Emmett, Ph.D., exercise physiologist and associate professor of physical education at Eastern Illinois University in Charleston.

Proper Shoveling Technique ▶

ⓐ With one hand, hold onto the end of the shovel handle. Place your other hand about 18 inches up from the point where the handle meets the blade. If your hands are a little more than shoulder-width apart, you have the right-size tool for you. Push the shovel straight ahead into the snow—don't shove it off to the left or right, where you might have to twist to pick it up.

ⓑ Scoop up a small load of snow, not a heavy pile—that only puts more of a strain on your heart and back. Take your time and shovel light loads. "This isn't a weight-lifting contest," says Dr. Spodick.

ⓒ Don't lift with your back. Instead, rise up, using mostly your arms and legs to lift the load.

Flipping your snowy load to the side or over your shoulder only pulls muscles and damages lower backs. Turn your whole body to dump the snow, pivoting with your feet, not twisting at the waist.

Finally, take lots of breaks. Stand up straight, walk around—this will keep your spine and your heart happy. If exertion causes any new unpleasantness or pain, discontinue the activity, says Dr. Spodick.

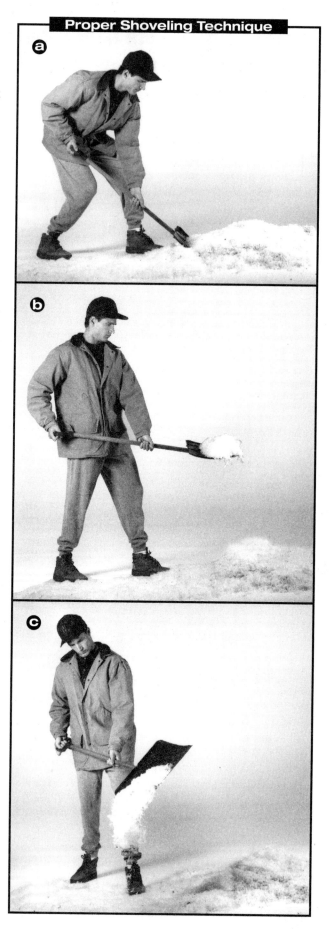

Proper Shoveling Technique

Hot Weather

After a long, cold winter, nothing's more glorious than being outside on that first 70-degree day.

Problem is, 70 degrees all too soon becomes 80 or 90 or even (gasp!) 100 degrees. Spring becomes summer and summer becomes an oven. The outdoor workout that left you invigorated in April now has you panting like a dog in July. Your feet burn. Your legs ache from heat cramps. Your vision blurs from the quarts of sweat streaming off your brow and the waves of heat shimmering ahead of you. If this is what being one of the boys of summer is like, you'd just as soon be a fall guy. And you will be if you don't take steps to minimize the effect of hot weather on your athletic performance.

"Hot weather puts all kinds of stresses on your body that aren't nearly as problematic in cooler situations," says Al Paolone, Ed.D., professor of exercise physiology in the physical education department at Temple University in Philadelphia. First, when we get hot, we sweat—a lot. Sweating results in large water losses. That's nothing to take lightly—dehydration kills. So does heatstroke, which happens when heat, fluid loss and physical exertion overwhelm your body's natural cooling system, causing your temperature to skyrocket. Your body could literally cook itself to death.

In hot weather, as in life, it's the cooler heads that will prevail. "The more you can do to minimize heat and the harmful effects of the sun, the better off you are. That means deflecting sunlight away from you as well as replacing the fluids your body is getting rid of in an effort to keep you cool," says Anthony D. Mahon, Ph.D., associate professor of exercise physiology in the Human Performance Lab at Ball State University in Muncie, Indiana.

Gearing Up for Warm Weather

When it's 80-plus degrees and the sun's out, you're probably thinking all you need to work out is a T-shirt and shorts. Think again. If you don't prepare yourself adequately to deal with hot weather, you could be facing sunburn, blisters and muscle cramps at a minimum, and heatstroke and skin cancer at a maximum. So take a moment to equip yourself for a hot time. Here's all you need.

- A water bottle. You can lose up to two quarts of fluid an hour when you're training in the heat. If you don't replace that fluid, you can suffer fatigue, headaches, muscle cramps, nausea, dizziness—just some of the signs of dehydration. As it is, you should be drinking six to eight eight-ounce glasses of water a day, at the very least. In addition, drink at least six ounces of fluid for every 15 minutes you're exercising in the heat, suggests Dr. Mahon. And we don't mean fluids that contain caffeine or alcohol—those ingredients will actually cause you to lose more fluid. It is also a good idea to be well-hydrated before you start exercising.

- Light, loose clothing. Light-colored, loose-fitting clothing will help keep you cool. Yeah, you were right—wearing a T-shirt and shorts is just fine for the outdoors. But avoid wearing any black or dark

Heat-Beating Beverages

Thanks to good promotion and perhaps their intriguingly salty and sugary taste, sports beverages are jumping off the shelves of grocery stores. The experts we talked with don't completely believe in them, however. It's not that they are bad for you; they're perfectly fine. It's just that it takes an enormous amount of exertion to become depleted in the things that sports drinks boast most about replenishing.

Many of these sports beverages contain electrolytes like sodium and potassium that offset sodium losses through sweat and help keep muscles from cramping up. But it is a rare guy who gets depleted of sodium; our salty diets more than take care of our needs, even when we lose a lot of sodium via sweat. In addition, many of these drinks are high in carbo-

hydrates (mostly sugar), which may give you an energy boost to help you exercise longer. Still, if your workout is an hour or less, water or orange juice is your best bet for rehydrating yourself. We took a look at some of the most popular sports drinks to see how they measured up.

Sports Drink (8-oz. serving)	Sodium	Potassium	Calories
10-K	55 mg.	30 mg.	60
All Sport	55 mg.	50 mg.	70
Exceed	50 mg.	45 mg.	70
Gatorade	110 mg.	30 mg.	50
Powerade	28 mg.	32 mg.	70
Hydra Fuel	25 mg.	50 mg.	64

colors—they absorb heat and will make you hotter, says Dr. Mahon.

• A brimmed hat. Light clothing is an important part of your warm-weather wardrobe, but a good hat is the real topper to any hot-weather exercise outfit. Make sure that hat is made of plastic mesh or straw— something with plenty of airholes to vent heat. It should also have a good-size brim to protect your eyes and give you extra coverage from the burning sun, suggests Dr. Mahon.

• Sunglasses. Don't want an eye burn, do you? If you're spending any time out in the sunshine, and particularly if you are at a place where light reflects easily off surfaces (like a beach or a baseball diamond), you'll need sunglasses to protect your eyes from retinal burns caused by ultraviolet (UV) rays. For safety's sake, buy a brand with UV blocking, which will help keep the sun's radiation from damaging your eyes, says Merrill Allen, O.D., Ph.D., professor emeritus of optometry at Indiana University in Bloomington.

• A layer of sunscreen. We can't guarantee that sunscreen will improve your athletic performance in hot weather, but it's probably the most important item you can wear under the sun. Sunscreen keeps the sun's ultraviolet radiation from penetrating your skin. Yes, that prevents you from getting a tan, but it can also keep you from getting skin cancer. Make sure it has a sun protection factor (SPF) of at least 15, suggests the American Institute for Cancer Research. And buy a brand that's waterproof, so you won't sweat the stuff off too quickly.

• Petroleum jelly. Nothing shortens a workout like the searing pain of a blister tearing open, exposing raw flesh to your burning sweat—talk about salt

in an open wound. You can keep blisters at bay with just a little dab of petroleum jelly. Rub some onto your heel, the pad of your foot or wherever you're prone to blisters, suggests Gary M. Gordon, D.P.M., director of the running and walking program at the Joe Torg Center for Sports Medicine at Hahnemann Hospital in Philadelphia. It feels a little slimy at first, but you'll get used to it.

How to Take the Heat

Even with proper preparation, you're bound to face some harsh realities of exercising in hot weather.

"Men who are very careful about exercising in hot weather can still end up in the hospital with heatstroke or a heart attack. They may have been in fairly good shape, but the heat got the better of them," says David Spodick, M.D., professor of medicine at the University of Massachusetts Medical School and director of the cardiac fellowship program at St. Vincent Hospital, both in Worcester. Now, you could avoid this fate by, say, joining an air-conditioned gym or taking up swimming as your full-time exercise. Of course, you may be the type who just has to exercise outside, no matter that tar roads are bubbling or trees are spontaneously bursting into flames. In that case, take heed.

Start slow. When you first begin working out in hot weather, be sure to pace yourself, says Dr. Paolone. Keep your workout to about 15 to 20 minutes. Each day, gradually increase your workout time by about 5 to 10 minutes. This will get your body acclimated to hotter weather and decrease your likelihood of suffering a heat-induced injury.

Stay off the tar. Avoid exercising on tracks or streets with tarred surfaces, says Dr. Mahon. Black tar absorbs incredible amounts of heat. That heat will radiate back up off the tar and only make you hotter. Stick to the sidewalk or seek out dirt tracks.

Seek the shade. Try to find places to exercise where there's shade or shelter from direct sunlight, suggests Dr. Mahon. Running along a tree-covered track will keep you much cooler than running in direct, glaring sun.

Check the climate. When you're hot, you're hot, but different kinds of heat will affect your performance in different ways. Humid heat, which can make running feel like swimming, is especially hard on your heart and lungs. Before you go out for exercise, check the humidity—the closer it is to 100 percent, the more you should think about shortening your run.

Conversely, dry heat, so often associated with the arid Southwest, may seem easier to deal with, but it, too, takes its toll. "The problem with dry heat is that you may not realize just how hot it is until it's too late," explains Dr. Spodick. With dry heat, our sweat evaporates off us as fast as we can perspire it. Consequently, we don't notice how much fluid we're losing; that leaves us wide open for dehydration and heatstroke. Either condition could kill you if left unchecked. So if you decide to exercise in dry heat, be sure to bring along plenty of water. Drink it often—and drink before you feel thirsty.

Pepper yourself with salt—cautiously. If you don't have heart or kidney disease, crunch on a few pretzels or low-fat potato chips after your workout. According to Dr. Spodick, in healthy individuals, eating salty foods after a dehydrating workout can help you retain fluids and increase blood volume. Don't overdo it—a handful of chips ought to suffice. Warning: If you have high blood pressure or are on a low-salt diet, talk with your doctor first.

Time your workout. Remember that the hottest time of the day is between 10 A.M. and 3 P.M.—that's also the time when UV radiation from the sun is at its most cancer-causing intense, warns the American Institute for Cancer Research. Try to time your workouts before or after these hours.

Know when to quit. Many of the more dangerous heat-induced ailments are downright insidious. "By the time you feel thirsty, you're already pretty dehydrated. And a lot of people never spot the signs of heatstroke until they're lying in the emergency room," says Dr. Spodick. Don't be one of the numbers. Dizziness, nausea, headaches, diarrhea, irritability, muscle cramps—these are all signs that the heat is getting to you. Stop what you're doing, get yourself to some place cool and take a breather.

The 3-Month Program

You know you should be working year-round on fitness, but real life isn't always about how things ought to be. That's why you're where you are right now—a few months away from the big event you promised to get in shape for last year.

Maybe it's a high school reunion, and you want to burn off the gut you built after your wild years ended. Or maybe your fitter-than-thou colleague down the hall roped you into some corporate challenge triathlon, and there's no backing out. Either way, you need to power up and slim down, and you only have a handful of weeks to do it. Don't waste time going to the gym and blindly trying to pump as much iron as you can in the time you have left.

"You can't just go in and lift and lift and hope for the best. That's how guys injure themselves," says Doug Lentz, Pennsylvania state director of the National Strength and Conditioning Association and owner of the Chambersburg Sports Medicine and Rehabilitation Center in Pennsylvania. "You have to go in with a game plan."

With the help of Lentz and other exercise experts, we've mapped out that 12-week plan. Like the most effective training programs, it focuses on building powerful aerobic benefits for your heart and lungs as well as offering routines for building calorie-burning muscle to help you look and perform great. Be warned: We're asking for a serious time commitment here. If you want to get in good trim in a relatively short span of time, you're going to have to do a lot of something towards your goal every day.

Ninety Days to Fitness

"You'll want to space out your weight training, do it every other day. That gives your muscles a chance to recover," says John Porcari, Ph.D., executive director of the LaCrosse Exercise and Health Program and professor of exercise and sport science at the University of Wisconsin in LaCrosse. As Dr. Porcari explains, it's during the resting phase, not the actual lifting, that your body builds more muscle.

Meanwhile, you can do aerobic exercise almost every day. "I'd try to do something aerobic five or six days a week. It's important to have that strong cardiovascular base," says Dr. Porcari. Plus, five days of aerobic exercise means five days that your body will be working extra hard to burn off some of the excess fat you've been accumulating.

If you haven't followed a regular exercise routine in a while, you may find this program rather grueling. If it's been a few years since you've exercised seriously, or if you've had medical problems, you should get an okay from your doctor before embarking on an exercise program as serious as this one, states Lentz. In addition, if you find this program leaves you too sore to do

Reference Points

The Do's and Don'ts of Diet

Your three months of diligent aerobic and weight training won't do you a lick of good if you don't modify your eating habits over the same period of time.

"First and foremost, cut out the fats," says Peter Lemon, Ph.D., professor of applied physiology at Kent State University in Ohio. "Although the American Heart Association says we should be getting no more than 30 percent of our calories from fat, you should try to shoot for an even lower percentage—20 to 25 percent."

The way to do that, he suggests, is to first set yourself a fat budget—for most men, that will be between 40 and 50 grams of fat per day.

Second, substitute your fat-laden favorites—steaks, doughnuts or deep-dish pepperoni pizza—for lower-fat fare that's just as filling—pasta, bagels or thin-crust pizza with low-fat cheese, mushrooms, peppers and onions.

Whatever you do, don't try to go on a crash diet to drop weight over your three-month training period. "You'll just undermine your workout goals," says Dr. Lemon. When you deprive yourself of food, your body will start burning some of its own stored fuels, but fat won't be the first fuel source—muscle tissue will be. "You might lose weight, but it will be muscle mass. And that's completely opposite of what you want to do," says Dr. Lemon. Instead, focus on aerobic exercise to burn the fat you have, and weight training to build muscle mass. The more muscle mass you have, the more calories you burn, and the less you'll need to diet.

Finally, if you've been able to switch to a low-fat diet during your three-month program, do your body a favor and stick with it for the next three months. And the next. And the next. "You want to avoid a mentality where, after three months, it's okay to go back to old eating habits," says Dr. Lemon. "So many people do it and end up putting on more weight than when they began."

---

the exercises effectively, or you just can't seem to get your body to operate at this level of intensity, there's no shame in admitting it.

"Everyone's different. Your recovery time might be longer than someone else's; you may not be able to do as many reps at the suggested intensity level. That's okay. Don't get discouraged," says Lentz. If Wednesday finds you still sore from Monday's workout, feel free to take an extra day to recover, or lift weights at a slightly lower intensity. Keep in mind that sore muscles mean the muscle tissue is rebuilding, coming back even bigger and stronger than before.

Don't focus so much on trying to do the exact number of sets and reps we recommend, Lentz says, but try to adhere to the basic principles we established in our Weight Lifting chapter. If we recommend two to three sets of 12 to 15 reps of light weights, and you can only stay at the low end of that range, that's fine—so long as you're still doing lots of reps of a light weight. Whatever you do, try to stick to your routine in some fashion—and don't give up.

As you'll see, in the first two months this intensive program focuses on getting your aerobic fitness to a high performance level while building significant muscle. The last month of the program is designed to help you take your strength to a new level. If you're working toward a more aerobic goal or you're planning to compete in an endurance sport, like a race, follow the first two months of the plan as shown. In the last month, spend just one day a week in the gym doing muscle-maintenance; the rest of the time, focus on preparing for the event. The sport-specific chapters in this part of the book will provide you with dozens of workout options you can use in that final month of preparation.

But first, you have to start your three-month program. Follow it faithfully and you'll find yourself fit and firm fast. That's our 90-day guarantee.

The First Month

Goals

Build a strong cardiovascular base by getting your aerobic capacity up to 30 minutes a day. Get right into a weight-training regimen. Lentz recommends using light weights and doing high reps, with roughly a minute's rest between sets.

Exercises

For your first month's weight training, Dr. Porcari suggests focusing on your chest, shoulders and calves. "These muscles take longer to build than most others, so start right away on them," he says. We factored that into your first-month workout. Do all exercises in the order listed.

- Legs: Leg press   page   95
- Legs: Leg curls   page   100
- Legs: Standing heel raises   page   100
- Chest: Wide-grip bench press   page   70
- Chest: Dumbbell flies   page   71

- Back: Bent-over rows page 88
- Back: Back extensions page 85
- Shoulders: Shrugs page 64
- Shoulders: Military press page 66
- Arms: Barbell curls page 48
- Arms: Overhead triceps extensions page 51
- Abs: Crunches page 77
- Abs: Oblique crunches page 83

Week 1

Start off with 10 to 15 minutes of aerobic exercise at about 65 percent of your maximum heart rate—this is the low end of your aerobic training zone.

Determining how much weight to lift takes a little guesswork at the beginning, Lentz explains. Experiment to find out how much weight you can lift with good form and still stay within the numbers of sets and reps required for your workout. The logic is a little circular, but a light weight is one that you can lift for 12 to 15 reps, a moderate weight, one you can lift for 8 to 10 reps, and a heavy weight, one you can lift for 3 to 5 reps. If you can do more than the highest number of reps, the weight is too light. Increase the weight by the smallest increment possible to get back into your zone. If you can't manage the lowest number of reps, cut back on the weight until you are back in your zone. You have the right amount of weight if you can complete the required sets and reps and still feel challenged.

In the first week, start with light weights. Do two to three sets of each exercise listed, lifting 12 to 15 reps per set.

Week 2

Add another five minutes to your aerobic workout—15 to 20 minutes—at 65 to 70 percent of your max. Increase your weight-training sets so you're now rising to the high end of the same range as week one: two to three sets of light weights, 12 to 15 reps per set.

Week 3

Move your aerobic workout up to 20 to 25 minutes, continuing at the same intensity as last week. As for weight lifting, this week increase the number of sets. Do three to four sets, 12 to 15 reps of light weights per set. You should start out at the low end of this scale—don't try to do four sets of 15 reps from the beginning.

Week 4

Thanks to your five-minute-a-week plan, you should have doubled your aerobic workout by now—exercising for 25 to 30 minutes at about 70 percent of your maximum heart rate. Continue to lift light weights, but now you should move your weight training to the higher end of the three- to four-set, 12- to 15-rep range.

The Second Month

Goals

This month, you'll want to add ten minutes to your aerobic workout. Keep building strength by lifting heavier weights—you should be noticing some definite physical improvement this month. To avoid injuring yourself as you move to progressively heavier weights, increase your rest from one to two minutes between sets.

Exercises

Here's a new batch of exercises for the month. You can alternate them with last month's exercise list. Varying the exercises you do will help keep you from getting bored and dropping out of your routine, says Anthony D. Mahon, Ph.D., associate professor of exercise physiology in the Human Performance Lab at Ball State University in Muncie, Indiana.

- Legs: Dumbbell step-ups and step-downs page 97
- Legs: Squats page 96
- Chest: Decline bench press page 73
- Chest: Alternating dumbbell press page 71
- Back: Rumanian dead lifts page 86
- Back: Lat pull-downs page 128
- Shoulders: Upright rows page 64
- Shoulders: Side lateral raises page 65
- Arms: Hammer curls page 49
- Arms: Seated triceps press page 51
- Abs: Crossover crunches page 78
- Abs: Oblique twists page 82

Week 5

Your aerobic workout time will level off this week, but up the intensity—do 30 minutes at 75 percent of your max. When you hit the weights, do three to five sets of eight to ten reps of moderate weights.

Week 6

Keep your aerobic exercise to 30 minutes, 75 percent of your max. For the weights, keep doing three to five sets of eight to ten reps of moderate weights.

Week 7

Add five minutes to your aerobic exercise, and keep up the heart rate. Meanwhile, consistently continue to do three to five sets of eight to ten reps of moderate weights. Remember: Increase your weight level one notch when you are able to surpass both the maximum set and rep counts.

Week 8

Move your aerobic exercise up to a full 40 minutes per session at the same intensity as last week. Meanwhile, keep doing moderate lifting—shoot for three to five sets of eight to ten reps.

The Third Month

Goals

You're in the homestretch now. If you're working toward a specific goal or event, now's the time to focus on that. Spend most of your workout time doing the activity you'll be doing in the event—running, cycling, whatever you choose. Do get to the gym at least one day a week for weight training, and stick to lifting moderate weights, roughly three to five sets of eight to ten reps.

But if you want to stay with the general program, here's the plan for your final four weeks. First, get your aerobic workout up to 45 minutes. Second, start maximizing your strength by lifting short sets of heavy weights. You'll be resting two to three minutes between sets.

Exercises

The same routine: Mix in these new exercises to keep your workout interesting.

- Legs: Barbell step-ups and step-downs   page 98
- Legs: Dumbbell lunges   page 96
- Chest: Inclined bench press   page 70
- Chest: Decline push-ups   page 74
- Back: Good-morning exercises   page 86
- Back: Bent-over rows   page 88
- Shoulders: Alternating front lateral raises   page 65
- Shoulders: Alternating press with dumbbells   page 66
- Arms: Concentration curls   page 50
- Arms: One-arm triceps pull-downs   page 52
- Abs: Hanging single-knee raises   page 79
- Abs: Sidebends with dumbbells   page 83

Week 9

Your aerobic routine is the same as last week—40 minutes at 75 percent intensity. Weight-wise, lift three to five sets of heavy weights, three to five reps per set.

Week 10

Keep your aerobic workout between 40 and 45 minutes at 75 percent intensity. Repeat your weight-training routine of three to five sets of three to five reps of heavy weights.

Week 11

Your aerobic workout is the same as last week, and keep doing three to five sets of three to five reps of heavy weights, increasing your weight levels when you can surpass those levels.

Week 12

For your last week, do all five or six days of aerobic exercise at 45 minutes per session, 75 percent intensity. Your weight-lifting routine remains the same as the previous three weeks. You should be fit enough for any reunion or sporting event. You look great; you feel great. Why lose your momentum? On Monday, get back to the gym.

The 12-Month Program

Peak Points

- **Set short-term fitness goals.**
- **Factor nutrition into your fitness program.**
- **Vary your workout to ward off boredom.**
- **Think. Plan. You can't reach your peak without a strategy.**

Maybe it was a New Year's resolution. Or a landmark birthday. Whatever the milestone, it's given you a chance to look back over the year, and the view ain't pretty. Long hours at work, short hours at the gym, one too many beers or big meals and—why be delicate?—sheer laziness have conspired against you. You feel dull and sluggish. Gazing into the mirror, you see that you *look* dull and sluggish.

Something in you snaps. With steely resolve, you stare down the corpulent apparition in the mirror. Your mind is made up: By this time next year, that lackluster leadbutt looking back at you will be gone, replaced by the image—no, replaced by the *reality*—of a firmer, fitter you.

Twelve months is a nice chunk of time to get in terrific shape, but it's also a long time in which you could lose your way. If you're going to stay committed to a year of fitness, you'll need a month-by-month plan, one that's flexible enough that you can build in your own goals and favorite exercises, yet specific enough that you won't have to wonder what to do next to stay in shape.

Scoring with Goals

Since you should be working out year-round anyway—not just doing crash training where you give yourself a month to get in shape—most experts agree that a 12-month regimen is one of the best formats for planning a lifetime of fitness. There are some motivational pitfalls to this approach, however.

"Most men want to see results right away—a year is too long for them. The danger here is doing too much too soon and injuring yourself. Or worse, you slog along aimlessly for a few weeks, and you don't see any results, so you give up," says

Anthony D. Mahon, Ph.D., associate professor of exercise physiology in the Human Performance Lab at Ball State University in Muncie, Indiana.

That's why it's important to set some goals in the short term, says Doug Lentz, Pennsylvania state director of the National Strength and Conditioning Association and owner of the Chambersburg Sports Medicine and Rehabilitation Center in Pennsylvania. If you go off saying, "This time next year, I'm going to be 40 pounds lighter and have 10 pounds of new muscle," you're setting yourself up to fail, says Lentz.

"It's too long a time from setting the goal to achieving it. You'll go for weeks without seeing a definitive landmark. And that's why so many men just give up," he says. Instead, give yourself interim goals and reach for those. "Some people set weekly or monthly goals. At the very least, set a quarterly goal," says Lentz. Build a program that pays incentives often and early, and you'll keep yourself on the fitness payroll this year and beyond.

Re-tooling Your Fueling

As you embark on your yearlong quest, don't just think exercise—think nutrition. "If you're eating badly, you're sabotaging your own fitness goals," says Peter Lemon, Ph.D., professor of applied physiology at Kent State University in Ohio. Fatty foods will clog the heart you're trying to improve. Or if you're not getting the recommended daily amounts of essential foods—6 to 11 servings of grains, 2 to 4 servings of fruit, 3 to 5 servings of vegetables—you're robbing those hardworking muscles of the fuel they need for exercise. Make sure your workout mentality extends from the gym to the kitchen.

Goal-setting, nutrition-balancing, exercising—they are all part of the 12-month exercise plan we've designed with input from some of the top fitness experts in the country. Although different experts have different theories about how much weight training and aerobic exercise you should be doing every week, we've grounded this program in a simple, standard format—the three-day-a-week plan. At varying points in the exercise routine, we'll suggest a certain number of reps and sets to help you build strength, size or muscle endurance. Do your best to stay in the ranges we recommend, or at least adhere to the principles, suggests John Graham, director of the Human Performance Center at the Allentown Sports Medicine and Human Performance Center in Pennsylvania.

- Warm-up (5 to 10 minutes)
- Weight training (30 minutes minimum, or as prescribed in the program)
- Aerobic workout (15 minutes minimum, or as prescribed in the program)
- Cooldown and stretching (5 minutes of each)

For obvious reasons, we've built this program on the January-through-December calendar year. If you're reading this in July, though, that doesn't mean you have to wait until the new year to start the regimen. Most of the routines and goals you'll be setting can be accomplished year-round, so feel free to jump in at any time—starting with the January workouts, of course.

The First Quarter

Goals

Fitness: Building cardiovascular fitness by getting your heart operating comfortably in the aerobic training zone—65 percent of your maximum heart rate; building basic muscle tone.

Nutrition: Start working to cut fat consumption to 30 percent or less of your daily calorie intake. Keep your diet high in carbohydrates—they're your muscles' preferred fuel. Spread your meals out, too. Instead of three big ones, eat five or six smaller ones over the course of the day. "This keeps your energy levels more consistent. That will help your performance," says Dr. Lemon. Otherwise, you could "bonk"—lose energy in the middle of the workout. Do that a couple of times, and pretty soon you won't feel like hitting the gym.

Got More Time?

Every once in a blue moon, it happens: You find yourself with a few extra hours during the week—could be a lunch hour, could be an afternoon off. If you find yourself with some time to spare and want to build that time into your workout, you can. It won't throw your month-by-month schedule off, and you won't overtrain or injure yourself. Here are two great things to do.

- Abs-work. The one area of the body most men would like to improve can be worked out on a daily basis. If you have a few extra minutes to spare every day, say first thing in the morning, spend about five minutes doing crunches. "Abs take longer to strengthen, so if you can, really try to work them out every day," says John Porcari, Ph.D., executive director of the LaCrosse Exercise and Health Program and professor of exercise and sport science at the University of Wisconsin in LaCrosse. Strong abs are important for good posture and strengthening your back.

- Aerobic exercise. Expand your aerobic workouts to five days a week. "It doesn't have to be a lot—just an extra 15 or 20 minutes. But you'll build your cardiovascular base that much faster—and you'll feel great," says Dr. Porcari.

January

For the first month of your fitness program, the important thing is to just go and do what you can. "Don't rush in and overdo it. You'll either end up injuring yourself or feel so sore that you'll give up. Either way, you're finished before you've started," warns Dr. Mahon. Instead, make this your orientation period. First, spend some time getting familiar with the machines and finding out what your maximum lift levels are—especially your one-rep max. By knowing the most you can lift in one rep, you'll be able to determine what percentage of this max you need to be lifting later in the program.

"The idea is to start laying a solid foundation that you can build on for the rest of the year," says John Porcari, Ph.D., executive director of the LaCrosse Exercise and Health Program and professor of exercise and sport science at the University of Wisconsin in LaCrosse. Spend at least half your allotted time doing aerobic exercise—stair-climbing, stationary cycling, running, whatever you like. The important thing is to get your heart rate up and keep it to at least 55 percent of your max.

At first, you'll be spending a minimal amount of time lifting weights. "Start off easy," says Graham. Focus on light weights—about 50 to 60 percent of your max—and one to two sets of 12 to 20 reps. To maximize strength gains over the next year, we've modified the Core Routine slightly, adding a couple of extra exercises and making it a little more involved. Here's the workout.

- Legs: Dumbbell lunges   page 96
- Legs: Leg press   page 95
- Chest: Bench press   page 69
- Back: One-arm dumbbell rows   page 88
- Shoulders: Lateral raises   page 123
- Arms: Barbell curls   page 48
- Arms: Overhead triceps extensions   page 51
- Abs: Crunches   page 77
- Abs: Oblique twists   page 82

February

Aerobic exercise will still be the mainstay of your workout, but now you should be upping the intensity so your heart rate is at 65 percent of your max. You should still be lifting relatively light weights, but make some slight increases. Lift at 50 to 60 percent of your max, and do two sets of 12 to 20 reps.

March

Keep increasing the intensity of your aerobic exercise; by now you should be at 70 percent of your maximum heart rate—well into the aerobic training zone. Now that you're familiar with the weights and are comfortable with pumping iron, start working on enhancing muscle development. Do that by dropping the number of reps while increasing the weight you lift. Start doing three to five sets of 8 to 12 reps of

moderate weights—Graham says that's roughly 60 to 70 percent of your max.

To keep things interesting, Lentz recommends varying your workout a little. "It doesn't matter what you do, as long as you're still working out the same major muscle groups." Consider trying these exercises—rotate them with the exercises in the January workout.

- Legs: Squats   page 96
- Legs: Leg curls   page 100
- Chest: Dumbbell flies   page 71
- Back: Back extensions   page 85
- Shoulders: Shoulder shrugs   page 64
- Arms: Inclined alternating
  dumbbell curls   page 129
- Arms: One-arm triceps pull-downs   page 52
- Abs: Frog-leg crunches   page 79
- Abs: Oblique crunches   page 83

The Second Quarter

Goals

Fitness: Start gaining weight—in the form of muscle. Shoot for five pounds of new muscle, and look for signs of muscular definition in your arms, shoulders and chest. Begin training for summer sports.

Nutrition: Continue to squeeze fat out of your diet. Focus more on proteins, which Dr. Lemon says help you build muscle. You'll find protein in lean meats and fish, beans and legumes, and low-fat dairy products.

Got Less Time?

If work deadlines and family obligations are squeezing your workout time down to a minimum, there are some proven ways to safely cut a few corners.

- The one-set workout. Carlos DeJesus, a fitness trainer and bodybuilding champion, recommends that his time-pressed clients do one set of 8 to 12 reps of heavy weights for each exercise in their workout routine. "I've seen the studies, and I've seen the strength gains in my clients. If you go all out on one set of reps, it's better than if you pace yourself for three traditional sets," he asserts. But be aware, this is an intense workout, cautions DeJesus. The key is to go all out, to work to momentary exhaustion. That means you'll probably need a spotter on some of your lifts. Before you start, you should be completely warmed up and stretched out. Finally, don't do a one-set workout more than three times per week.

- Merge warm-ups with aerobic exercise. You can cut 5 or 10 minutes out of your routine by combining your warm-up and your aerobic workout. This will require some minor re-ordering of your routine—instead of the 10-minute warm-up, weight-training, 15 minutes of aerobic exercise, then a cooldown, do 15 to 20 minutes of aerobic exercise at the start of the workout. Begin at a slow pace for the first 5 minutes, then get your heart up into the training zone (the exact intensity will depend on what point you're at in the program). Then do your weight training as usual and a 10-minute cooldown.

"The aerobic activities get the heart pumping and warm up the muscles for weight training just as a warm-up would. And you'll still get the benefit of your normal aerobic workout," says Anthony D. Mahon, Ph.D., associate professor of exercise physiology in the Human Performance Lab at Ball State University in Muncie, Indiana.

But as a reward for reaching your first quarter goals, go ahead and have that burger or beer you promised yourself. Just don't go crazy.

April

As you sense the first hint of spring, you'll be tempted to blow off your workouts. Don't give in to spring fever—instead, start transferring your aerobic workout to the outdoors. Instead of stair-climbing, try speed-walking or running. Instead of stationary cycling, do the real thing. Just remember that you're out there with a specific goal in mind—to keep your heart rate in the aerobic training zone. By now, you should be working firmly at 70 to 75 percent of your max.

Weight-wise, do three sets of eight reps at 65 to 80 percent of the one-rep max you set at the beginning of this program, says Graham. To keep your strength gains from leveling off, vary your exercise program by using the exercises listed in the January and March programs. Alternate the exercises with each workout session. By working the same muscles differently every time you work out, you'll increase your strength gains. "Not only that, you'll keep the workout from becoming too boring—that could kill any workout," says Dr. Mahon.

May

Now's the time to start training for your favorite summer sports. Using the sport-specific chapters in this book as your guide, start adding at least a couple of new sport-specific exercises to your routine every week. Ideally, these are exercises that will increase your lateral movement, explosive power and general strength, speed and mobility. Here are some examples.

- Legs: Box jumps   page 235
- Legs: Tuck jumps   page 224
- Chest: Alternating dumbbell press   page 71
- Back: Back extensions with weights   page 87
- Shoulders: Alternating front lateral
  raises   page 65
- Arms: Wrist rolls   page 56
- Arms: Forearm curls   page 59
- Abs: Raised-leg crunches   page 78
- Abs: Vacuums   page 80

June

You've spent the spring building muscle, now you can start relaxing your building regimen and focus more on maintenance. Cut back your weight training to twice a week. During that time, do two sets of 12 reps at 55 to 65 percent of your max. Then devote your third day entirely to an activity with some aerobic component—your favorite sport, for example (continue to do the minimum 15 minutes of aerobic exercise on your weight-training days, too).

Third Quarter
Goals

Fitness: Work toward a specific sporting or athletic event that's going to put all the gains you've made to the test—a 10-K race, a bicycle century, a swim meet.

Nutrition: Stay the course with less fat and more carbohydrate. In the warmer months, be sure that you're getting enough fluids, says Dr. Lemon. Carry a water bottle with you everywhere you go, and especially during a workout.

July

Increase the time of your aerobic workout so you're doing 30 minutes of aerobic exercise every time you work out. And just as you were varying your weight training to keep from getting bored, vary the aerobic exercise—cycling one day, running the next, maybe some tennis or racquetball thrown in for good measure. To give yourself an excellent short-term goal, Dr. Porcari suggests working toward a specific sports event in late summer—a 10-K running race or a 40-mile bicycling ride, for example.

Move your weight training back up to three days a week, 30 minutes per session. Focus on maintenance—three sets, 12 to 20 reps, 50 to 60 percent of your max. For a benchmark, compare how much you can lift now to what you were lifting in January.

August

More of the same. But now, begin tailoring your aerobic workout to the event you're planning to compete in. If you've signed up for a road race, make sure you're doing plenty of running. If it's a long bike ride, work on your cycling. You get the idea.

September

Extend your aerobic exercise a little more each week—try to add 10 minutes by the end of the month. By now, you're doing at least 40 minutes of aerobic exercise each session. Of course, you may have an actual life to lead, so go ahead and move one of your workout days to the weekend, if you haven't already. Keep working toward that event. Visualize the medal hanging on your wall or the framed eight-by-ten of your gasping self crossing the finish line. Now that's an accomplishment.

Fourth Quarter
Goals

Fitness: Prepare for the winter by packing on a couple of extra pounds of muscle and keeping your aerobic fitness well into the aerobic training zone.

Nutrition: You're approaching the holiday season, a time of stuffed birds, rich desserts and holiday parties. In other words, a fat orgy. Steady on, man.

Try to keep your eating habits consistent. For example, don't starve before a big holiday feed, otherwise you'll pig out on all the wrong foods, Dr. Lemon advises. And should you indulge, don't sit around feeling slovenly about it; get to the gym that much earlier the next day.

October

What with all your fun-in-the-summer antics, you have probably missed a few weight-training workouts, so you'll want to work on muscle development for the remainder of the year. When the holidays roll around, you're going to need that extra muscle to help burn off all the extra food you'll probably be eating. Keep your weight-training schedule at three days a week—three sets of 12 to 20 reps at 50 to 60 percent of your max. And while the weather is still nice, keep doing your aerobic exercise outdoors. Continue doing 40 or more minutes per session.

November

Build up your weight-training intensity—three sets, three to eight reps at 70 to 80 percent of your max. With your emphasis shifting to muscle building, you can reduce your aerobic exercise to 15 to 20 minutes per workout, though more is fine, too. Be sure to keep your heart rate around 75 percent of

your max. To keep a little variety in your weight-lifting workout, add these exercises to your repertoire and alternate them with the other exercises for the various muscle groups.

- Legs: Front squats   page 99
- Legs: Leg curls   page 100
- Chest: Inclined bench press   page 70
- Back: Rumanian dead lifts   page 86
- Shoulders: Alternating press
  with dumbbells   page 66
- Arms: Concentration curls   page 50
- Arms: Seated triceps press   page 51
- Abs: Crossover crunches   page 78
- Abs: Hanging single-knee raises   page 79

December

As you finish up the year and the holidays start to take a big bite out of your schedule, you may find it tougher and tougher to stick to a workout. Sure, it would be easy to skip a few workouts. But we don't call this the ultimate plan for nothing. Do your best to get to the gym three times a week. Try to push the envelope this month—shoot for three sets of six to eight reps at 70 to 80 percent of your max. That way, when the New Year rolls around and you gaze in the mirror again, you won't have to resolve to get fit—you'll only have to resolve to stay fit.

Preventing Injuries

By now, most of us know it's a mistake to think that striving for power and stamina means gasping and grunting during workouts and suffering with throbbing muscle aches later. "No pain, no gain" has become such a thoroughly discredited piffle of an axiom, it hurts just to mention it.

And yet, there's no escaping the fact that gains make pain more likely, if not from overexertion, then from injuries that all too often accompany sports and exercise. It's not that we're willfully trashing ourselves, it's that stuff, you know, happens. But injuries aren't just happenstance: Most of the time, we set ourselves up for them. "A vast number of injuries are completely preventable," says David Janda, M.D., director of the Institute for Preventative Sports Medicine in Ann Arbor, Michigan.

Most injuries involve damage to what we think of as hard muscles, but what doctors refer to as soft tissue—namely pulls and strains. "Soft" refers to the fact that muscles are pliable, stretchable and bendable, which overall makes them pretty forgiving. Still, you have to respect their limits, not only to avoid short-term pain and inconvenience but also unforeseen trouble down the road. "Many injuries can have long-term ramifications physically and economically," Dr. Janda says. "I see people all the time who complain about injuries they got 25 years ago." If you avoid injuring muscles, you'll likely avoid damaging tougher parts of the body as well, such as bones, tendons and ligaments.

Becoming Injury-Resistant

If you've read most of the other chapters in this book, you realize that respect for the body's limits drives a lot of the concepts and principles we've discussed throughout. Here's a roundup of the most crucial ways to keep your body in action and your program on track.

Progress gradually. None of us likes being told to take things easy, but you simply can't rush your gains. Pushing your body harder than it's ready to be pushed results in damage, whether it's tiny tears that make your muscles sore, or larger traumas like lower-back spasms. This is a critical point to remember for anyone beginning a new routine or sport. "For example, on a long-distance, multi-day bicycle tour, we found that people with the least amount of training had the most injuries," says Andrew Dannenberg, M.D., assistant professor at the Injury Prevention Center of Johns Hopkins University School of Hygiene and Public Health in Baltimore.

Warm up. "Without question, inadequate warm-up is the major cause of injury," says Allan M. Levy, M.D., team physician for the New York Giants, partner at the Sports Medicine Center in Fort Lee, New Jersey, and co-author of the *Sports Injury Handbook*. Muscle fibers are like rubber bands: When they're cold, they're stiff and liable to tear. Warm muscles up, and they're not only more pliable but they also contract faster and, in effect, become stronger. Higher body temperature also lubricates joints better and improves muscle cells' ability to convert oxygen and glucose to energy. You just need to raise your body temperature about two degrees—enough to break into a light sweat—by doing light calisthenics, jogging, riding an exercise bike, walking briskly or whatever it takes.

Then stretch. Warming up and stretching go hand-in-hand, Dr. Levy says, and should be considered two parts of a single process. Once muscles are warmed, stretching them increases flexibility, further reducing risk of injury. (For more on stretching, see Flexibility on page 32.)

Use safety gear. A lot of injuries come from a lapse of common sense, Dr. Janda says: not wearing a helmet, for example, when doing sports in which it's common to crack your head. It's an obvious point, but one that's often lost in the interests of feeling the wind in your hair, avoiding hassles, not looking dorky or what have you. The sheer number of headbangers dragged into hospitals every year shows that such temptations take far too great a toll on basic safety measures.

Learn the right moves. Dr. Janda believes that if we all possessed the fundamental skills and understood the basic forms and techniques of our sports, the vast majority of sports injuries would vanish overnight. True, you have to learn by doing,

Part Five
Body
Maintenance

but you can also learn by watching more seasoned participants or reading books and magazines.

When muscles talk, listen. "Don't work through a pain," Dr. Levy says. "If it's persistent, something's wrong and you need rest or treatment." Underline persistent for those times when a little discomfort is part of the deal. "If you're running and feel lousy for the first mile, you can stick it out if you feel better in the second mile," Dr. Levy says. "If you feel worse in the second mile, go home."

Training Pain-Free

The fact that different sports require specific forms of training means that each also involves particular types of injuries—and particular ways to avoid them. Here's how to protect yourself when doing three popular forms of exercise in which speed, balance, high impact or a combination of the three results in an unusually steep rate of injury.

Running

Take a freeze-frame of a runner in midstride and what do you have? A guy who's airborne. A guy who's about to land on one foot with all his body weight, multiplied two to three times by the forces of gravity and forward momentum. With this kind of hammering, it's no surprise that when a study followed participants in an Atlanta 10-K race for ten years, 53 percent reported being injured. Here are some things you can do to improve your odds.

Factor in some walking. Being much easier on muscles, joints and tendons, walking is a smart addition to a running routine, especially if you're just starting. "Think in terms of time, not distance," Dr. Janda advises. "Alternate a fast walk for five minutes

with a light run for five minutes, then walk again. The next time you go out, alternate running seven minutes and walking five, and gradually increase your intensity that way."

Wear true running shoes. Running is one of the few sports that cries out for sport-specific footwear. Running shoes cushion the impact of planting your feet and help keep you rolling smoothly from one stride to the next, Dr. Dannenberg believes. (See Buying Shoes on page 320.)

Think smooth and soft. Try to run on even surfaces; running on a pitted, pitched or gnarly path is an invitation to ankle twists and sprains. Also, when possible, run on soft surfaces such as dirt, groomed grass or packed wood chips, which cushion the stresses of running more than hard surfaces like asphalt, says Dr. Dannenberg.

Bicycling

"There are between 800 and 1,000 bike-related deaths a year, but these are the tip of the iceberg in terms of total injuries," says Dr. Dannenberg. Here's how to ride safe.

Don't flip your lid. Most of the deaths Dr. Dannenberg refers to are from head injuries sustained in crashes. Insurance against this ugly eventuality comes in two parts. The first, of course, is not to take your head for a ride while your helmet languishes in your hatchback. The second is not to crash. Keep loose items (bags, shoestrings, arms of outerwear you've removed) out of spokes and chain rings. If you're riding on the pavement, watch out for unexpected obstacles such as opening car doors; if you're off-road, keep your speed within your abilities.

Pedal fast. Common sense says straining against

Body-Temperature Injuries

You don't need to smash, twist or grind your body to get it into trouble. There's also danger of damage that starts from the inside out. Let your body temperature swing too far to either end of the thermostat and you'll be facing potentially deadly problems. Here's how to keep your thermostat set in the temperate zone.

• Hypothermia comes about when low internal temperature interferes with the body's ability to regulate vital machinery like metabolism and heartbeat. One key factor is getting wet, which vastly increases heat loss in the cold. Wear clothes that wick moisture away from the body rather than holding it close to the skin. Polypropylene underwear is better than cotton in cool weather. "Avoid cotton—it's miserable when wet," says Andrew Dannenberg, M.D., assistant

professor at the Injury Prevention Center of Johns Hopkins University School of Hygiene and Public Health in Baltimore. Another key factor is loss of energy. When you're active, body heat generally makes up for lost warmth, but you should head for shelter once intensity—and body heat—dwindles.

• Heat exhaustion is a supply-and-demand problem: Muscles and skin, which compete for fluids from the blood, become understocked in the face of extreme heat and/or humidity. Obviously, not exercising in extreme heat or humidity will solve a lot of problems. Schedule hot-day activity before 10 A.M. or after 3 P.M. Wear loose-fitting clothes, drink lots of fluids and realize that muscle cramps, goose bumps, fatigue and lightheadedness are some of the first signs of trouble.

The Perfect First-Aid Kit

It's part of the nature of accidents and mishaps that you're not prepared for them. After all, if you knew it was going to happen, it *wouldn't* have happened. That's why it makes sense to have handy a kit of ointments, balms and patches at all times: While wincing at the stupidity (and it's always something stupid, isn't it?) that left you with an abrasion, contusion or unintended incision, you can draw some comfort in the fact that you were smart enough to bring tools. Here's what to include, as recommended by Eric A. Weiss, M.D., associate professor of medicine at Stanford Medical Center and board member of the Wilderness Medical Society.

For Relieving
- Ibuprofen tablets (Motrin, Advil), for reducing inflammation from sprains and strains, and reducing the pain of headache and sunburn
- Benadryl or other antihistamines for hay fever, poison ivy, rashes and bee stings
- Pepto-Bismol or (if allergic to aspirin) Imodium for sudden stomach trouble
- Aloe vera gel for minor burns and frostbite
- Spenco 2nd Skin Dressings, moleskin and molefoam, for blisters

For Cleaning
- A ten cubic centimeter irrigation syringe with an 18-gauge catheter tip, for use as a squirt gun to flush dirt and microorganisms
- Neosporin or another triple antibiotic ointment
- Antiseptic towelettes with benzalkonium chloride, for swabbing

For Patching
- Sterile dressings (two- by two-, three- by three-, and four- by four-inch)
- Sterile eye pads
- Sterile gauze bandage
- Assorted adhesive bandages
- Elastic bandage
- Wound closure strips or butterfly closures for pulling wound edges together
- Tincture of benzoin for making adhesive bandages, wound closure strips and moleskin all stick better

For Technical Assistance
- Tweezers
- Tape
- Safety pins
- Blunt-tip bandage scissors, for cutting cloth
- Waterproof matches
- A pencil and writing paper in a sealed plastic pouch
- Small first-aid book
- Epi-Pen, for injecting a single dose of epinephrine in case of severe allergic reaction to bee stings or food (prescription required)
- Latex surgical gloves and CPR Microshield, to protect against infectious diseases like AIDS

---

the resistance of a high gear could make you more susceptible to overuse injuries. Spinning at lower gears tends to reduce strain and propel you more efficiently. Save the high gears for when you have sufficient speed to keep each pedal moving at the recommended 80 to 100 revolutions per minute for non-racers and 100 to 150 for racers, says Dale Hughes, director of the Walden School of Cycling in Rochester, Michigan, and chairman of the National Off-Road Bicycling Association.

Have a fit. If you do a lot of riding, it's common to experience knee and back pain from improper positioning on the bike. Ask a bike shop mechanic to check the position of your saddle, handlebars and pedals, says Dr. Janda.

Support your back. The leaned-over stance used when riding both road and mountain bikes can put strain on your lower back. To shore up your torso, strengthen your gut muscles (which provide most of the spine's support) with abdominal exercises such as crunches two or three times a week, says Dr. Janda.

In-Line Skating

Before taking up in-line skating, "make sure your primary medical bills are paid," says Bob Gollwitzer, owner of the Skaters Edge shops in Philadelphia and director of the Sport and Competition Council of the International In-Line Skating Association (IISA). He's joking, sort of. "It can be a dangerous sport, no doubt about it," he says, not laughing this time. The most recent IISA figures put the annual injury tally at 76,000. According to the National Center for Injury Prevention and Control at the Centers for Disease Control and Prevention (CDC) in Atlanta, almost 70 percent of in-line skating injuries are fractures, dislocations, sprains, strains and "avulsion," a fancy term for being torn limb from limb. Here's how not to be.

Wear a helmet. Only about 5 percent of in-line skating injuries involve head damage, but no type of trauma poses a higher risk of lasting disability.

Be well-padded. Don't stop with the helmet. "In-line skating is one activity where appropriate protective gear really involves a whole range of

The Swaddle Factor

You've seen these guys in locker rooms, whipping out their roll of cloth tape and swathing their knees, ankles, elbows until they look like an extra from *The Mummy*. Looks impressive, but does it do any good?

"The idea is that by restricting motion, you reduce your risk of injury," says David Janda, M.D., director of the Institute for Preventative Sports Medicine in Ann Arbor, Michigan. But wrapping is useless on knees and elbows. "There's no indication that wrapping these joints has been of value to any athlete I'm aware of," Dr. Janda says. The only place wrapping really works is the ankle, which is particularly vulnerable to sudden, traumatic movements in a number of different directions.

Still, Dr. Janda is cautious about advising anyone to wrap his own ankles, because the protection you assume you're gaining may simply not be there. "You need to take the structure of the joint into account," he says. "Besides being difficult to do it properly on yourself, there's a method and a technique to wrapping, and it really needs to be done by a second, trained individual."

The best form of injury protection, he emphasizes, is strengthening and stretching exercises that keep muscles well-conditioned. With any luck, you'll never need a wrap for what they can actually be useful for: *treating* injuries.

---

things," Dr. Dannenberg says. In fact, what really gets massacred in falls is the wrist, which accounts for a whopping 37 percent of injuries—a rate four times higher than the next-most-common injury site, the elbow. Research at the CDC finds that wearing wrist protectors cuts your odds of injuries such as lacerations, sprains and strains considerably. The other parts of the recommended ensemble are elbow and knee pads.

Take a lesson. "The backward fall is the most dangerous kind, and it's most common in beginners," says Gollwitzer. "Braking, striding, gliding and falling are four critical things every skater needs to know how to do, and taking a lesson at the start will instantly push your skills two weeks ahead of where you'd be on your own."

Keep your head up. Looking at the horizon gives a power-assist to your sense of balance and keeps your center of gravity over your toes. "If you watch your feet, you completely throw off your balance," Gollwitzer says.

Stay off the streets. If you don't have a local park to skate in, take to the access roads that feed corporate or industrial parks, which are largely traffic-free after-hours and are usually laid out in circular paths or loops.

Caring for Injuries

Even the man who takes to heart all the reasonable precautions outlined in the last chapter will at some point find himself wincing with pain. It's the nature of athletics. You're moving your body, exerting force, building speed, pushing your limits. When things are at their best, conscious thought melts away and the intuitive intelligence of muscles and nerves takes the controls. When you're lost in the flow of movement, a conscious thought like, "Be more careful!" is not only unwelcome, it's often counterproductive.

Then something goes wrong, the world blurs sideways, flow spatters into chaos and suddenly you're looking up at what seems a strangely peaceful sky. Your intellect barges in on your subconscious neural party and asks what the hell is going on. "You've done enough harm," the brain tells the body. "Let me handle this."

What happens next is important. The brain has to know what to do, and the body has to go along with the plan—not just because you want the pain to stop but also because you want to repair whatever is damaged as soon as possible. To not deal with injuries actively is to risk not being able to do anything actively. "Most men who stop running permanently do so because of injuries," says Susan Kalish, executive director of the American Running and Fitness Association in Bethesda, Maryland.

The Big Picture

The two most common sports-injury categories are muscle injuries and tendon and ligament injuries, says four-time Mr. Universe Bill Pearl, trainer of ten Mr. Universes and eight Mr. Americas and co-author of *Getting Stronger*.

We'll remind you of the basics.

• Muscles are groups of fibers that contract to cause movement. Muscles are attached to bones, other muscles or skin (contracting muscles is what makes you smile) and are responsible for all bodily movements and force. When abused, misused, overused or put to use without first being warmed up, muscles can tear, go into spasms or do any number of painful things.

A lot of blood flows through muscles to supply them with sufficient oxygen and nutrients to do their jobs, and also to sweep away waste products. This blood flow helps muscles heal quickly—in minutes, hours, days, weeks—depending upon the extent of the strain they were under.

• Tendons are among the body's toughest materials. They are connective bands and cords that attach muscles to bones. Connective tissue doesn't have much give, isn't very rubbery, doesn't care to stretch. So, when overly stressed, tendons rip loose from bone, or they tear.

• Ligaments—also made of tough connective tissue—envelop joint sockets, lashing opposing bones together firmly. As with tendons, ligaments can tear or separate from bone.

Tendons and ligaments have weak blood supplies, so they take much longer to heal when badly injured—as long as six months in some cases. Severe tears might take surgery to fix.

If you suffer a serious tendon or ligament injury, you must quit exercising the injured area. And you must be particularly careful when you resume exercising. And you can't even think about restarting early, if you want to rebound quickly. "Injured ligaments and tendons often are pain-free long before they are completely healed," says E. Davis Ryan, P.T., owner of Community Physical Therapists in Fort Lee, New Jersey, and co-author of *The Lazy Person's Guide to Fitness*. They need to be babied for at least six weeks, he says.

The Core Healing Routine

All injuries are unique and deserve lots of individual attention, but they're also much the same. Because the body's response to insult is fairly consistent, the steps a wounded warrior should take are similar from one injury site to another, notes David Janda, M.D., director of the Institute for Preventative Sports Medicine in Ann Arbor, Michigan. Even when a doctor's attention is called for, you'll usually want to first try these forms of aid to get some immediate relief.

Use the RICE stuff. It's a classic, familiar formula for reducing swelling and pain, this acronym for Rest, Ice, Compression and Elevation (RICE). What's less appreciated is that these four courses of action are grouped together because each takes a different approach to counteracting a single problem: the spilling of blood and fluids into the injured body part. This bloat-provoking leakage and the pressure it exerts—especially when it's in a joint—can severely limit mobility and curtail your return to active life long after the pain has subsided, says Allan M. Levy, M.D., team physician for the New York Giants, partner at the Sports Medicine Center in Fort Lee, New Jersey, and co-author of the *Sports Injury Handbook*. Keep swelling down, and you'll be back in action faster, with less pain and aggravation. According to Dr. Levy, the reason RICE works is that:

• Rest of the injured area keeps circulation to a minimum so that less fluid trickles out of broken or damaged blood vessels. It also reduces wear and tear on vessels, allowing them to heal and seal more quickly. "Rest" doesn't mean just avoiding exercise, it means keeping the injured area as still as possible at all times, since even small movements will boost blood circulation.

• Ice constricts blood vessels, curtailing the flow of blood to the injury (and also deadening pain). Dr. Levy recommends filling a zip-lock storage bag with a mixture of ice and water: The ice keeps the injury cold, but the water keeps the temperature above 32 degrees, reducing risk of frostbite. Strap it on with an Ace bandage and leave it there no longer than a half-hour: Research at the University of Chicago finds that the healing effect of ice peaks after 25 minutes; after 30 minutes, there's danger of damaging tissue and nerves. Avoid applying heat: "The current feeling is that you should only use heat when loosening something up immediately before going back into action after the injury has healed," Dr. Levy says.

• Compression squeezes the area, keeps blood from moving outside of the vein walls and also stanches the flow of fluid to keep swelling down. A snug bandage does the trick.

• Elevation makes it more difficult for blood to reach the damaged area. It also allows fluid that has accumulated at the injury site to flow down and away. Elevating the injury doesn't just mean raising it higher than normal, but to a level higher than your heart.

Stretch for the future. Stretching is a foundation of prevention and treatment alike, for similar reasons: Tight muscles curtail movement, effectively reduce strength and, significantly, leave themselves vulnerable to becoming injured again, says Dr. Levy. The problem here is that when you damage muscles, they react involuntarily by contracting, or shortening. It's a protective mechanism short-term, but long-term, muscles that aren't gradually lengthened again will heal in their shortened state. When you resume activity, these shortened muscles will more easily tear than when you first got injured—that is, unless you stretch. As a rule of thumb, you'll know you're ready to resume activity when you can stretch the injured muscle as far as you can the same, uninjured muscle on the other side of your body without pain, says Levy.

Pop the right pill. You're in pain, you want relief, you open the medicine cabinet. What to choose? For injuries, the pain reliever of choice is ibuprofen, the main ingredient of familiar brands such as Advil, Nuprin and Motrin IB, says Dr. Janda. Ibuprofen is an anti-inflammatory, which means it reduces swelling and with it, pain. If you don't have any on hand, try aspirin, because it also has anti-inflammatory properties, suggests Dr. Janda. Aspirin interferes with blood clotting, however, so it shouldn't be taken in large doses during contact sports, Dr. Levy notes. The last choice is acetaminophen medications such as Tylenol, which kill pain, but do little to reduce inflammation. (They do, however, provoke less stomach irritation, if that's an issue for you.)

Serious or Minor

Some injuries sideline you for a day, a week. But with smart care, you're back in business fast enough that you've lost hardly a step.

And then there are *injuries*. Broken bones, ligament tears, repetitive stress injuries that threaten to sideline you long enough to degrade your overall fitness level, not to mention your mental state, says Dr. Levy.

The strategy for dealing with small and big injuries is the same. You use the same first-aid method in the moments after the injury: RICE. Applied quickly, RICE greatly lessens the damage and recovery time required in most cases, says Dr. Levy.

You also use the same recuperation strategy: Do everything you can to let the injury heal as quickly as possible, then do everything you can to get the injured part back to where it was, or even better, in terms of flexibility and strength, says Dr. Janda.

Other truisms exist for injuries, no matter where they occur: For example, a pulled muscle needs to be worked—stretched—as it heals; torn ligaments or tendons need to be left alone, advises Dr. Janda.

The final truism is that while each injury should be treated uniquely, the same dozen or so happen over and over and over. "Most of the injuries I see are in just a handful of areas," says Dr. Janda. We bet you know right where they are. Here are some specific healing techniques for those places that typically take the most punishment.

Rehab Programs for Weight Lifters

At age 65, four-time Mr. Universe Bill Pearl, trainer of ten Mr. Universes and eight Mr. Americas, still gets up at 3 A.M. and begins a 2½-hour workout. "I only train six days a week; I don't want to get fanatical about it," he jokes.

Training six days a week, Pearl knows that injuries are inevitable. And he knows how to use weight training to speed rehabilitation from injuries. Below are two programs: one for injured muscles, one for injured tendons or ligaments. Muscle injuries take less time to heal than injuries of connective tissues. Plan accordingly.

Rebounding from Muscle Injuries

Don't do any strenuous exercise until the swelling has gone down. The amount of time this takes will vary based on the extent of the muscle pull or tear. Once the swelling and pain have diminished, Pearl advises full-range-of-motion exercises, mimicking the weight-lifting movements of a well-rounded lifting program, like our Core Routine, but without any weights. Only when you can do that without pain should you begin weight lifting again.

Of course, begin with lighter than usual weights, lifted a few days a week. Select a weight in the light to medium range for your training level. This program, he says, causes injured muscles to flush with fresh blood, rebuild tissue and clear away wastes. The intention in this training program, he says, is to rebuild strength first, then endurance.

• First week. Do one to three sets of 15 reps with lighter than usual weights. When this is comfortable, increase weight to rebuild the strength you lost during the time the injury had you sidelined.

• Second to fourth weeks. Increase weight again until you're above your former strength level. Just getting back to the former level is not the goal. "You weren't strong enough then to prevent the injury, so now you must make the muscles stronger to prevent further injuries," Pearl says.

For serious weight lifters, move up to six sets—the first three sets at ten, eight and six reps, the next three at eight, six and four.

After a month, you can work back into your regular program.

Rebounding from Tendon/Ligament Injuries

You must listen closely to your body in this program, so that what you do is healing and not hurting. Tendon and ligament injuries are easily irritated. The key in this training is to avoid straining and to do only a few reps, says Pearl.

As with the muscle program, only begin working with weights when the swelling has subsided and you can go through the full range of motion without pain. This is a six-week program, three days a week, of a well-rounded program like our Core Routine.

• First two weeks. Do one to three sets of eight to ten reps with medium weights. Don't overdo it and don't strain. You need to quit while feeling you could do at least two or three more reps.

You may experience some tenderness and swelling after this workout. If it doesn't ease up before the next workout, lay off until it does. Then reduce the weight and number of sets and try again.

• Third and fourth weeks. Slowly up the weight and number of sets. Do three to six sets of reps in this order: ten, eight, six, ten, eight, six. Stay with these until you have nearly no injury-related swelling or soreness after the exercise.

• Fifth and sixth weeks. Build strength. Increase weight and effort to the point where it is difficult to reach the targeted number of reps for each set. Do three to six sets of reps in this order: ten, eight, six, ten, eight, four.

At the end of the program, return to your regular routine.

A couple more general pointers from a weight-lifting pro who not once, but four times, ruled the body-building universe:

• Always warm up, get the blood circulating, raise the body temperature, work through range of motion before tackling the heavy weights.

• Always start small. Begin with a light weight and add resistance with each set. The world champions do. They don't head for the big weights on their first set.

Wrist

Let's see, how could you possibly injure your wrist? Does the alphabet start with A? There's aerobics, baseball, basketball, boxing, carrying, discus throwing, egg tossing, football, golf . . . you get the point.

Wrists are particularly prone to overuse injuries and repetitive-motion injuries, says Dr. Levy, as well as sprains and even fractures from sticking your hand

out to break an unexpected fall.

Sprains are the most common wrist injury, says Dr. Levy. He x-rays all but the mildest wrist sprains because a sprained ligament sometimes pulls loose a bit of bone, causing a fracture. A fractured wrist needs to be encased in a cast. A sprained wrist usually heals well in a soft splint.

Primary treatment of a sprained wrist is the standard RICE prescription. A wrist-support splint available in drugstores helps immobilize it during the rest phase. Then, as it heals, begin building strength and flexibility with these range-of-motion exercises. Dr. Levy recommends taking an anti-inflammatory medication through the first ten days of physical therapy. Among the exercises he advises:

Grip Strengtheners

Squeeze a small, soft rubber ball, putty or a not-too-resistant grip strengthener until your hand is fatigued, suggests Dr. Levy.

Wrist Rolls

This exercise was also described in Arm Joints on page 56. Tie a light dumbbell to a three-foot long rope or chain. Firmly tie the other end of the rope to the center of a broom handle or hefty dowel. Stand upright with your feet shoulder-width apart. Hold the handle at shoulder height, with your hands shoulder-width apart, palms down, and roll the rope up on the handle, using the handle as a spool. When the weight has reached the top, lower it back down again. Continue until fatigued.

Tennis elbow doesn't sound like a wrist injury, does it? But actually it is an inflammation of muscles in the forearm—the muscles involved in moving the wrist—and an inflammation of the tendon tying the muscles to the elbow, says Dr. Levy. When you have a serious case of tennis elbow, you can't open a jar, turn a faucet, lift a cup of coffee, clench anything or squeeze with your hand without hot pain shooting up the inside of your arm or radiating around your wrist and elbow.

Baseball pitchers get something similar to tennis

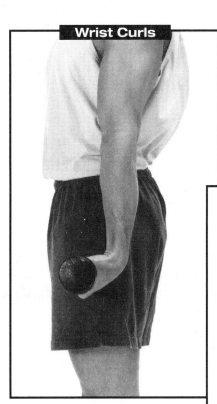

Wrist Curls ►

This is a variation of the forearm curls described in part 2. In the *Sports Injury Handbook*, Dr. Levy recommends holding a comfortable weight (five pounds or less) at your side. With your elbow locked and your palm facing forward, roll your wrist as far forward as it will go comfortably and then let it back down slowly. Repeat to muscle exhaustion.

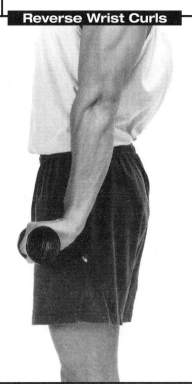

Reverse Wrist Curls ►

Same as above, except your palm faces backward. Flex your wrist forward as far as it will go comfortably, then let it down.

elbow from snapping the ball. But in this case, it's on the inside of the elbow. (Sometimes they get much more serious pitcher's elbow—a bone injury—which requires arthroscopic surgery and takes up to a year to heal.) Golfers get tennis elbow, too, but on their nondominant side. A right-handed golfer will find his left side affected.

The treatment for tennis elbow is exactly the same as that used for a wrist sprain, which is described above.

When to see a doctor: As Dr. Levy notes, even a minor wrist sprain should be looked at, given the possibility of it developing into something worse. If you have any pain that is recurring in your wrists, you could have a repetitive stress injury. Given the delicacy of the joint and the importance of your hands to all existence as you know it, when it comes to wrists, don't play tough—get to a doctor if you suspect anything is wrong.

Elbows

If you've ever spent an afternoon on the tennis court, golf green or baseball diamond, you appreciate how susceptible this versatile joint is to overuse injury. Use the following stretches as soon as you begin to feel any soreness or pain in your elbow, says Dr. Levy. You don't have to wait until pain strikes to do them, however. These and other exercises can precondition your elbow and help you avoid painful joint problems entirely. Check it out.

When to see a doctor: Severe problems are usually the result of a hard blow (or a series of traumas). Get checked out if you have a persistent "funny bone" feeling of numbness or tingling at the tip of your elbow: It may indicate a nerve injury, says Dr. Janda. Also seek attention if you develop small bumps that protrude from your elbows (Popeye had this problem): You may have fluid buildup from a form of acute bursitis.

Elbow Relief Stretches

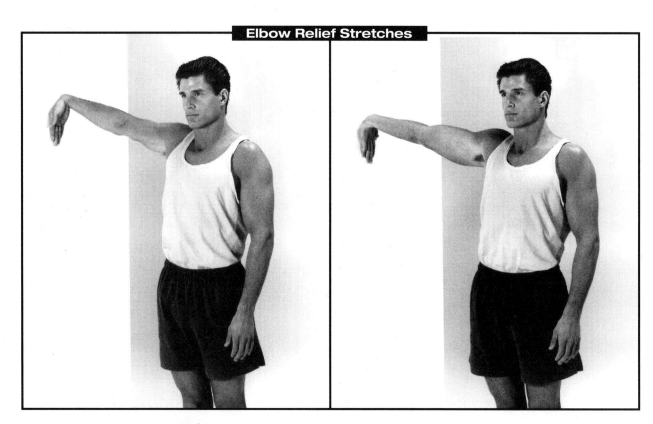

Elbow Relief Stretches ▲

Regardless of what side of your elbow hurts, do both of the following stretches. This will balance the muscles, says Dr. Levy. Stand alongside a wall and extend your arm straight to the side. Press the back of your hand against the wall, fingers pointing down. Keeping your hand pressed down, raise your arm higher on the wall until you feel a stretch in your forearm. Hold 20 to 30 seconds.

Next, place your palm against the wall, elbow straight, fingers pointing down. Keeping your palm pressed down, raise your arm higher on the wall until you feel a gentle stretch.

Here's an alternative wrist stretch: Extend your arm straight out in front of you so that it's parallel to the floor. Your elbow should be locked, your palm facing down. Use your other hand to pull your extended hand down toward the floor.

Knees

Because it's such a complex joint that depends on bone, ligaments, tendons and fluid to work properly, the knee is one of the most frequently injured parts of the body.

The most common form of overuse injury is runner's knee, in which the kneecap, which normally rides in a groove when the knee bends, becomes misaligned and rubs on the side of the groove. The problem is caused by overpronation of the foot, which may require orthotics to correct.

In the meantime, if you are exercising and your knee starts to hurt, immediately stop and call it quits for the day. If there's swelling or pain, apply the RICE method. You can remedy a minor case of runner's knee yourself by strengthening your quadriceps muscles to better support your knee and gradually pull your kneecap back into alignment. To do this, you'll need to do modified leg extensions, says Dr. Levy.

A second common knee problem is a ligament sprain from making a too-quick pivot, landing wrong from a jump or twisting your leg in a gopher hole. Sprains take time to heal. In the short term, use the RICE method to aid the healing process. If it's a minor sprain, it will heal on its own, but you will want to put the knee through its full range of motion and work on strengthening your leg muscles to prevent a recurrence, says Dr. Janda.

For a good stretch, use your hand to pull the foot of your injured leg up so that the heel presses your buttocks. Also, do modified leg extensions.

When to see a doctor: There are a number of knee injuries that are every bit as nasty as they sound: torn cartilage or ligament, a dislocated or broken kneecap. To separate the serious from the merely painful, Dr. Levy offers this rule of thumb: "If you receive a blow," he says, "and the pain is on the same side of the knee that was hit, it's probably just a bruise, and the pain will go away rapidly. If the pain is on the opposite side, consider it a serious injury." That means get to a doctor.

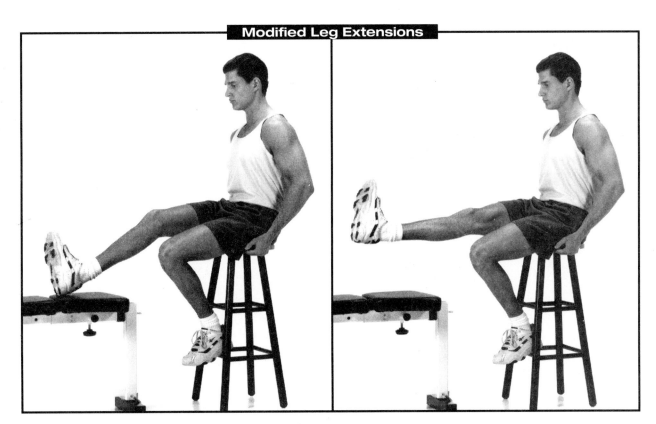

Modified Leg Extensions

Modified Leg Extensions ⏶

Sit in a chair and extend your injured leg straight in front of you, parallel to the floor. Next, place a footstool, box, bucket or similar object under your foot to prevent your leg from dropping any lower than six to eight inches when lowered. Why? Doing a leg extension through the knee's full range of motion will make the problem worse, while doing just the uppermost 30 degrees of motion will make it better. If you wish to add resistance, put some ankle or free weights in a gym bag and slide your foot through the handle so you can use the bag as a weight.

Ankles

The ankle's strengths are also its weaknesses. It provides movement in lots of different directions: up, down, back, forward, side-to-side. That allows crucial mobility for the feet and legs, but in a rare instance of seemingly careless design, it also makes a critical component of balance and stability inherently unstable.

The ankle injury you can do something about is the mild sprain, in which the fibers of the ligament become partially torn, usually from rolling too far off the outer part of your foot. Immediately apply the RICE method.

One method of icing involves dunking the foot in a bucket or small trash can of ice water. This isn't necessarily a pleasant prospect, but it's good medicine, says Dr. Levy. Another makeshift method is to use an athletic bandage to wrap and hold a bag of frozen peas around your ankle. Ice for 20 minutes on, 20 minutes off, for two days or until the swelling is gone.

Between icings, and while sleeping, keep your ankle compressed with an athletic bandage, but not so tight that you completely restrict blood flow, says Dr. Janda. Prop it up with pillows to elevate it above the level of the heart.

As with the knee, begin putting your ankle through range-of-motion and light strengthening exercises as soon as possible, says Dr. Levy.

When to see a doctor: Ankle sprains and breaks are difficult to differentiate (the more dire fractures sometimes feel less painful), so everything but the most mild sprains should be taken to a doctor for an x-ray. Clues that the injury is serious include swelling that keeps getting worse or doesn't go away after 72 hours, or not being able to walk, says Dr. Levy.

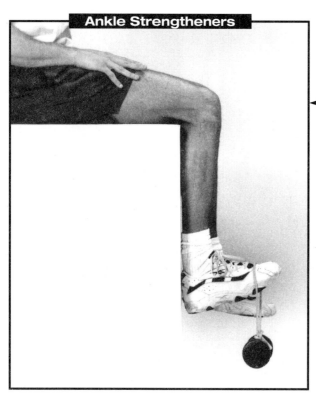

Ankle Strengtheners

◄ Ankle Strengtheners

Tie a piece of rope about 1½ feet long in a loop through a ten-pound weight and drape the loop over your foot (make sure you have shoes on). While sitting on a counter or stool, use your ankle to lift the weight as many times as you can. If you can, also try moving the weighted foot from side to side.

Alphabet Stretch

For improved range of motion, sit on a high chair or with your legs crossed so that the injured ankle is off the floor. Trace the letters of the alphabet with your foot, keeping your toes straight so all motion comes from the ankle.

Shoulders

Apparently, if God had meant for us to swim and play tennis, football, baseball and volleyball, he would have given us more shoulder ligaments. As it is, the few that exist are weak, so there's little support for the shoulder when you make forceful movements with your arm over your head.

The common microtraumas that give us sore shoulders are easily remedied with some gentle stretching, icing and anti-inflammatories, says Dr. Janda.

The main overuse shoulder problem is a rotator cuff injury, an inflammation of the tendons that help hold the shoulder in place. If pain is flaring up, stop what you are doing and, if you sense an injury, apply the RICE method, advises Dr. Levy.

The main treatment for *minor* rotator cuff injuries

is conditioning the shoulder muscles with any number of exercises, says Dr. Levy. If you do any kind of regular workout, the format of these exercises will sccm comfortably familiar.

But remember: When you're dealing with a shoulder injury, you want to use *light* weights—15 pounds or less—much lighter than the moderate to heavy weights you normally would use. Once you've repaired the damage and conditioned your shoulders, then you can slowly start adding more weight, Dr. Levy says.

When to see a doctor: You should see your doctor if it feels as if your shoulder has come out of its socket or you can't move your shoulder or raise your arms above your head.

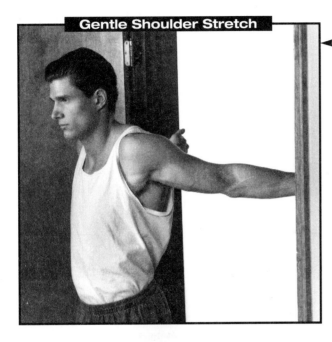

Gentle Shoulder Stretch

◄ Gentle Shoulder Stretch

Stand in a doorway and hold onto the doorjamb at about shoulder height with both hands. Move forward through the door so that your arms are pulled behind you and your elbows are straight. When you feel a gentle stretch in your shoulders, hold for 30 seconds. This is a very versatile stretch that you can do anywhere. Plus, by slightly modifying this exercise, you can also stretch your chest muscles (see City Living on page 257).

Biceps Curls

Do a biceps curl, holding a light dumbbell at your side with your palm facing forward. Bend your elbow to bring the weight to your shoulder, then slowly lower to the starting position. Repeat 50 times or until fatigue sets in. Next, try the same move, but with your palm facing rearward at the starting position.

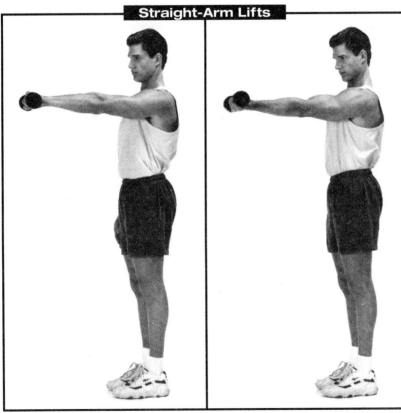

Straight-Arm Lifts

◄ Straight-Arm Lifts

Hold a dumbbell at your side, your palm facing rearward. Keeping your arm straight, lift the dumbbell in front of you, raising your arm no higher than parallel to the floor. Slowly return to the starting position. Then try the same move, but with your palm facing forward at the starting position.

Side Lateral Lifts

Hold a dumbbell at your side, your palm facing your body. Keeping your arm straight, lift the weight out to your side, raising your arm no higher than parallel to the floor, then return to the starting position. Repeat 50 times or until you tire.

Back

Back problems tend to feel worse than they are. You may swear you have a blown disk and need sophisticated surgery, but actually at least 90 percent of cases are nothing more than spasms of weak or overloaded muscles. The fact that you can usually treat yourself is the somewhat tarnished silver lining in what's otherwise a state of abject misery.

When back muscles spasm, the immediate goal is to get them to relax. Try the postures and stretches below, says Dr. Levy. RICE may also work, as might anti-inflammatories and muscle relaxants prescribed by a medical doctor. If the problem does not resolve quickly, consider manipulation therapy from a chiropractor or osteopath. Many recent scientific studies have established the effectiveness of manipulation for lower-back pain.

A back injury does not necessarily mean you should lay off exercising, says Dr. Levy. "In fact,"

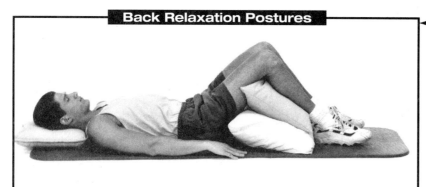

Back Relaxation Postures

◄ Back Relaxation Postures

Lie on your back with your knees bent and your feet flat on the floor. This tilts the pelvis backward and flattens out the back. Put a soft pillow or rolled towel under your neck to support its natural curvature, and place another support under your knees. This posture puts the spine in a neutral position so that muscles are fully at rest.

Seated Back Stretch

◄ Seated Back Stretch

When you're able to move around more, sit in a chair and spread your legs so that your knees extend beyond shoulder-width apart. Lean forward with your hands on your knees and gently rock from side to side to give your back a gentle stretch.

Slowly let your torso drop between your knees while you slide your hands down to grip your ankles. For an added stretch, raise one arm over your head. Hold for 15 seconds; repeat with your other arm.

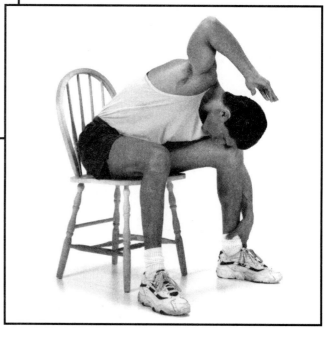

Back Stretch

This stretch is described in the Back chapter on page 85. Lie on your back and pull one knee slowly toward your chest as far as pain allows. Hold for 30 seconds. Then do the same with the other leg.

Easing Dings and Irritations

The body is like a small child: Even the most innocuous offenses make it scream for attention. You know the problem is minor, but pain makes the situation impossible to ignore. This is good, because sometimes little problems, left untreated, become big ones. Here's how to pacify pain from:

• A jammed finger. Next time a flying ball goes head-to-head with an extended digit, grab the injured finger with your thumb and index finger and pull for five seconds, rest five seconds, then pull again, suggests David Janda, M.D., director of the Institute for Preventative Sports Medicine in Ann Arbor, Michigan. That will stretch compressed tissue, align the joint better and allow squished-out fluids to flow back in.

• A whacked thumb. You can handle a hammer, but it's the rock you use to pound a tent stake that will get you. Lift the smashed thumb above the level of your heart and gently squeeze the tip for five minutes to reduce swelling, bruising and pain, suggests Dr. Janda.

• A low blow. Everybody may be laughing, but it's no joke. Lie down and put a rolled towel or T-shirt under your testicles, resting the ends of the roll on each thigh. "That will support the scrotum so your testicles aren't hanging down and will also help get blood flowing to the area," says William Forgey, M.D., author of *Wilderness Medicine: Beyond First Aid.*

• A bleeding gash. Loss of blood is dangerous because you don't have that much to spare. To stanch its outward flow, raise the wound above the level of your heart and put direct pressure on it with the heel of your hand, using a clean gauze pad or washcloth, suggests Dr. Janda. After about ten minutes, dress the wound with a clean, soft, bulky material—like a shirt, towel, handkerchief, pillowcase, whatever works to spread pressure over a large area around the wound. Now bind the dressing in place with cloth strips (torn, if necessary), belts, cord or string, tying the knot so that it rests directly over the wound for a snug fit. Don't tie it so tight that you cut off blood circulation. If your wound is serious, Dr. Janda advises that you get to an emergency facility for a proper evaluation.

• A speck in the eye. When rubbing your eyes and crying tears won't dislodge grit, locate the speck with the help of a mirror or friend, then flush the eye with a steady stream of water from a water bottle, suggests Dr. Janda. Failing that, try pulling the top eyelid over the lower lid: The lower lashes may sweep the grit out from under the upper eyelid.

• Bruises. Got smacked in the thigh with a softball and it's turning blue? Ice bruises, 20 minutes on, 20 off, until the swelling goes down, says Allan M. Levy, M.D., team physician for the New York Giants and partner at the Sports Medicine Center in Fort Lee, New Jersey. Use the rest of the RICE program as well.

• Scrapes. Clean and disinfect them, treat with an antibiotic cream, then bandage, says Dr. Janda.

---

notes Warren A. Scott, M.D., chief of sports medicine at Kaiser Permanente Medical Center in Santa Clara, California, "exercise, rather than rest, is recommended for most patients with back problems." But you must back down from sports that involve twisting or jolting your back or that require quick, sharp, sudden movements, the doctors caution.

Some activities that Dr. Levy considers relatively pain-free for those with back problems are bicycling, walking, swimming, cross-country skiing and water aerobics.

Runners, Dr. Levy says, need to cut down a bit and run only on softer surfaces. Don't run if it makes your back pain worse, he says.

When to see a doctor: See your doctor if pain radiates below your knee or is accompanied by any numbness or loss of coordination or body control.

Hamstrings

Pulled hamstring muscles are particularly common with runners. You might have this injury if you feel debilitatingly sore muscles in the back of one or both of your thighs.

For relief, ice the pained muscle three to four times a day for about 20 minutes each time until the swelling goes down. This could be two or three days, says Dr. Levy.

Unless you have a major rip, you can begin gently stretching your hamstring muscles as early as the second day. Stretch slowly—don't bounce or jerk—and push only to where it feels uncomfortable. Stop before reaching the point of pain, says Dr. Levy. He recommends doing the following stretch.

Hurdler's Stretch

Begin by sitting on the floor with your injured leg fully extended and the other leg bent at the knee and resting flat on the floor, the bottom of its foot against the inside of the injured leg's thigh. Gently lean forward and grasp the extended foot with both hands. Hold the stretch for 20 seconds. For balanced conditioning, repeat with the other leg extended.

Neck

A neck injury can be a strain, sprain, rupture or major compression causing paralysis, notes Dr. Levy. If a person exhibits numbness in or the inability to move a body part following a blow to the neck or head, don't move them, says Dr. Janda. Call for paramedics who know how to limit or avoid further injury in such situations.

Waking up with a painful or stiff neck after exercising or heavy lifting is another matter. If this is a common occurrence, ask a physical trainer for a neck-strengthening routine. In the short-term, here's how to rebound quickly from the injury, as suggested by Dr. Levy: Ice the area for 20 minutes on, 20 off. An anti-inflammatory medication can help bring down swelling and ease pain. Begin restoring flexibility with the following gentle stretching exercises.

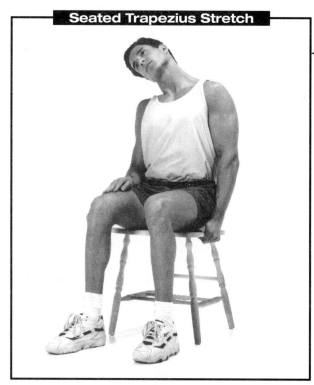

Seated Trapezius Stretch

◄ Seated Trapezius Stretch

Sitting in a chair, grasp the seat of the chair on the side where you are feeling pain, and slowly and gently bend your upper body and neck to the opposite side.

Shrugs

Lift your shoulders toward your ears as high as possible, then drop them as low as they will go. Do five repetitions.

Shoulder Rolls

Standing with your arms at your sides, lift and roll your shoulders in a circle, five times forward, five times backward.

Neck Turns

While sitting, body facing forward, slowly turn your head to one side, gazing out over your shoulder, and then turn to the other. Do five reps.

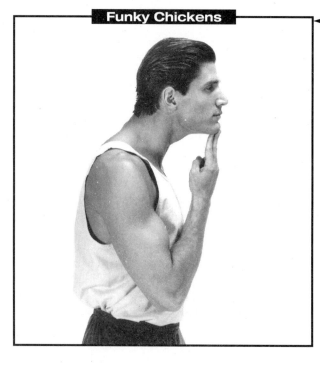

Funky Chickens

◄ Funky Chickens

After doing the neck turns described in the previous exercise, jut your head and chin forward and back five times. (Guitarists sometimes do this, keeping rhythm.)

Head

Any blow to the head that causes disorientation or any loss of consciousness—even momentary—is considered a concussion and should be taken seriously. If recovery is not rapid and progressive, get to the hospital fast. Immediate treatment is rest and observation, so long as the victim has been checked by a doctor and seems okay, says Dr. Levy. Watch for nausea, headache and further loss of consciousness, all danger signs of possible internal bleeding.

In a concussion, the brain swells. That makes it particularly prone to a second injury from even the slightest glancing blow. So avoid risky physical activity for at least seven days or until all symptoms—dizziness, confusion, headache, fatigue, overall weakness—clear up, recommends Dr. Levy.

Massage

Your gym offers a massage service and you've never had a massage. You think, "Who couldn't use a massage? I could use a massage. I'll get a massage." You make an appointment with a woman named Terry, a therapist certified by the Associated Bodywork and Massage Professionals. She has you fill out a medical history form like you get at the doctor's office, except that in the fine print above your signature it reads, "any illicit or sexually suggestive remarks or advances by me will result in immediate termination of the session, and I will be liable for payment of the scheduled appointment."

In a room that can be accessed through both the men's and women's locker rooms, she asks you (in so many words) to get naked, lie face down and cover yourself with a towel while she finds something else to do in another room. The light is low and the air is warm and moist, while wind-chimey, New Age music drifts softly from a tape deck. You're paying about a buck a minute for this experience. "Some people consider massage a luxury," she says when she returns. "Some consider it an essential way to relax physically, mentally or spiritually." She advises you to let go of thoughts about all the things you need to do. She begins with a touch so delicate it's difficult to tell she's there. Then, she presses more firmly. . . .

The True Benefits

What happens next is unique to the dynamic between your therapist and her methods, and your body's particular mix of kinks. At the end, you are a little poorer and a lot more relaxed.

What else have you gained? That depends a little on who you talk to. The medical establishment traditionally has been skeptical about some of the many benefits that legions of therapists and lots of their clients ascribe to massage. In particular, the notion that massage "cleanses" the body of harmful "toxins" is unsubstantiated at best. "One major benefit is that massage stimulates circulation," says Robert King, co-founder and co-director of the Chicago School of Massage Therapy and author of *Performance Massage.* This is a fact that's not in dispute. Massage will even help squeegee muscles of lactic acid, a waste product produced during exercise that contributes to soreness, but whether this provides any inherent benefit is unclear.

One problem (at least from a scientific point of view) is that the joys of massage are subjective in nature: If you say it makes you less sore or enhances your wellness, nobody can argue, but nobody can objectively measure these effects either. Still, tracking what people say can be compelling. In one study, for example, sufferers of chronic back pain who failed to respond to drugs, physical therapy or chiropractic treatments said they felt better after getting two massages each week for four weeks.

Stick to a subjective burden of proof and you'll find plenty of satisfied athletes who will extol massage's workout benefits. During heavy training, Triathlon legend and three-time Ironman champion Scott Tinley gets one or two 60- to 90-minute massages a week, to cite one example. "Massage enhances body awareness," says Joan Johnson, proprietor of Sports Massage of the Rockies in Boulder, Colorado, who has worked with U.S. Olympic teams in cycling, figure skating, swimming and track and field. "It helps identify tender, tight areas that athletes may not be aware of but may be prone to injury." In her book *The Healing Art of Sports Massage,* Johnson also says massage keeps muscles supple and elastic (which improves range of motion and strength) and stimulates delivery of nutrients in blood (which accelerates healing of post-workout muscle damage).

How to Do It

All of which is fine if you can bankroll a regular regimen of pricey sessions with a therapist or coax a partner into laboring with what is, after all, known as bodywork. "Using professionals can get expensive," Johnson admits, which is why she advocates and designs programs of self-massage. "It's not quite as pleasurable as having someone else work on you, but it can provide the same kinds of benefits," she says. "As a therapist, I can tell the difference between the muscles of people who work on themselves and the muscles of people who don't."

While many therapists advocate (and can deliver) full-body massage, Johnson says five areas usually need the most attention. Here are some simple ways to attend to them.

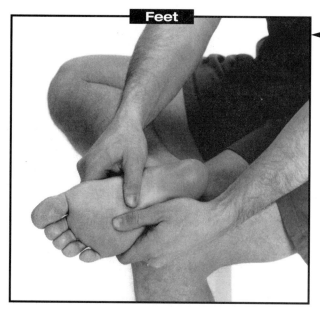

Feet

◄ Feet

They're easy to reach and they respond readily to stimulation: Just take your shoes off and they're already saying "Aaah." Massaging the feet can make the entire body relax, says Johnson, pointing out that one specialized bodywork technique, reflexology, deals largely with things podiatric.

Sit down and cross one foot over the opposite thigh. Massage up and down the bottom of the foot using your thumbs, fingers and palms to stroke lengthwise or make circular motions, concentrating on the arch. Massage the toes individually, squeezing, rolling, rotating each one, then pulling each gently away from the foot. On the top of the foot, use your thumbs to stroke the furrows between the tendons, moving the pressure from the base of the toes up toward your ankle.

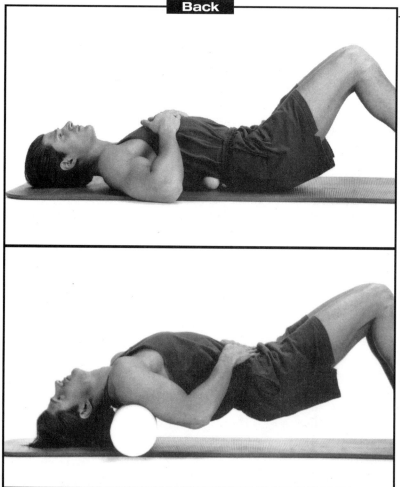

Back

◄ Back

The back, being particularly prone to stress and pain, is also particularly in need of massage. It figures: The part of the body you need to stroke most is least strokeable. To reach it, you'll need the help of a tool or two.

To reach the lower back, the easiest solution is to lie on a tennis ball on a firm surface such as a carpeted floor or firm mat, using your body weight to exert pressure on the areas you want to hit.

For the upper back, try using a cylinder of pliable foam, available from packaging businesses that stock them for padding (ask them to cut you a three-foot section) or from The Massage Store, 1-800-728-2426. Start by putting the roller under your shoulder blades, arching your back slightly with your head near the floor. Press your back over the foam in small, slow movements. For the middle back, raise your head and contract your abdominals to keep your back flat and straight. Slowly roll from mid-ribs to lower back, favoring the muscles along one side of the spine. Next, roll along the other side of the spine; then emphasize whatever side you feel needs the most work.

A Bevy of Bodyworkers

What's your pleasure? There seem to be as many different massage techniques as there are aches they're designed to alleviate. Since not all techniques feel great while you're getting them, it's wise to find out what a therapist practices before he or she lays his or her hands on you and yours. Here's a rundown of basic methods.

• Swedish massage is most familiar. It's a feel-good technique in which your oiled body is kneaded, stroked and vibrated.

• Shiatsu is a form of acupuncture without needles in which the therapist puts pressure at specific points for purposes of releasing or redirecting "energy" that's said to flow along a network of meridians.

• Reflexology is similar to shiatsu, except that it concentrates on the feet and hands, where pressure points are said to affect other locations in the body.

• Rolfing perhaps is best known for its deep-tissue work. Its creator, a biochemist named Ida Rolf, theorized that mental and physical balance are a function of structural alignment. Rolfers dig deep to straighten out body and mind. Variations designed by Rolf disciples include Aston-Patterning and Hellerwork.

• Feldenkrais builds on the idea that body and brain continuously send signals back and forth: Tension comes from the brain telling the body how to behave because of what the body tells the brain. Theoretically, interrupting this circular communication with systematic physical manipulation healthfully reprograms the brain's instructions.

• Trager Work delves even deeper into the mind-body thing, attempting to reach subconscious triggers for tension and pain through rhythmic rocking, rolling, jiggling and wiggling.

• Alexander Technique aims to overcome poor posture habits that interfere with coordination and performance, by feathering the body with light, subtle touches.

• Lymphatic massage uses light strokes purported to unclog the lymph glands (which manufacture cells for the immune system), freeing the release of toxin terminators and supposedly boosting overall immunity.

Using a Thera Cane

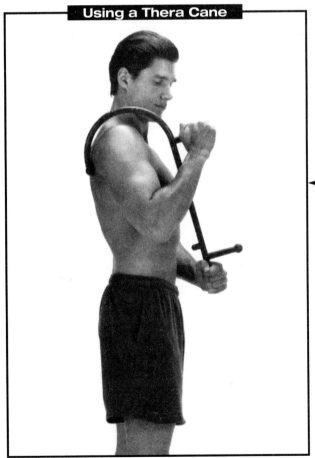

◄ Using a Thera Cane

For a more sophisticated tool that reaches the unreachable, Johnson speaks highly of the Thera Cane, a J-shaped rod equipped with handles and an array of jawbreaker-size balls for pressing into the back. It's available at medical or physical therapy supply stores, or from The Massage Store.

Neck

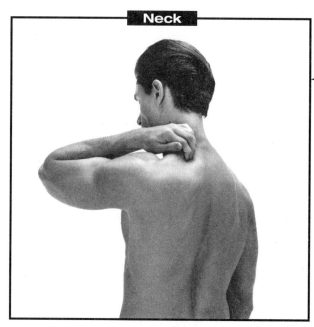

◄ Neck

The neck is subject to plenty of stresses even when you're not exercising. Reading about massage in a book, for example, requires you to tilt your eyes forward, meaning the 16-pound ball your eyes are anchored into is being held up by your neck muscles. You do this kind of thing all day.

Reach your left hand over your left shoulder and dig your fingers into the trapezius muscle at the base of your neck. Tilt your head away from your hand while dragging your fingers toward your left shoulder. Repeat on the other side.

Shoulders

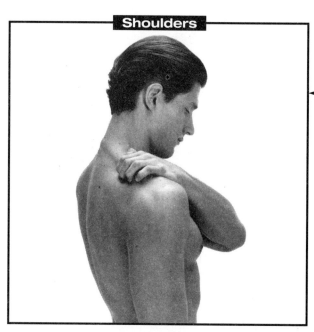

◄ Shoulders

They're the neck, continued. But shoulders also bear the burden of muscling and moving the arms. Whether you're throwing a ball or using a computer, sustained motion is tough on shoulders.

In a move similar to that for the neck, reach over your right shoulder with your left hand (so that your right shoulder muscles stay relaxed), pressing your fingers into the muscle at the top of your shoulder. Press and squeeze the muscle, rocking your fingers back and forth. Repeat on the other side.

Was It Good for You?

This ain't brain surgery, so maybe you're not inclined to grill a massage therapist about qualifications beforehand. The proof is in the putting of hands and the way that business is conducted. Here are some signs of a good therapist, according to Robert King, co-founder and co-director of the Chicago School of Massage Therapy and author of *Performance Massage.*

• You're asked to fill out a medical history form beforehand, identifying potential problems such as high blood pressure, back pain, numbness and epilepsy.

• Your therapist always keeps you draped appropriately, with the genitals covered at all times.

• The therapist varies the pressure depending on your ability to handle it. If it hurts too much, a therapist should never say, "I have to work this out." That puts her agenda ahead of yours.

• She can always explain why she's doing what she's doing.

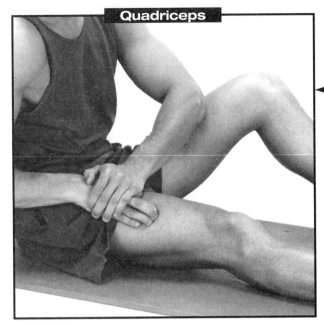

Quadriceps

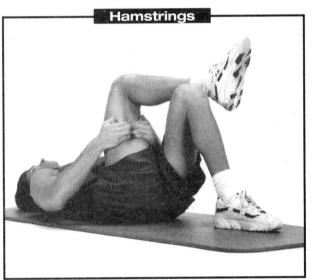

Hamstrings

◄ Upper Legs

The upper legs are prone to soreness in most sports and outdoor activities. Running, climbing, bicycling, skating, basketball, tennis—all are tough on quadriceps and hamstrings.

For the quads, while sitting on the floor or a mat, first loosen things up by shaking, squeezing and kneading muscles. Rest one hand on either side of your thigh so that your thumbs meet at the top of your leg. Press both thumbs into the top of your leg, pushing them toward your knee. Then, on either side of your thigh, press the middle three fingers of one hand into your leg muscle. (You can press the top of the stroking hand with your other hand to help apply pressure and control the movement.) While pressing, push your fingers toward your knee. Repeat on the other leg.

For the hamstrings, sit against a wall with one leg extended and the other bent so that the foot is flat on the floor. Use your hands to shake, squeeze and knead the back of the bent leg, working the entire length of the muscle. Repeat on the other leg. Next, lie flat on your back with your left leg bent, the foot flat on the floor. Raise your right knee toward your chest, resting your right foot or ankle on your left leg. Grab the back of your right leg with both hands, pressing with fingers bent so that the backs of the fingers on one hand make contact with the backs of the fingers on the other hand; then move your fingers toward your buttocks.

How to Find a Massage Therapist

Massage therapy is burdened by licentious connotations, not without reason. In the 1960s and 1970s, so-called massage parlors provided sex, not massage. The massage profession has since gained respectability, not least because of professional standards that legitimate practitioners impose upon themselves. Here's how King suggests you evaluate a therapist's qualifications beforehand.

Get a referral. There's no better recommendation than that of a satisfied client, especially if it's a friend. If the therapist's services are fronted by your gym, ask other members for a critique.

Check affiliations. Most good therapists belong to at least one of any number of nonprofit professional organizations such as the American Massage Therapy Association or the American Oriental Bodywork Therapy Association, which set professional standards for membership. Ask about it, or check the therapist's card or forms.

Glance at the wall. That's probably where you'll find the piece of paper that shows your therapist has been greenlighted by a national certifying authority, such as the National Certification Board for Therapeutic Massage and Bodywork, or the training credentials showing how many hours this person spent learning the craft. The hours of training are not as important as the accreditation status of the school, he adds.

Does a lack of any of the above mean you'll have a lousy or sordid experience? Not at all, King says. But your chances of being satisfied (assuming you don't want a lousy or sordid experience) are greater with at least some of these elements in place.

Preventing Disease

Feeling sick and tired too often?

Suffering chronic bouts with illness and infections?

Have high blood pressure? Unhealthy cholesterol readings? Diabetes? Are you stressed out?

Ready to do something about it?

Take the exercise prescription.

Okay, okay. It's true. Yes, even men who exercise religiously get sick at times. Some bully bacteria or virulent virus pounces when their guard is down.

But, you know what? Men who exercise get sick much less often than men who do not.

They have fewer sniffles, fewer aches, pains, fevers, colds, flus, infections, heart attacks and so on.

They feel better, more vibrant. Their minds, muscles and moods all function more effectively. Stressful situations don't faze them much. Their immune systems are stronger and more efficient.

And when they get sick, they bounce back fast.

We haven't created a special workout for disease prevention, since most any regular exercise routine will bolster your immune system. Instead, we'll explain how exercise affects your body's disease-fighting tools. If you are convinced—and may we say the arguments are most persuasive—and you haven't exercised in a long time, turn to The Inactive Man chapter on page 139 for information on how to launch a new routine.

The Exercise Prescription

In 1995, two of the nation's preeminent health watchdog groups—the federal government's Centers for Disease Control and Prevention (CDC) in Atlanta and the American College of Sports Medicine—issued a joint statement that gave formal endorsement to the exercise prescription. The statement formally marked a fundamental shift in the way the medical community views the role of exercise.

"They examined a persuasive body of scientific evidence and concluded that regular moderate physical activity is an important component of a healthy lifestyle—helping to prevent disease and enhance quality of life," says Jonathan Robison, Ph.D., an exercise physiologist, nutritionist and executive co-director of the Michigan Center for Preventive Medicine in Lansing.

The exercise prescription is flexible, says Dr. Robison. You don't have to buy a stair-climber or take part in sports you don't like. All you have to do is accumulate a minimum of 30 minutes of moderate-intensity physical activity several days per week, he says.

"Let people know that they can garden, walk the dog and so forth—they don't have to work out on stair-climbers and stationary bikes and treadmills to be healthy," says Dr. Robison.

The CDC and American College of Sports Medicine doctors determined that just 30 minutes of exercise—even if gathered in little snippets throughout the day—is enough to make us healthier and more disease resistant if done regularly.

"For the general population, we can probably be a little less obsessive about how high our heart rates are while we exercise or how long we're going for at a time, and focus more on just moving and having a good time and getting our breathing and heart rates up a bit," says Dr. Robison. "The recommendation for maintaining health is to accumulate 30 minutes of moderate physical activity most days of the week. All that really matters is that it's movement and that it is burning calories. You can walk for 30 minutes three times a week, or walk for 10 minutes nine times a week and probably get similar health benefits."

This is a recommendation for general health and, for instance, should not replace rehabilitative exercise routines prescribed for men following heart attacks or other specific conditions, notes Dr. Robison.

Throughout this book we've emphasized that the best fitness routine mixes up lots of exercise types to make sure you achieve all three tenets of fitness: strength, endurance and flexibility. It turns out that that apparently is the best formula for disease resistance as well. "Mixing aerobic and resistance training may offer the greatest, long-term health benefits," says Dr. Robison.

But don't overdo it, cautions Charles Swencionis, Ph.D., head of the health psychology program at Yeshiva University in

Postpone Crippling Old Age

Once we thought that getting weaker, fatter, dimmer and slower were natural effects of aging. Now we realize that they are natural effects of aging and inactivity (and poor diet plays a complicating role).

Regular exercise, including strength training, not only postpones debilitating symptoms associated with aging but can reverse many as well, researchers at Tufts University have conclusively shown. Exercise, in other words, can turn back the clock. Some examples:

• More brainpower. Research with seniors shows that fit folks fare better on tests of mental agility. They think faster and more clearly.

To gain and maintain this benefit—at any age—you need to get your blood pumping regularly, as in aerobic exercise, experts say. This draws more oxygen into the bloodstream and to the brain, which needs lots of oxygen to work well. Also, aerobic exercise is believed to contribute to the health and fitness of the parts of the brain responsible for motor activities.

• Stronger bones. A study with older women showed strength training actually resulted in increased bone mass and improved balance.

To assure strong bones, include weight-bearing and impact-loading activities in your routine, says Sydney Lou Bonnick, M.D., director of osteoporosis services at the Center for Research on Women's Health at Texas Woman's University in Denton and author of *The Osteoporosis Handbook*. A weight-bearing activity is one in which you stand, letting your skeleton support your weight. Impact-loading refers to any activity in which your bones are jarred. Walking counts. When your heel strikes the pavement, an impact passes upward through your skeleton.

• Greater sexual vitality. Aerobic exercise that keeps plaque from forming in heart arteries also keeps pathways open in arteries that pump blood into the penis, says Dudley Seth Danoff, M.D., in his book *Superpotency*.

• Less creakiness. Regular stretching and strength training restore flexibility and range of motion in seniors, says Dr. Robison.

New York City and co-author of *The Lazy Person's Guide to Fitness*. "Exercise that is moderate will increase resistance to disease. But overdoing it to the point of exhaustion is not going to help the immune system," he says.

And, he cautions, don't overwork the heart when exercising. We offer a formula for calculating the proper heart rate range on page 27. But, as Dr. Swencionis says, you don't really need to count with a stopwatch in your hand. If your heart is pumping faster than usual—fast enough that you start to sweat in a few minutes—and yet not so hard that you can't breathe comfortably or carry on a conversation, you're in the right zone.

Why It Works

Here's why the exercise prescription works.

• Quite simply, "exercise is what the body is designed to do," says Dr. Swencionis. "It is not designed to sit at a desk, or use a computer, or ride in a bus or drive a car. It's made for walking around, hunting game on the plains of Africa. That's really the kind of thing the body needs to do. When you deprive it of adequate physical activity, it develops all kinds of illnesses."

• The chemistry of the body is affected by exercise. The type and quantity of brain chemicals and hormones released changes—for the better—in a regularly exercised body. That, in turn, affects all sorts of systems. We produce more of a blood-clot dissolving substance. Our cholesterol balance changes, making our blood thinner and easier for our heart to pump. Our blood also is redder, more pumped up with fresh oxygen, bringing more life to each cell. We tax our immune system less, thus it is more prepared for a major fight. And on and on and on.

• We make energy differently, more efficiently, when we're fit. We also tap into different fuel stores, particularly the fat stored around the belly.

• We lose weight, and that makes a difference in how our body works. "Aerobic exercise (combined with a low-fat diet) lowers high blood pressure and cholesterol and controls diabetes. Just a loss of 10 to 15 pounds can mean you can stop taking drugs for these conditions, or take much lower doses," says Dr. Swencionis.

• Aerobic exercise increases our sense of well-being, lessens tendencies toward depression and anxiety, and puts the brakes on immune-dampening reactions to stress.

Want even more compelling evidence of how exercise will help your health? Read on.

Improve Cholesterol Levels

You probably know that HDL cholesterol wears the white hat and LDL wears the black one. But it's really not quite that simple, explains Covert Bailey, a popular fitness writer, in his book *Smart Exercise*.

Our bodies *need* cholesterol to digest fat and to manufacture male and female hormones, he says. But too high of an LDL cholesterol level is damaging. And too low of an HDL level is not good either. Physicians, says Bailey, recognize high levels of HDL cholesterol as a sign of good health.

So that's our goal with the exercise prescription—to raise the HDL and, maybe, to lower the LDL. If you have trouble keeping track of which is which, think of H as standing for healthy, and L as standing for lousy. It's a bit of an oversimplification, but a good memory trick.

The more unfit you are, the quicker and more dramatic improvement you will see in your cholesterol levels when you start exercising, Bailey says. That's encouraging. People who exercise all the time have to work hard to keep improving their cholesterol counts. Out-of-shape people will see improvement if they just start walking.

Low intensity exercise won't produce great gains in HDL levels, Bailey says, but it will quickly lower LDL levels. And, by getting into the habit of shaking your booty, you may find it easier to make the transition to more vigorous exercise—which *will* raise your HDL, he says.

Lessen Stress Damage

Our bodies are equipped to snap into emergency supercharged mode in an instant in response to stressful situations. Glucose stores are released from the liver, the heart pumps faster, blood vessels to the muscles open wide, as do our pupils—so we can get a better look at what we're confronting or the path on which we're fleeing, notes Dr. Robison. Amino acids are sucked from tissues and burned for fuel.

All this is in response to hormones—like adrenaline—that spurt in response to stress, says Dr. Robison. In an emergency situation, the physical changes give us a tremendous edge. They're sometimes referred to as the fight or flight response.

The same physical changes occur, though, in response to emotional stress. Ideally, in an emergency, we use all that energy. We slay the dragon, save the maiden, outrun the attacker, whatever. But, with emotional stress, we just stew. If the stress is chronic, the physiologic changes can be debilitating and destructive to the immune system. Stressed-out people get sick more easily. Add unfit to the equation and you have a real whammy.

The good news, say the experts, is that regular exercise alters how our bodies respond to stressors. Studies show fit people are less flustered by emotional stressors and actually secrete less stress hormones in day-to-day stressful situations, says Bailey.

Even better, fit people produce an even more powerful response to unusual stressors, like real danger, than do nonexercisers.

And even better yet, says Dr. Robison, people who exercise regularly are more resistant to depression and anxiety.

Also important, Dr. Robison adds, are rest and relaxation. Exercise, rest and relaxation all are crucial for optimal functioning of mind, body and spirit—and optimal functioning is crucial for maximum immunity. The beauty is, it is within our control and reach.

Listening to the Heart

Exercisers have stronger, healthier hearts.

Regular aerobic workouts build powerful, resilient heart muscles. And regular exercise causes the body to create more of its blood-clot dissolving substance and slightly less of its clotting factor. Hearts celebrate both developments. Our hearts don't have to push so hard to pump thinner, cleaner blood.

Are we listening to our hearts? Our hearts want us to exercise.

A program of exercise is carefully designed and prescribed when a man is rebounding from a heart attack. Why wait? A little exercise now, and we may avoid heart trouble altogether.

Just remember Dr. Swencionis's caution not to overdo it—especially if you are not now in the exercise habit. Start slowly and carefully. "Enjoy yourself," says Dr. Robison.

Rebounding from Disease

When we're sick, we fall off the exercise wagon. If we don't, our bodies tell us to. They moan, they gasp, they beg. They say, "Puhleeze. Don't force me to do this!"

Your exercise routine can be a part of the healing process, or it can be a hindrance. Here, we'll talk about how to recognize when to exercise and when to take it easy.

Mustering Strength

When your body is battling a bacterial infection, it needs every calorie of energy it can muster for infection-fighting and healing, says Charles Swencionis, Ph.D., head of the health psychology program at Yeshiva University in New York City.

During the acute period of the infection, lay off exercise completely, says David Nieman, Dr. P.H., professor of health and exercise science at Appalachian State University in Boone, North Carolina. You probably won't feel like working out anyway, so don't force yourself. Instead, conserve energy, he says. When your symptoms move to a point where you seem to be in the recovery phase—usually in a week to ten days or after any fever has passed—try resuming gentle exercise.

Viruses require a slightly different approach.

"If you just have a cold—runny nose, sore throat, the usual—then it's okay to engage in moderate activity," says Dr. Nieman. In fact, sweating a bit may lift your spirits. "A leisurely stroll may help you psychologically; it may make you feel better," says world-class runner Bob Glover, who runs a New York City fitness consulting firm and is author of *The Runners Handbook.*

But don't mess with the flu or other serious sickness. If you're feverish and achy or if your throat is ticklish, skip exertion. It can make you a good deal sicker, says Dr. Nieman.

"There have been instances where people pushed themselves when they had an illness, and the infection ended up spreading to the heart muscle," says Dr. Nieman. "It could be dangerous, and possibly even fatal, to exercise strenuously if you're seriously ill."

On the other hand, exercise *is* the prescription—or an important part of it—for rebounding from certain debilitating long-term diseases, such as arthritis, many heart problems, chronic pain, depression, chronic stress, chronic constipation and much more, says Dr. Swencionis. Just remember that an exercise program for getting the upper hand on any serious ailment—such as heart disease—should be designed only in consultation with a qualified doctor or therapist, he says.

Restarting the Exercise Engine

As we begin to get well—or in the case of a long-term disease, as we begin to adjust to life with it—we're faced with the daunting task of restarting our exercise program. Often, the first thing that needs to be kick-started is our exercise motivation.

Restarting can be tough. We can do it right, or we can do it wrong. If we do it wrong, we're likely to become discouraged and lose interest in exercise. Or worse, we could make ourselves even sicker. Here are a few pointers from experts to help make sure that doesn't happen.

Stick to the "neck rule." If you have a cold and you still want to work out, it's probably okay to do that. "Just follow the neck rule: If your symptoms are from the neck up—sniffles, headache, runny nose—then a light to moderate workout won't hurt," says Dr. Nieman. If your symptoms involve the chest or include body aches, or if you have a fever, do not work out. "Just rest—working out when you have more systemic, body-wide symptoms can actually be harmful," says Dr. Nieman.

Use the 30-second rule. For aerobic exercise or sustained activities, Dr. Swencionis swears by his 30-second formula. It's simple: If you've been unable to exercise for a long time, subtract 30 seconds from your regular exercise routine for each day, beyond three, that you were laid up. Then restart at that lesser level and add 30 seconds per day until you're back to the ideal. Remember, if your symptoms get worse, back off.

Be a lightweight. If you were working out three days a week before your cold, don't expect to jump right back in at the same level of intensity. You'll probably still

Rebounding from Chronic Illness

Chronic ailments and diseases put a damper on life in general, not to mention exercise. And yet, there are numerous symptoms of serious and chronic illnesses that exercise can minimize or eliminate. Below we've listed a few diseases in which exercise has been proven to make a difference.

If you have these or any other serious illness, you should, of course, consult your doctor or specialist before exercising, says Thomas M. Petro, Ph.D., associate professor of microbiology and immunology in the Department of Oral Biology at the University of Nebraska Medical Center in Lincoln. He may be able to offer additional or modified exercises to help you work out with your specific condition.

• AIDS. People who test positive for HIV or who have full-blown AIDS can benefit greatly from exercise, especially a muscle-building regimen. "It's been shown that the more lean muscle mass you have, the longer you can resist the disease," says Dr. Petro. "And weight training can help you build and maintain lean muscle mass."

On the other hand, sufferers should rest during those periods when their bodies are fighting off the opportunistic viruses that can attack during AIDS. "Rest during those times, so your body can marshal its forces to fight the disease. Then, when you feel well enough, you can resume exercising," states Dr. Petro.

• Arthritis. Research shows that regular, vigorous exercise has a healing effect on stiff, painful joints and helps men and women beat common osteoarthritis symptoms.

Exercise, says James Fries, M.D., associate professor of medicine at Stanford University, actually feeds cartilage with needed nutrients it wouldn't get otherwise. Exercises that move painful joints through their full range of motion are best, according to Dr. Fries. For example, walking, rowing, cross-country skiing and cycling are best for arthritis in the knees and hips, he says. Swimming is an excellent exercise for arthritis of all types. There is no such thing as too much exercise for overcoming arthritis, he notes. The

minimum, he says, is about 30 minutes a session, three or more days a week.

• Cancer. Dr. Petro says the more physically fit you are, the better you can resist the ravages of certain types of cancer—and the better you can withstand the effects of cancer treatments like chemotherapy. In addition, exercise has been shown to limit your risk for other types of cancer, including colon and testicular cancer.

• Diabetes. Roughly six million men suffer from diabetes, usually a variety known as adult-onset or Type II diabetes. As we get older or put on more weight, we become more prone to diabetes. But studies have shown that aerobic exercise—five or more times a week, 30 minutes per session—can reduce your risk of developing Type II diabetes by more than 40 percent. And if you already have Type II diabetes, you know controlling your blood sugar is key to controlling the disease. Studies show that exercise—especially walking—can be helpful as part of an overall plan to control blood sugar.

• Depression. David Nieman, Dr. P.H., professor of health and exercise science at Appalachian State University in Boone, North Carolina, says that exercise has always been one of the best ways to cope with stress, a leading cause of depression among men. Studies have also shown that regular exercise doesn't just improve mood, it creates a high-energy state that makes active people in general feel more optimistic and positive than sedentary people.

• Heart disease. If you've had a heart attack, your doctor will probably recommend a specific program of regular, brisk exercise. This can reduce your chances of having another heart attack, says the American Heart Association. And if you've never had a heart attack, this sort of exercise is one of the best ways to ensure you never have one. Not only does exercise make you feel and look better but it also improves your chances of survival. If you've had recent heart disease, it's important that your program be monitored and assessed by a doctor to make sure you aren't causing further damage through overexertion.

feel a little weak, says Dr. Nieman. "Once your symptoms subside, it's okay to start working out again, but keep your weight training to one day a week for a couple weeks, then resume your normal schedule," he says. For your first week back, do just one set for each exercise, and use a light to moderate weight.

Ease into stretching. Ligaments tend to overstretch when you're running a fever. That's part of why you feel so achy when you're sick, says Dr.

Swencionis. This capacity to overstretch makes ligaments particularly prone to injury if you work out when you have a fever. Don't resume stretching until your body has kicked the bug and lost its achiness.

Carry a bottle. Illness makes us sweat. Exercise makes us sweat. Put the two together, and you're looking at one dried-out body.

"It's for a very good reason that doctors tell you to drink lots of fluids when you're sick," says Thomas

Germs in the Gym

You still have the sniffles, but you want to work out. Public-spirited soul that you are, you don't want to get your germs all over the equipment and infect the next guy. Consider this the expert's germ-free gym guide to post-cold etiquette.

Wait three days. Even after your cold symptoms have subsided, you can still infect others with your cold germs. As a general rule, postpone your return to the gym until three days after your symptoms have subsided, suggests David Nieman, Dr. P.H., professor of health and exercise science at Appalachian State University in Boone, North Carolina. Meanwhile, exercise by yourself, either with weights at home or by running, walking or cycling.

Wash up before the workout. We often trans-mit cold germs with our hands, so after you change into your workout togs, eradicate the germs on your paws by soaping up and washing with hot water. "It can greatly minimize the amount of germs you spread," says Dr. Nieman.

Carry two towels. One towel is for you—to wipe off all the sweat and other fluids that are likely to be leaking out of you while you're recovering from a cold, says Dr. Petro. Do not use this towel to wipe off the equipment. If you're really considerate, use a second towel exclusively for wiping off the equipment before the next guy. "You could even go so far as to spray that towel with some kind of antiseptic," he says. "Just don't forget which towel is which."

M. Petro, Ph.D., associate professor of microbiology and immunology in the Department of Oral Biology at the University of Nebraska Medical Center in Lincoln. It's not just to flush a cold out of your system. When you're sick and feverish, your body temperature is raised in an attempt to kill off whatever's infecting you. Even if you're on the mend, you're probably still sweating a lot more than usual, so be sure to carry a water bottle with you and drink from it every couple of minutes while you exercise. "Dehydration not only inhibits your performance in exercise but it also makes you weaker and more prone to relapse," says Dr. Petro.

Soothe the savage throat. When you're just getting over a cold, especially one that has affected your throat, suck on a cough drop or hard candy a few minutes before your workout, says Dr. Petro.

"Exercise is going to be hard on a throat that's just recovering from sickness," says Dr. Petro. "Even if your throat isn't sore, take the cough drop. It will pre-soothe your throat and prepare it for all the heavy breathing you're about to do."

Cough it up. Aerobic activity can be part of the healing process, says Dr. Petro. "Once you're past the point of fever and you're starting to feel better, you'll probably still be coughing and hacking a lot, especially when you exercise." And that's okay—increased physical activity will help you bring up phlegm and mucus and clear out your passages. "Just keep a handkerchief or some tissues handy," he says.

If your cough becomes dry, your throat starts to feel scratchy or your coughing starts to sound more like a goose honking, stop exercising. "When this happens, you're irritating your airways, which can expose you to infections like bronchitis and sinusitis," warns Dr. Petro. Take it easy for another day or two,

then resume your workout.

Watch your meds. Cold medicines may keep your head clear, but their active ingredients—antihistamines and decongestants—can affect your balance and concentration. Keep that in mind before you go pounding away at the stair-climber or treadmill, both of which require a little balance to use safely, says Dr. Petro.

Check the side of your medicine bottle. That warning about operating heavy equipment applies to weights, too. Make sure you have a spotter with you during your first few days back at weight training, suggests Dr. Nieman. He'll keep your attention focused on the weights and help you out if your concentration—or the weight—slips.

Although it's generally safe to exercise while you're taking most antibiotics and cold medications, check with your doctor if you're on medication for a specific chronic disease, advises Dr. Nieman. Certain heart medications, for example, can affect your blood pressure, and exercising while you're on them could lead to serious injury, or even death.

Monitor your vital signs. During your first few days back in the gym, pay close attention to your body, says Dr. Swencionis. If you sense your symptoms getting worse with exercise, if your heart works harder than normal, if you feel dizzy or find yourself short of breath, or if you develop serious discomfort, back off, he says. You probably returned too soon.

If it feels good, do it. If you're coping with a long-term illness, it's important to remember that *you* have the disease, says Dr. Petro; it doesn't have you.

"With a chronic illness, it's easy to slip into the mode of, 'I'm sick, I shouldn't exercise.' But often, exercise can be very good both mentally and physically when you're dealing with an illness," says Dr. Petro.

Rebounding from Arthritis

Arthritis needn't put a stop to your active lifestyle. Research shows that regular, vigorous exercise has a healing effect on stiff, painful joints and helps men (and women) beat common arthritis symptoms.

Exercise, says James Fries, M.D., professor of medicine at Stanford University, feeds cartilage with nutrients it wouldn't get otherwise. Cartilage has no blood supply, unlike most other tissues.

How does exercise feed joints? When a runner bears weight on a knee joint, for example, it squeezes out all the water and waste products from the cartilage—"just like water squeezes out of a sponge when you press down on it," Dr. Fries says. "When you let up on the pressure, it fills up again with water and oxygen. That exchange nourishes the cartilage cells and keeps them alive."

The Arthritis Foundation recommends the same three exercise types for overcoming the disabling effects of arthritis as we've been pushing throughout this book: range-of-motion flexibility exercises, strengthening exercises and endurance exercises. Data now suggest endurance exercise as particularly important.

Much of this book covers strength and endurance training. But here are some specific range-of-motion movements suggested by the Arthritis Foundation for various body parts. Understand that these don't add up to a workout program; rather, they are highly specific stretches that should be plugged in as needed to a broader routine. Finally, if you have arthritis, check with your doctor before beginning any exercise program. Start each of the following exercises lying on your back. Do these exercises once or twice per day, three to ten times each. Don't bounce. Move slowly and remember to keep breathing. If you have severe pain, stop.

- Knee and hip: Bend one knee, so your foot rests flat on the floor. Extend and lift the other leg. Then bend the knee of the lifted leg, and using your hands behind your knee, pull it toward your chest. Next push the leg into the air, straightening it. Finally, lower it slowly to the floor. Don't kick it into the air if you feel pain in the knee. Repeat with the other leg.

- Hip: Avoid this exercise if you have lower-back problems, a hip replacement or osteoporosis. With your feet about six inches apart, legs straight, point your toes upward. Slide one leg out to the side, keeping the toes pointing up. Don't lift the leg, just slide it. Then slide it back and do the other leg.

- Hip and knee: With your legs as straight as possible and your toes pointed upward, roll your hips and knees so your left toes point to the left and your right toes point to the right. Your heels should pivot but essentially remain in the same place. Return to the starting position and repeat. When you finish with that motion exercise, and with your legs still straight, push one knee down toward the floor by tightening the muscles on the front of the thigh for a slow count of five. Relax. Then repeat with the other leg.

- Shoulder: Lie with your arms close to your sides, fingers pointing to your feet. Raise one arm in a smooth motion, keeping the elbow straight, moving it through a circular arc until your hand reaches the floor beyond your head. Then smoothly return it to the side of your leg, going through the same arc, elbow still straight. Repeat with the other arm.

- Fingers: Stretch and spread the fingers of each hand. Next bend all the finger joints except the knuckles. With your bent fingertips, touch the top of your palm. Then reach your thumb over until it contacts the second joint of your little finger. Next stretch out the thumb. Finally, stretch all your fingers again. Repeat.

Want more assistance? You can call the Arthritis Foundation at 1-800-283-7800 for a free copy of "Exercise and Your Arthritis." Or check into "The ROM Dance" (ROM stands for Range of Motion). This is a great, oft-prescribed form of stretching that generates relief from arthritis pain and enhances the mind-body connection. If your doctor or therapist suggests that you try ROM, you might check with adult schools, recreation programs and occupational or physical therapists in your area to see if "The ROM Dance" is available. For a list of ROM certified therapists, contact The ROM Dance Network, P.O. Box 3332, Madison, WI 53704-0332.

Always consult your doctor first to make sure physical activity is okay, says Dr. Petro. Then, if you feel up to a little activity—even if it's just getting out of bed and walking around the house, do it. "Don't set yourself a strict fitness regimen; try to go with the flow. Some days you'll feel too weak to do anything—so don't, and don't feel guilty about it. Know that on your better days, you can get up, get a little exercise, maybe get a change of scenery in the bargain. That will make you feel better," says Dr. Petro.

Part Six
Getting Equipped

Setting Up a Home Gym

Gyms are scarce near your home or work. You don't want yet another spigot on your wallet. You can't spare the time it takes to get to a gym and back. You fail to see the need for tons of fancy equipment to achieve your fitness goals. You're not at ease with the spandex crowd.

Those are just a few reasons we could come up with for not joining a gym. No doubt you can think of a few of your own. But let's not be negative. If you can't find happiness among the maddening crowd in a brightly lit hall of chrome and mirrors, you may be a candidate for a home gym. The minuses of health clubs are exactly the pluses of a home gym—and a home gym has some advantages all its own.

"Mainly, it's convenient," says Liz Neporent, president of Frontline Fitness, a consulting firm that sets up private and corporate gyms in New York City. "You're open 24 hours a day." It's also more private and more under your control. There's no waiting for equipment. You can listen to jazz instead of top 40, or watch *Gilligan's Island* instead of CNN. And, for the man who just wants to retreat to his castle after a strenuous workday spent fighting barbarians, there's less time away from the bosom of the family.

Still, a home gym costs money, time and effort just like a health club. If you want to make your investment worthwhile, you have to do it right. It all comes down to two things: equipment and a place to put it.

The Real Estate

As a rule, you need the space before you can furnish it, so don't go rushing off to a fitness supplier until you've come to an understanding about domestic property values and usage restrictions.

Consult the Board of Significant Others. Gain approval from the woman in your life, and even your small fry, says Neporent, before proceeding with any major expansion or even minor renovation. Will you have to move other stuff to make room for equipment? Where will you put what's displaced? Did anyone else have designs on the space? Knowing this stuff beforehand saves trouble in the long run.

Choose an appealing spot. "If the space isn't inviting, you won't go to it," says Neporent. More likely than not, the best available location is lit by a bare 40-watt bulb, with cobwebs hanging off crates jammed with half-empty paint cans. A charming spot if you're Gomez Addams. You, however, had better brighten things up. Lamps with shades, a carpet, some clear floor space to move around in— use them all to create a turf boundary between you and the spiders, she says.

Measure everything. Get a reading on floor space and, just as important, *ceiling* space before you buy anything, says Neporent. Also measure doorways, stairwells or any other feature of interior geography you'll have to negotiate to get your gear where it's going.

The Equipment

How much equipment do you need in order to qualify your setup as a bona fide gym? "What people call a home gym often amounts to just one piece of equipment," says Cathy McNeil, spokesperson for the International Health, Racquet and Sportsclub Association. In her opinion, that's not enough. And she's right.

Let's be clear: Having a single piece of equipment is better than having none at all. But if you're seriously construing your home arrangement as a club alternative, there need to be some genuine equivalencies. That means you ideally should have gear for both strength and aerobic training—in other words, free weights or a resistance-training machine, along with a cardiovascular device such as a treadmill, stationary cycle, stair-climber, rower or cross-country skier. "A stationary bike thrown in the basement is not a gym," Neporent states.

What you choose for equipment is entirely a matter of personal preference. But preferences are always swayed by the winds of enlightenment. For additional

Let Your Wallet Be Your Guide

You're on a budget, but you still want quality. What can you afford? We asked Liz Neporent, president of Frontline Fitness, a consulting firm that sets up private and corporate gyms in New York City, to tell us what to purchase if you can spend:

$100: A good aerobic step that's adjustable to different heights and comes with a video workout guide, and rubber tubing or rubber bands for resistance training.

$100 to $700: A noncomputerized stationary bike or a trackstand for mounting your road or mountain bike, and an inexpensive set of free weights. "Inexpensive" doesn't have to mean cheaply made. When buying gear without moving parts,

check out used-equipment stores, where good weights can be found at a fraction of their original cost.

$700 to $2,000: A treadmill or stair-climber, stationary bike, rower or ski machine; and possibly a multistation machine, but more likely free weights. "With free weights you could equip yourself like a king and still have money for a bench," Neporent says.

$2,000 to $3,000: A piece of health club–quality equipment in any aerobic category—maybe two, and a superior multistation machine with two stacks of weight plates instead of just one.

---

input on this score, we consulted Charles Kuntzleman, Ed.D., adjunct associate professor of kinesiology at the University of Michigan in Ann Arbor. He recently conducted a massive evaluation of 130 pieces of indoor exercise equipment for *Consumers Digest*, coordinating reports from 50 testers, including exercise physiologists, bodybuilders, runners, cyclists, doctors, nurses and coaches. Here's a wrap-up of what he says you need to know to be an educated buyer of home-gym equipment.

Free Weights

Think "gym" and you're likely to picture barbells and dumbbells. We covered the relative merits of free weights versus machines in Weight Lifting on page 22, but when you're lifting at home, there are a few other considerations to bear in mind about weights. One is the sight of them: If they're not properly stored, they have a tendency to make a merely cluttered space verge on Animal House ambiance. Another is the sound of them. If you live above your neighbors and have, say, bare wood floors, the thunder of falling iron plates won't earn you any friends. (It won't do the floor much good either.) But these matters are largely fixable by being diligently neat and using cushioning materials like a workout mat or rug, or weights with vinyl coverings, says Dr. Kuntzleman. On the purchasing front, you should:

Consider your needs. Unless you're seriously into bodybuilding (in which case you'd consider a 310-pound set of weights), a good starter set would include about 200 pounds of plates, with weight ranges from 1 to 25 pounds, along with bars to slide the plates onto, recommends Dr. Kuntzleman. Your set should include two bars for dumbbells and one for a barbell, he says.

Do a quality check. You'd think it would be

hard to go wrong buying slabs of metal, but quality is indeed an issue. "On the low end, it's unfortunately common to find weights that aren't true," Dr. Kuntzleman says. "It might be labeled 5 pounds, but actually be 4½." Other cheapness giveaways are poorly baked paint that chips, and sharp edges in the metal. For the good stuff, expect to pay from $1 to $1.50 per pound. Quality brand names include Ivanko, York, Universal and Sonata, he says.

Get a good collar. "You have to be careful that the plates stay in place," Neporent says. There are a number of ways in which these weight-holding gizmos, or collars, work. Some just screw on like a big nut holding an oversized washer. The best, however, include some form of self-locking mechanism, usually held in place with springs that let loose only when you manually release them.

Invest in a bench. "The most common mistake is buying one that's too narrow," Dr. Kuntzleman says. He recommends a width of at least 36 inches. Anything less won't provide good support for your shoulders and may be downright unstable. Better benches include a number of features that are probably worth the money, he says, such as the ability to set the bench at an incline and adjust the barbell rack up and down. For materials, look for steel tubing at least two inches square and a bench covering of quality vinyl such as Naugahyde.

Multistation Machines

As we've said elsewhere, machines have their advantages, but at home, they have some handicaps, too. For one thing, they take up a lot of space. Not just side-to-side space, but up-and-down space. "For some machines, you need close to seven feet of overhead clearance," Dr. Kuntzleman says.

There are two basic types of home machines: the

Equipment-Buying Made Easy

Every piece of equipment is different, but the way you buy them should be pretty much the same. Even when faced with an overwhelming selection of products, keeping a few key considerations in mind will help guide you to gear that won't do you wrong, says Charles Kuntzleman, Ed.D., adjunct associate professor of kinesiology at the University of Michigan in Ann Arbor.

Spend enough. You're making an investment—something that should hold up to years of use, if not abuse. If you skimp on cash up front, you'll be disappointed with performance later. And you just won't use something you don't like.

Buy from specialty stores. "Don't go to a place that sells a bazillion other things," advises Dr. Kuntzleman. Specialty retailers have what discount and department stores don't: higher-end products, knowledgeable sales staff and service for products after you buy them.

Test out different models. "Buy only what you can see and touch yourself," says Liz Neporent, president of Frontline Fitness, a consulting firm that sets up private and corporate gyms in New York City. "Any reputable dealer will let you try out equipment on the sales floor."

Avoid assembly hassles. "Assembling things like multistation machines can be extremely time-consuming," Neporent says. "If you buy from a gym equipment dealer, they should deliver it assembled and installed."

Ask who will repair it. Ideally, suppliers will honor warranties and do repairs themselves. If they don't, make sure there's a servicer available in your county—or at least in your state. "I once bought a stationary bike that had an excellent warranty, but there was only one guy who serviced a four-state area," Neporent says.

---

kind that uses cables to raise metal plates and the kind that forgos weight stacks in favor of some other form of resistance. These forms include oversize rubber bands or bungee cords, springs and cylinders that create resistance using air (pneumatic) or liquid (hydraulic). Non-weight-stack machines tend to be lighter, smaller and less expensive than plate-and-cable gear, but they're sometimes not as sturdy or biomechanically sound as weight-stack units. Beyond that, consider these factors, says Dr. Kuntzleman.

Know the value of numbers. If you like knowing just how much weight you're lifting, gravitate to machines with plates, in which you increase weight by moving a pin. With non-weight-stack machines, there's no way of telling how upping the resistance translates to pounds.

Gauge the fuss factor. Sure, multistation gyms are designed to let you do multiple exercises, but if you have to pull something apart, change cables or otherwise reconfigure the machine for each station, you're going to waste time. "A machine like that can add up to 45 minutes to your workout," Neporent says.

Consider safety. If there are children in the house, that alone might be a reason to avoid weight-stack machines, unless the stacks are covered by a shield that protects small fingers from getting caught between plates.

Treadmills

There are two categories of treadmills, but only one type is worth considering—motorized. With these, a small motor drives the belt on which you're walking or running, providing a close simulation of actual outdoor locomotion. With nonmotorized units, *you* drive the belt, sliding it along with your feet as you go through the motions of propelling yourself forward. This might sound like a better workout because it's more difficult, but in reality, it's just more difficult, period. "It's tough to get the belt moving at a consistent pace; you get tired quickly, and it's hell on your legs," Neporent says.

Motorized treadmills are a considerable investment: Expect to pay at least $1,000 for a good unit that features electronic programming; if you're a serious runner who will use your equipment three or more times a week, aim to spend in the $2,000 to $3,000 range. To make sure you're investing wisely, says Dr. Kuntzleman, follow these tips.

Get a good motor. When running, you hit the mat with two to four times your body weight—a force that momentarily slows or stops the motor. To keep up a steady seven- to eight-mile-per-hour pace (and to be able to start the tread moving without taking your weight off it), you'll need at least 1.5 horsepower. Make sure that number is labeled for "continuous duty," says Dr. Kuntzleman. Cheaper models use a sly "peak power" rating that undervalues the power available over a sustained period.

Ask for industrial strength. Welded frames of aircraft-quality aluminum or heavy steel (12-gauge or less) are de rigueur for both solidity and flexibility. Shy away from anything held together with too many bolts, says Dr. Kuntzleman, which tend to come loose and make the frame shake and squeak.

Go long. You want a surface with enough room on it, or you'll feel like you're running on a balance beam. Get a tread that's at least 50 inches long, says Dr. Kuntzleman. Make it wide enough, too—18 inches, minimum.

Raise your sights. Outdoors, hills provide half the challenge. To get the same thing indoors, you'll need a machine that can raise and lower the tread elevation while you're running on it. Good brands include Trotter, PaceMaster and Star Trac.

Stationary Bikes

It's a classic piece of gear, so tried and true it can be found in the basements of aging uncles and the common areas of senior centers as well as the most crowded corners of the trendiest health clubs. You can update the concept with new language (for example, "spinning"), but the basics are the same: You climb on something with a seat, a wheel, pedals and handlebars, and make like a latter-day Greg LeMond. As with most products, manufacturers are happy to tack on bells and whistles to drive the high-end market, but stationary bikes don't have to cost a lot to provide a good workout. Here's what should guide your purchase, according to Dr. Kuntzleman.

Choose your resistance. The bike has to work against you in some way, or you'll make the wheel spin faster than you're pedaling, creating a coasting effect. The choices for resistance mechanisms are:

• A weighted flywheel that's driven by a belt. It's inexpensive and simple but highly effective, smooth-feeling and extremely durable. Just make sure you get a wheel that's heavy enough, with a weight of 25 to 50 pounds.

• Caliper brakes, which hold the wheel back by applying pressure to the rim. Picture riding a real bike with the brakes on all the time and you'll understand why this mechanism feels awkward and tends to wear out relatively fast.

• Air resistance caused by fan-like aerodynamics of the wheel. It's genuinely cool: The fan blades create a breeze that gets stronger the harder you work. (Many models also have movable handlebars that keep the upper body moving, too.) Resistance increases with faster pedaling, which is an elegant concept, but you may want other resistance-changing options.

• Magnetic resistance, in which a thin flywheel passes between two magnets, which are moved closer or farther apart electronically to change resistance. It is smooth and quiet, generally comes with superior programming features and, not surprisingly, is expensive.

Examine your needs. You have the luxury of wide price options, since good-quality bikes can be had for less than $300 as well as for high-end prices of above $1,500. If all you're looking for is a decent workout that has the feel of outdoor riding, you don't need to spend more than a few hundred bucks, says Scott Schaeffer, fitness manager at Tom Schaeffer's Recreation and Sports Center in Shoemakersville, Pennsylvania.

As you move up the price scale, a basic bike becomes an ergometer—equipped with electronic displays that show you things like precise pedaling resistance, calories burned, heart rate and revolutions per minute. These are good for calibrating your workout to exact parameters, matching your performance on a different machine if you train elsewhere, grading yourself against national standards and competing against other bikers or a computerized opponent. But even basic bikes usually have a speedometer, odometer and timer. Do you need more? Your choice.

Focus on fundamentals. Whatever you choose, the most important qualities to look for are comfort and solidness, says Eric Holland, a sales representative at Bike Line in Emmaus, Pennsylvania. You don't want the bike rocking while you're rolling, and you don't want numb buns or a sore back. The seat and handlebars should be adjustable but firmly held in place with a pin that drives all the way through the seat tube and post, then locks into place. "There have been a couple of lawsuits about collapsing seats," Neporent says. "If you're a heavy rider and the seat fails, I'll leave it to your imagination where the pole goes."

Stair-Climbers

Why buy a machine when there are real stairs to climb? Well, if you're the retro-grouch type, maybe a stair-climber isn't for you. If, however, you want a great aerobic workout that's easy on bones and joints, trains muscles for familiar, real-life, day-to-day movements and gets you off your butt while you watch TV, this may be the thing for you. Go a step beyond, and your workout will seem more like mountain climbing: Technically, the market is divided into steppers, which work just the lower body, and climbers, which provide handles to grasp so that your motion is more akin to scaling a ladder. Here's what you need to consider, says Dr. Kuntzleman.

Vote on independence. The foot platforms on stair-climbers go up and down in two different ways. With one, the pedals move in tandem, so that when one foot goes down, the opposite pedal goes up automatically. It feels balanced and is easy to get the hang of. With the other, each pedal moves independently of the other, which theoretically provides a slightly better workout. Independent movement takes a bit more getting used to, but feels quite natural once you do. One isn't better than the other, just different. Try them both and decide for yourself.

Consider mechanics. As with stationary bikes, stair-climbers require you to work against a force. On the low end, resistance comes from pushing pedals against pressure from a hydraulic or pneumatic cylinder. Hydraulic cylinders are usually filled with oil, which keeps them lubricated and free of maintenance problems. Pneumatic cylinders are a bit more troublesome because inner friction and heat tends to wear them down.

Higher-end machines forsake cylinders altogether in favor of cables or chains that wrap around a flywheel. The extra cost buys you a quieter and smoother workout, for starters. Beyond that, "the higher-end machines have better railings along the sides or top, feel more substantial and have graphic displays that provide more information with greater accuracy," Neporent says. Bottom-line, acceptable units can be found for under $500, but our experts draw a "can't-go-wrong" line at around $1,200.

Judge by feel. Try out any machine you're considering for at least 10 to 15 minutes to make sure it feels comfortable. It shouldn't make your feet tingle or feel odd, or make you bend over while you exercise. The pedals should be wide enough to make your feet feel stable and secure, and the motion should feel smooth and steady, not sticky.

Rowers

All over the land, rowing machines are gathering cobwebs in dusty basements and attics, the detritus of yet another passing fitness fad, circa 1985. It's too bad, really, since rowers offer the unusual advantage of simultaneously working both the lower and upper body without putting undue strain on either. That's what sold people on them in the first place. So what happened? Mostly, manufacturers flooded the market with shoddy goods that turned buyers off. The majority of these provided resistance using hydraulic or pneumatic cylinders, which, beyond their technical liabilities, didn't feel at all like real rowing. Fortunately, there are plenty of good units still out there. Here's what to look for, says Dr. Kuntzleman.

Look for wheel resistance. Quality manufacturers dispensed with shock absorbers and turned to wheels: You pull on the handle, which spins a fanlike flywheel via a cable or belt. As with some exercise cycles, the harder you pull, the more resistance you get from the fan. Perhaps the best-known of these is the Concept II rower, but similar designs are offered by companies like Tunturi and Ross; all of these fall in the $700 range. The hands-down coolest rower, however (for a few hundred dollars more), is the WaterRower, in which the "wheel" is a tank of water containing a stainless steel paddle that rotates when you pull back on the handle. You can change the resistance by filling or draining the tank. Best of all, the paddle's motion produces the gratifying gurgling sound of swooshing water. You can find out more about the WaterRower by calling 1-800-852-2210.

Consider stowability. Some of these units seem to take up as much space as a rowing shell on the Charles—lengths of eight feet aren't uncommon. Check to see if it can be stood upright against a wall (even the WaterRower can be tipped without spilling), or easily broken down.

Cross-Country Skiers

Although it's not the only player in the market anymore, NordicTrack has been synonymous with this type of machine for years, with good reason: Their equipment has consistently been well-made and fairly priced. In fact, Dr. Kuntzleman's choices for best buys in this category are all NordicTrack models, ranging from $400 to $600. Says Neporent, "They're one of the best fitness bargains out there." Indoor skiing is an acquired taste, not to mention an acquired skill—difficult and awkward at first, but easily mastered after one or two practice sessions. More than in other categories, you can quickly narrow your candidates for purchase, says Dr. Kuntzleman, but you still need to evaluate a number of options.

Get the movement you want. A number of competing models offer "dependent" motion of the feet similar to some stair-climbers: Moving one foot moves the other the opposite way. NordicTrack has kept to independent foot movement, which is part of what makes you feel so gangly on the machines at first, but which more closely simulates real skiing. It's the same story with arm movement: Moving arms in tandem is easier, but working them independently is generally better. (With some models, you pull on cables or belts; with others, you hang on to poles.)

Determine the features you want. As usual, the higher you move up the price range, the more information you get from electronic displays, such as speed, distance and time. How much of this you need is a matter of taste.

Choosing a Gym

Somewhere in the 1970s and early 1980s, gyms changed. They became less the kind of place where a crusty Burgess Meredith coaches a down-on-his-luck Sly Stallone, and more the kind of place where a buff John Travolta meets a perfect Jamie Lee Curtis. Solid chunks of metal and leather in the form of barbells and punching bags were supplemented or replaced altogether with ergonomic, hydraulic, cantilevered, LEDed marvels of technology. Training sessions on how to land a left hook were transformed into classes in which women in leotards and leg warmers jumped around to perky tunes from Wham. Gyms became health clubs.

This sounds like a lament, but it's not. What the fitness boom has given men is options. In the old days, if a man wanted to go someplace with more equipment than he had at home, he had to surround himself with street fighters, kids at the field house of his alma mater or whomever the local YMCA attracted. He couldn't be guaranteed staff to help him, access to reasonably up-to-date equipment or a clientele with whom he felt comfortable. There are still no guarantees with health clubs, but there are plenty of choices, which means far more control over the environment in which you train. Just ask any of the 19.2 million people enrolled in the 15,000 health and sport clubs and YMCAs nationwide.

Perhaps paramount in the sheer proliferation of fitness establishments is the option to go someplace that's actually close to where you live or work. This, in fact, is the first element to look at when thinking about joining a gym. "The rule of thumb is that if it's more than a 10 or 15 minute drive away, or—if you're in the city—further than ten blocks, it's too far," says Liz Neporent, president of Frontline Fitness, a consulting firm that sets up private and corporate gyms in New York City. Most people won't regularly attend a club that's more distant.

Is This What You Want?

To further foster regular attendance, it helps to lay out clearly what you expect from a club and what you're willing to pay for. That way, you'll find the greatest support for your goals and be less inclined to squander your money.

Health clubs are categorized in two basic ways, according to Cathy McNeil, spokesperson for the International Health, Racquet and Sportsclub Association (IHRSA).

Fitness-only clubs provide the basic amenities you should expect from any commercial gym: resistance training equipment, often with both machines and free weights; cardiovascular equipment such as stationary cycles or stair-climbers, and an aerobics area where classes are offered.

Multipurpose clubs offer everything fitness clubs do, in addition to sports facilities such as swimming pools and/or tennis, racquetball, squash or basketball courts. These clubs are usually bigger and more expensive. Often, they're more oriented to family activities, some of which may be organized by the club (these might include after-school swimming lessons, summer camps and seasonal parties).

Do you need all of this? If you just need some of it, which features are you likely to use most? Are you just looking for a place to heft dumbbells or ride a stationary cycle? If so, investing in home equipment may be what you need (see Setting Up a Home Gym on page 312). Just don't overlook what McNeil identifies as the main advantage clubs have over home gyms: people. Trained staff will be able to help design your programs and make sure you're using equipment to maximum advantage. Plus, McNeil says, there's a benefit to being around other exercisers. "Exercise is harder to do on your own," she says. "The research suggests that even when you already have equipment at home, if you join a club, you're more likely to exercise in both places."

What to Look For

Location and cost aren't everything. After all, it's common to find several choices available within a given geographic area and price range. How to choose? One way is to personally visit each of the clubs you're considering, suggests McNeil. Only by being on site will you be able to conduct the following evaluation.

Appraise the staff. There was a time when just about any muscle-bound ape could get a job in a gym, but increasingly, you should expect club staffers to have credentials. Standards set by IHRSA require club supervisors to have at least a bachelor's degree in exercise science or certification by any of a number of organizations, says McNeil. The greater number of staff members that are certified, the better. Certifying agencies include the Aerobics and Fitness Association of America, the National Strength and Conditioning Association, the American College of Sports Medicine, the American Council on Exercise and the Cooper Fitness Institute. Beyond that, IHRSA requires that at least one staffer be trained in CPR. If the club is an IHRSA member, that's a good sign, she says.

Credentials are just the start. "The thing I see most clubs fall short in is service," says Neporent. If staffers answer the phone rudely or ignore clients so they can continue blathering to each other about last Saturday night, put a black mark in your mental book. Expect staff to be friendly, helpful and knowledgeable. And make sure that their first order of business is having you answer a questionnaire about your health and goals, which they should be eager to see if they're to tailor your program, says McNeil.

Inspect for cleanliness. Pay particular attention to showers and locker rooms, where moisture can foster growth of bacteria and fungi. Don't write off a funky smell as an unavoidable by-product of too much sweat and too little deodorant. Look to see that soap is available in dispensers (not bars) and that the dispensers aren't crusted over. Make sure that shower stalls are free of scum, drains aren't clogged with hair and countertops are wiped down. "There's no excuse for dirtiness," Neporent says. "Even the machines should gleam."

Note equipment condition. "Under Repair" signs on equipment aren't necessarily a bad sign: It may indicate management's swift response to even slightly out of whack machinery, says Barbara Baldwin, information services director for the American Running and Fitness Association. But it's wise to ask how often this happens, or how long equipment tends to be out of action. And check the free-weight area: Are plates returned to storage locations or left mounted or lying around, requiring you to search for what you need or undo somebody else's setup?

Check out the crowd. Visit the gym at the same time of day you'll be using it, to evaluate crowds, waiting time and atmosphere, which vary at different hours, says Baldwin. Ask the staff how many members use the gym, and find out when the place is most and least busy.

Talk to members. If possible, cut yourself loose from the guided tour and talk with club members out of staff earshot, Baldwin says. Ask for their honest impressions of the facility, equipment, staff and clientele.

Ask for a trial workout. Any club worth its salt will let prospective members take a free trial aerobics class, and most will allow you to work out on the equipment, under supervision, at least once before signing up. Be leery of any club that won't, says Baldwin.

Look at the child-care area. If you plan to bring tots, you may actually want to check this out first. Here, cleanliness standards should be extra high, says Baldwin. "Ask if there are rules for parents, like making sure younger children are diapered before coming in, or not allowing kids in if they're sick," she advises. Evaluate crowding in the child-care area separately: When the weight machines are lightly used, the aerobics classes—and the day care—may be jammed. Is there a limit to how many children are allowed in? If so, you could end up tending your kids instead of working out. Is there always a caregiver present, or do you have to call ahead? "I've seen instances where the caregiver didn't show up, so the kids were simply unattended," says Baldwin.

Doing Business

Most clubs relieve you of your money in two ways: First they charge an up-front enrollment fee (expect to pay at least $100), then monthly dues that generally range from $30 to $70. But there are plenty of variations on this scheme, says McNeil. Some clubs, for example, charge a much higher enrollment fee in exchange for much lower dues over an extended period. These are usually called lifetime memberships. Another twist is the "gold" membership, in which enrollees get more privileges than regular members (free access to racquetball courts, for example).

Many clubs will offer a choice of paying a year's dues from month to month or all at once. Some will deduct the funds directly from your bank, with your approval. As with any contractual agreement, there are good deals and not-so-good ones. Here's what the experts advise.

Ask about refunds. What happens if you move or get injured and want to revoke your membership? Some states require clubs to refund a portion of your enrollment fee if you move a certain distance away (anywhere from 15 to 50 miles) or are disabled. If there's no state law, ask what the club policy is, says McNeil. Do they have inactive memberships, in which you pay lower fees while you're living elsewhere but don't have to shell out another enrollment fee if you move back?

Manners for Muscleheads

We don't care how big you are. We still expect you to abide by these essential rules of gym decorum—and you should expect the same from us.

Don't hog the equipment. A weight bench isn't a chaise longue. If you're done with your set, move on, whether somebody's waiting or not. If you have more than one set to do, let somebody else work in with you while you rest between sets.

Bring clean clothes. Empty your gym bag as soon as you get home and throw your workout clothes into the laundry. That way, you won't find yourself stretching already-ripe duds through one last workout.

Cut the chatter. Be friendly, but never talk to anyone who's in the middle of a set, and, in fact, talk very little the rest of the time.

Tote a towel. Use it to wipe the equipment off when you're done using it, so someone else doesn't have to.

Pick up after yourself. It only takes a few seconds to take the plates off the bar and return them to their racks. If you don't do it, the next guy does. If everyone does it, everyone's happier.

Also, find out if the club is part of a network in which members can easily transfer from one club to another, says McNeil. Such transfers are a selling point for large organizations such as Bally. With other clubs, ask if they belong to IHRSA's Passport Program, which may not necessarily allow easy transfers from club to club, but will allow customers from member clubs to use other facilities in the network for a small daily fee when traveling.

Finally, many states allow signatories to change their minds about a contract within anywhere from 1 to 15 days after signing and still get their money back. With health clubs, however, you can't back out after you've started using the club.

Avoid lifetime memberships. "They're almost always a rip-off," says Neporent. "You don't know where you'll be three years from now." Consider the case of Jack, a corporate prole in Manhattan who put down upwards of $1,000 for a lifetime membership in a wonderful club in nearby Westchester County. Dues were a paltry $5 a month. But he moved out of state two years after joining. After that, he kept paying his monthly dues year after year because the club allowed him to sell his membership, and he hoped to find a buyer. "It's a wonderful marketing scheme," says McNeil, "because it makes members part of the sales force." Since Jack joined his gym, New York and many other states have set limits for health-club con-

tracts, usually to a maximum of 36 months.

Pay month to month. Never mind lifetime memberships; McNeil advises against paying even for one year in advance. "You're best off with the shortest contract you can get, unless you really know what you want and are sure you'll stick with it," she says. This isn't just to avoid blowing money on something you won't use; it's also protection against the club closing its doors and eating your prepaid dollars in bankruptcy court. "While some states have bond laws to protect consumers in the event of club closings, they are largely ineffective," says McNeil. "Individual members would actually only get a fraction of their money back."

Try to make a deal. Is there any way the club would charge you less? If you don't know, ask, suggests Neporent. Maybe there was a just-ended promotion that they'd be willing to extend. Or, some clubs are willing to charge you less if you agree only to use the club during the least busy hours of the day—an arrangement that allows the club to bring in new member dollars without aggravating the crowding during prime time.

Get it in writing. You've heard this before, but it bears repeating: Everything you've been told or promised verbally should be inked onto the contract—fees, payment terms and any understandings you have about refunds, buy-one-get-one-cheaper deals for couples or discounts of any kind, says McNeil. And if language is added to the contract, the salesperson should put his or her initials next to it.

Watch for red flags. The staff is friendly, appears knowledgeable, answers all your questions. It all seems nice. There's just one problem.

• They ask for your credit card number before you see the facility. This should set off your scam sensors, despite the smiles of the staff and their dismissing of this request as a silly formality. Even if they're willing to let you tour the gym later, says McNeil, your payment information shouldn't be an issue until you've told them payment is on *your* agenda.

• They won't let you try out the gym. Maybe they're especially sensitive to liability. Maybe you should wonder why.

• Staff is absent from the gym floor. What's the use of a staff if they're never on hand to help out members? You never know when you'll need a spotter quickly, or when a friendly pointer might keep you from hurting yourself, says Baldwin.

• Management reserves the right to sell your membership. Some clubs trade memberships like banks trade mortgages. The club gets a lump-sum payment and the buyer gets your monthly dues. "Now the club's financial incentive is to get new members, not to serve you," McNeil says.

Buying Shoes

When we were kids and the entire universe was simpler, it was easy to buy what were then called gym shoes or sneakers. You'd accompany a parental unit to JCPenney on Main Street, where you'd find maybe two different canvas/rubber models in the right size. You'd try them on, and Mom or Pop would press the tip of the shoe and ask, "Is that where your toe is? Do they feel okay?" Two yesses and you were gone. You'd wear your sneaks to school until they got holes in them, then wear them some more at home until stitches and laces could no longer keep them together.

Today, we go to discount megastores (they account for the largest share of sales by far), where we find walls and walls of "athletic footwear": running shoes, walking shoes, hiking shoes, basketball shoes, court shoes, aerobic shoes, cross-training shoes, uptown, downtown, all-around-the-town shoes. Who's responsible for this infernal diversity?

The shoemakers, of course, who, by segmenting the market for different uses, can sell us two or three pairs of shoes instead of one. But it's not entirely them. It's us, too. We enjoy footwear that caters to the specific abuses to which our tender peds are subjected. "Growth in the industry has mirrored the growth of athletic and active culture in general," says Gregg Hartley, executive director of the Athletic Footwear Association (AFA).

What the running and aerobic booms of the 1970s and early 1980s made apparent was that when feet are pounded repeatedly in the same manner, a sneaker just isn't enough. "Sprain your ankle, get a stress fracture, develop tendinitis—these are all things that can happen from wearing the wrong shoe for the activity," says Michael Lowe, D.P.M., team podiatrist for the Utah Jazz basketball team.

Selecting a Shoe Type

Which brings us back to those endless aisles of options. What'll you have: uppers of leather, canvas, soft nylon, mesh nylon or a combination? Soles of black carbon or styrene-butadiene rubber? Midsoles of polyurethane, EVA, air, silicone or honeycomb?

Enough already. To decide what's right for you, don't start with the shoe and what it offers but with yourself and what you need, realizing that a certain amount of the technical stuff is sheer marketing hype. "Features like air pumps or 'energy return systems' are largely gimmicks," says Carol Frey, M.D., associate professor of orthopaedic surgery at the University of Southern California School of Medicine and director of the Orthopaedic Foot and Ankle Center at Orthopaedic Hospital, both in Los Angeles, and a leading medical expert on athletic shoes. "If you can lace your shoes correctly, that's enough to give you an excellent fit. And energy return is something your feet provide naturally even when you're barefoot."

Sales gimmicks aside, the fundamental question to ask yourself is, do you need a different shoe for every activity that you participate in? For a lot of us, the answer is clearly no, says Dr. Frey. Just look at what people tend to buy and why. According to the AFA, the biggest slice of the sales pie—a full quarter of it—goes to basketball shoes. The next biggest categories are cross training (19 percent), walking (13 percent) and running (10 percent) shoes. (See "What Sells Best" on page 324 for more information on athletic shoe sales.) All of these shoes have lots of crossover appeal: You can wear them exercising, and you can wear them buying groceries. In fact, AFA surveys reveal that having a performance advantage only ranks third in consumer opinions about what's "very important" in an athletic shoe. Uppermost in priority are the more general qualities of "comfort, fit and feel" and "suits active lifestyle" (see "What Buyers Say Is Important in Athletic Shoes" on page 324).

"A cross-training shoe (which is designed to be used for multiple activities) does a perfectly good job of supporting and protecting the foot if you play a little tennis, walk or lift weights," says Dr. Lowe. Beyond that, the need for a specialty shoe is strictly a matter of how much time you spend at one thing.

Lacing for All Occasions

For the most part, we all lace our shoes the same way. Yet our feet are all different, with different problems and needs. Are you lacing your shoes the best possible way for your feet? Maybe not, says Carol Frey, M.D., associate professor of orthopaedic surgery at the University of Southern California School of Medicine and director of the Orthopaedic Foot and Ankle Center at Orthopaedic Hospital, both in Los Angeles. She points out that manufacturers actually design their shoes to provide lacing options, but we largely ignore them. Here are some innovative lacing patterns she recommends for a number of different problems.

ⓐ Narrow feet. Running laces through eyelets that are set more widely apart pulls the sides of the shoe more tightly over the top of the foot.

ⓑ Wide feet. Running laces through eyelets that are closer to the tongue of the shoe widens the lacing area and relieves binding.

ⓒ High arches. Lacing shoes straight across from eyelet to eyelet so that the laces never cross over one another eliminates pressure points on the tongue that can aggravate pain.

ⓓ Slipping heel. Lacing as you normally would, but then using the last two eyelets on both sides to form a tuggable loop closes the top of the shoe more snugly.

ⓔ Pain on the top of the foot. Eliminating lace crossover in spots where you have a bruise or tendon injury helps alleviate pain.

ⓕ Pain in the toes. By first running one side of the lace all the way to the top eyelet, you form a buffer between your foot and the remainder of the lace (which you run through all other eyelets), suspending the lace off ingrown toenails or corns.

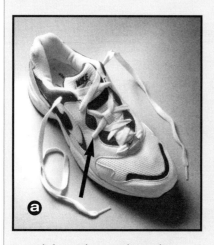
ⓐ Laced through outside eyelets

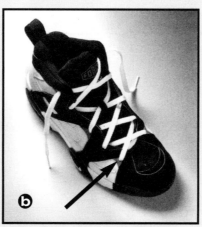
ⓑ Laced through inside eyelets

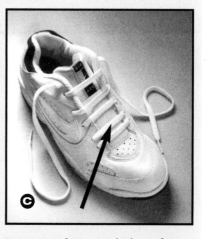
ⓒ Laces travel in straight lines from eyelet to eyelet

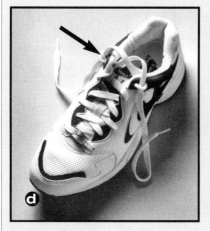
ⓓ Create a loop between the first and second eyelets on each side; then feed the laces across to the opposite loop

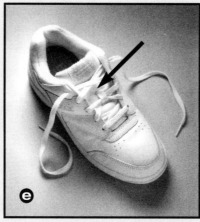
ⓔ Laces left uncrossed over injured area

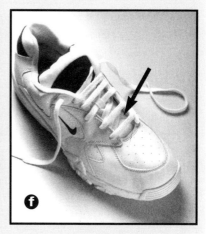
ⓕ First lace goes from top eyelet to bottom eyelet on opposite side; then work the one lace back to the top

"The rule of thumb is that if you do a given activity three or more times a week, you need a sport-specific shoe," says Dr. Frey. "The only exceptions are running and basketball, which are the two sports with the highest injury rates to the feet and knees. For those, you should buy special shoes even if you only do them once a week."

What Makes Shoes Different

Once you know what to look for, well, what do you look for? How is one type of shoe distinct from another? In what ways will your feet appreciate the differences? Here's a brief rundown of the qualities that characterize each major category as you browse the aisles, according to our experts.

Running. Even though it's not the best-selling category, most of the research and design innovations have occurred in running shoes, which require superior performance on a number of levels. First and foremost, a good running shoe needs plenty of cushioning to dampen the impact of feet striking the ground: You'll find extra padding in the heel and some form of shock-absorbing material in the midsole, such as air, gel, polyurethane or EVA (ethyl vinyl acetate, a plastic foam). In addition, the shoe needs to provide stability as the foot rolls from heel strike to pushoff, flexibility to allow the foot to bend and traction to maximize grip. The sole is key to all three. It should have lugs for traction and stability and lines at the forefoot for flexibility, and it should sweep up over the toe, also for traction and stability. Ideally, the shoe will also be lightweight, with uppers usually made of nylon.

Walking. Because the motions involved are similar, you'll find many elements of running shoes in walking shoes, particularly shock-absorbent heels and midsoles. There are differences, however. First, because weight is less an issue with walking shoes, uppers are often made of leather. The forefoot, while needing to be flexible, may be stiffer than that of a running shoe, which requires more toe bending, and the heel area may be stiffer as well. Soles generally have a less-prominently lugged, lower-profile tread, often with a herringbone pattern.

Basketball. The most obvious feature of a basketball shoe is the high-top design for stabilizing the ankle during jumps. (Some players wear low-cut models for the sake of superior agility, but Dr. Frey advises against this because ankle injuries are less common in high-tops.) Unlike running and walking shoes, whose soles are rounded to enhance the forward rolling of the feet, basketball soles are flat to accommodate quick stops and snap movements backwards and sideways. The treads are likely to have geometric patterns with multiple edges, such as squares and diamonds, to allow superior traction in

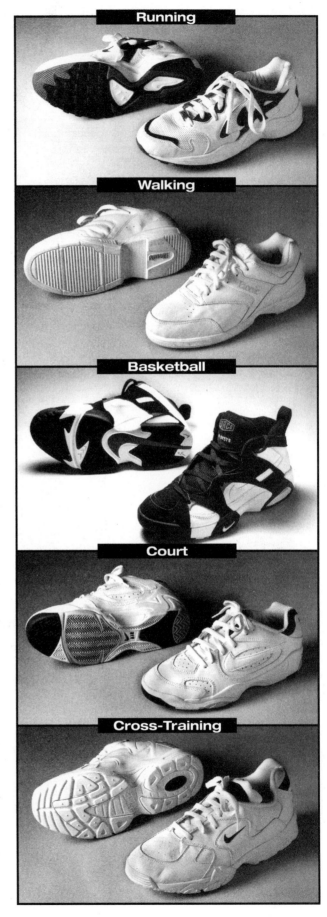

many different directions, along with a circular pivot point at the ball of the foot.

Court. Technically, a basketball shoe is a court shoe, since racquet sports and basketball demand similar movements, with one exception: Basketball requires more vertical jumping. "A court shoe often has harder composite materials on the bottom because it doesn't have to be as forgiving as a basketball shoe," says Dr. Lowe. Still, a court shoe will have cushioning in the midsole and insole, with a firm heel structure and roomy toe area that has reinforcement across the front. You don't need a high-top, but it's important to have good ankle support, says Dr. Frey, which is why some models offer mid-cut styling.

Cross-training. The Great Compromise. Cross-trainers offer some of everything for the casual exerciser but not enough of anything for the serious athlete. "It's a category that's tough to categorize," says Dr. Frey. "Some are designed to combine running and walking, others running and hiking, others are more court cross-trainers. There are all kinds." Generally, though, cross-trainers are mid-cut, with a look that's closest to court shoes. The toe area and toe cap are less substantial than a basketball shoe's, but more substantial than a running shoe's. They're less flexible than running shoes, but they provide more lateral stability for activities such as stepping or aerobics.

Aerobic. This is one category that may be largely lost on men, since we don't exactly flock to jazzercize and "Sweatin' to the Oldies" classes. For all practical purposes, there's nothing an aerobics shoe provides that you won't find in a cross-trainer. In fact, Dr. Frey notes, an aerobic shoe really *is* a kind of cross-trainer, since it combines the light weight and shock absorption of a running shoe with the stability and toe/heel reinforcement of a court shoe.

Hiking/outdoors. At last count, hiking boots and outdoor shoes only comprised 7 percent of the athletic footwear market, but it's the fastest growing category of all. The distinction between walking and hiking is largely a matter of toughness and terrain. Hiking boots and shoes place a premium on water resistance, so they're put together using few seams where water might trickle in. The heel is reinforced, the ankles are supported with a padded high-top structure and the toes are given plenty of room. Soles are firm and heavily lugged for traction and durability.

How to Make the Perfect Purchase

When buying athletic shoes, you are on your own. Assuming there's a salesperson to advise you (hardly something you can count on), he or she won't necessarily be knowledgeable about shoes or (especially) about your feet. Even the professionals have a

tough time of it. "Getting a proper fit is one of the major battles we deal with all the time," explains Dr. Lowe of his work with the Utah Jazz. "You can have a shoe that has all the fancy bells and whistles, but if it doesn't fit, you'll still have sprained ankles, stress fractures and tendinitis."

The first rule is to spend enough. Buying a $70 shoe instead of a $30 one will generally get you more support, lighter weight and better materials in greater quantity. But whatever your budget, it'll be easier to make a regrets-free purchase if you follow these tips.

Check where there's wear. The ways you've eroded your old shoes can help guide you to new ones. If, for example, the back of the heel is worn toward the outside of the foot, you tend to roll along the outer edge when you run (this is known as underpronating). Underpronators have rigid, immobile feet; they should buy shoes that are heavily cushioned and feature soft midsoles and less medial support. These shoes are usually built on a curved form to encourage foot motion.

Overpronators roll their weight to the inside of the foot, so the heel will be more worn toward the inside. It is the more common problem. Overpronators should buy motion-control shoes: rigid, heavy and durable. Such shoes might include features such as a medial post, a polyurethane midsole and a carbon rubber outsole. Many are built on a straight shoe form to offer more stability and support.

Examine the new shoe. You need a shoe that will stay comfortable and in one piece for the duration. Feel the inside for places where stitching is raised or coming loose. If you find any, select another shoe. Look at where the sole and upper come together and try peeling the pieces back from each other. "If I can stick a credit card between them, I don't like that shoe," Dr. Frey says.

Try different sizes. Numbers on boxes mean nothing. A size 11 from three different makers will fit three different ways. You will find what you need comfort-wise only through trial and error. Avoid ordering through the mail unless the supplier has a terrific return policy, advises Dr. Frey.

Get a three-way fit. To get good comfort and support, pay attention to three primary parameters, says Dr. Frey.

- The longest of your *toes* should clear the end of the shoe by ⅜ to ½ inch—about the width of your thumb.
- The *ball* of the foot should fit comfortably into the widest part of the shoe.
- The *heel* should fit snugly without any slippage.

Put on both shoes. Typically, one of your feet is slightly larger than the other. Getting a perfect fit only

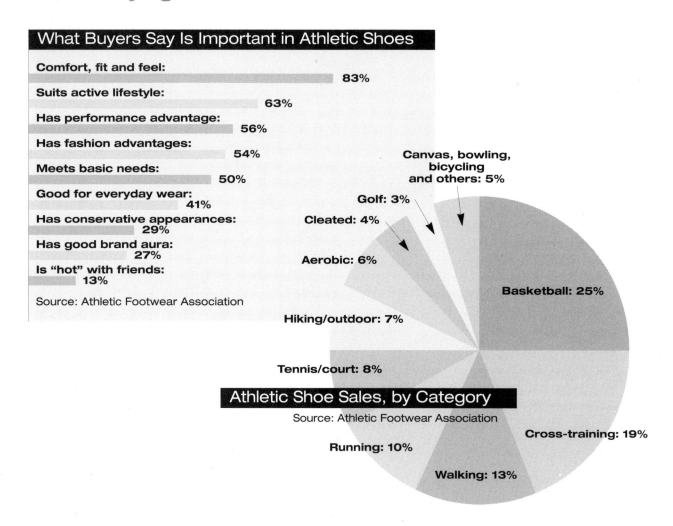

What Buyers Say Is Important in Athletic Shoes

Comfort, fit and feel: 83%

Suits active lifestyle: 63%

Has performance advantage: 56%

Has fashion advantages: 54%

Meets basic needs: 50%

Good for everyday wear: 41%

Has conservative appearances: 29%

Has good brand aura: 27%

Is "hot" with friends: 13%

Source: Athletic Footwear Association

Athletic Shoe Sales, by Category

Source: Athletic Footwear Association

- Canvas, bowling, bicycling and others: 5%
- Golf: 3%
- Cleated: 4%
- Aerobic: 6%
- Hiking/outdoor: 7%
- Tennis/court: 8%
- Running: 10%
- Walking: 13%
- Cross-training: 19%
- Basketball: 25%

on the smaller foot means the larger one may be cramped. If you already know which foot is biggest, base your purchase on how that foot fits, recommends Dr. Frey. And stand up after lacing to let your foot spread out.

Shop late. Feet swell by as much as 5 percent between morning and evening, says William Rossi, D.P.M., a consultant to the footwear industry. Fitting too early in the day could get you a shoe that pinches.

Don't force it. There are lots of tricks and traplines a salesperson may use to rationalize a purchase. Don't fall for:

- "That's a good, snug fit." Snug means tight, maybe too tight, says Dr. Rossi. Snug in the heel is good. Snug anywhere else is a prescription for pain.
- "It will stretch out." No it won't. Shoes may become more comfortable as they conform to your gait, but you should never compromise on the three-way fit (front-to-back, side-to-side, top-to-bottom). "It either fits or it doesn't," Dr. Lowe says.
- "If you wear thicker socks, it'll be perfect." So you need a new sock wardrobe, too? Before

going to the store, put on the socks you plan to wear with the shoe. If you can't fit those socks, look elsewhere, says Dr. Frey.

When to Replace Shoes

It's tough to say good-bye to an old friend, especially one that still looks so good for its age. But used shoes are like used cars: They can look great on the outside but be trashed where it counts. Here are some guidelines on when to relegate shoes to garden duty.

For running, measure miles. Repeated pounding eventually compresses the cushioning materials that are running shoes' reason for being. Replacement is partly a matter of your weight and the surface you run on. If you tend to run on hard surfaces like concrete or plant your feet heavily, replace running shoes every 300 miles. If you run on soft surfaces or are light on your feet, get a new pair every 500 miles, recommends Dr. Frey.

For others, clock hours. A sturdy cross-trainer can withstand 100 to 125 hours of wear and tear from a 185-pound man who exercises four or five days a week, according to Tom Brunick, director of the Athlete's Foot WearTest Center at North Central College

What Is a Shoe?

Uppers. Soles. Stabilizing bar. What are they talking about? Here's a visual glossary of the parts of a shoe.

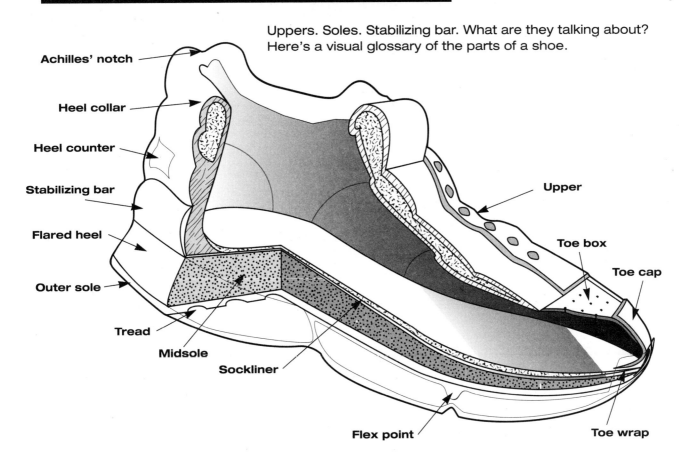

Achilles' notch
Heel collar
Heel counter
Stabilizing bar
Flared heel
Outer sole
Tread
Midsole
Sockliner
Flex point
Upper
Toe box
Toe cap
Toe wrap

in Naperville, Illinois, and a technical editor for *Runner's World* magazine. A man weighing less than 170 pounds could eke out an additional 25 hours or so. That translates to four to six months of use. Note, however, that this assumes a fairly intense exercise schedule, with shoes getting pounded almost every day. If you allow more of a break between exercise sessions, either by working out less or rotating different pairs of shoes, cushioning materials may decompress slightly, providing perhaps another month of wear, he says.

Get a rear view. Put your shoes on a counter and look at them from behind. If they list to one side or the other, the midsole cushioning is probably shot, says Brunick.

Compare for wear. Go to a store and try on a new pair of the model you're currently wearing, recommends Brunick. If the cushioning of your old shoes feels dead compared to the new ones, it probably is.

Don't ignore the obvious. If the upper is worn through or the lugs on the bottom are fading away, you're pulling a Norman Bates: keeping in your closet a cherished shell whose sole has long since departed.

Outdoor Equipment

It's hard to explain the allure of well-crafted sporting gear, just like it's hard to put into words the feelings you might have for a lithe, intelligent, good-humored woman whose long legs slide past the refined patterns of a silk dress, whose hair rakes without pretense over one eye, whose body shape suggests sublime physical pleasures, whose sharp wit promises intriguing verbal jousts. . . .

Come to think of it, it's a lot more difficult to explain rationally the allure of equipment. But hardware definitely holds seductive appeal. We've heard from men, for example, who say they sleep with their mountain bikes. Whether or not it's true, the fact that any man would voice such a claim and expect other men to understand goes a long way toward suggesting the depths of the male desire for extremely cool and probably expensive toys.

As with other objects of desire, when the time comes to commit financially and emotionally to years, if not decades, of shared experiences, you want to know you've made the right choice. There's only one way to do that, and that's to know what you're looking for before you do the looking. We covered indoor exercise equipment in Setting Up a Home Gym on page 312. Now it's time to head for the great outdoors.

How to Buy

Before getting into the particulars of specific types of equipment, we should note that the experts we spoke with had one bit of advice in common (which they share with experts of indoor equipment): Buy from an outfitter or specialty store. Salespeople there are best qualified to match good equipment to your needs, abilities and physical potential. Unfortunately, it's maddeningly easy to find specialized salespeople who can't find the words to express what they know, or choose to intimidate customers rather than show them the way. Dealing with the inarticulate or the snooty is another reason to be prepared with the following when you buy sports equipment.

Bicycles

The great thing about bikes is that we learned most of the essential skills necessary to use them when we were still forming lines behind Teacher to use the potty. The machine you learned on, however, likely resembled nothing you'll find in stores today. True, all bikes have two wheels, pedals and a handlebar, but to outfit yourself, you'll need to look beyond these basics and make some decisions.

Survey the terrain. The major choice is between road bikes, which have smooth, skinny tires to minimize resistance on paved surfaces, and mountain bikes, which have knobby, fat tires to improve traction and absorb impact on off-road trails. The road bike, once known as the ten-speed, was the standard for years. Then, in the 1990s, the astonishing ascendance of mountain bikes pushed most road bikes off dealers' racks, just like CDs replaced vinyl in record stores.

Because of their overwhelming popularity, assume from here on that we're talking about mountain bikes, but don't give up on the idea of buying a road model. Think first and foremost about where you'll do most of your riding. Aside from a certain of-the-moment cachet, there's no reason to buy a mountain bike if you won't be riding it off-road: With their thick tires and low gears (for hauling up steep, scrabbly hills), mountain bikes are sluggards on asphalt.

A third category of bike, called the hybrid, combines features of mountain and road bikes (tires, for example, are thicker and knobbier than a road bike's, but thinner and less grippy than a mountain bike's). Most serious riders consider hybrids a sorry compromise, however: They're not rugged enough for real off-road riding and not efficient enough to perform well on extended road rides.

Rate the rattle factor. Much of the go-anywhere excitement of mountain biking hinges on the ability to bounce across rocks, jump over stumps and dive off small cliffs. Basically, there's a whole lot o' shakin' going on, and you'll need to decide how badly you need shock absorbers to handle it. Your need will depend on the kind of riding you do. A person who does

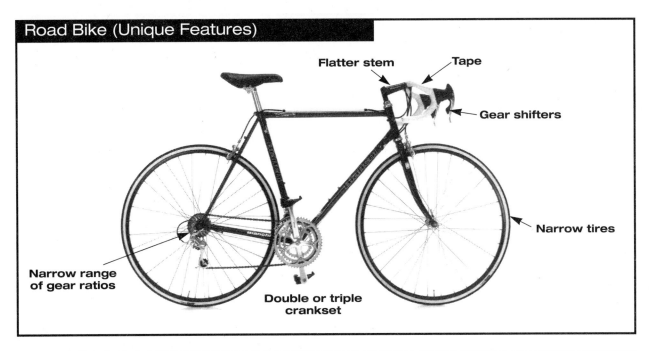

Road Bike (Unique Features)

Flatter stem

Tape

Gear shifters

Narrow tires

Narrow range of gear ratios

Double or triple crankset

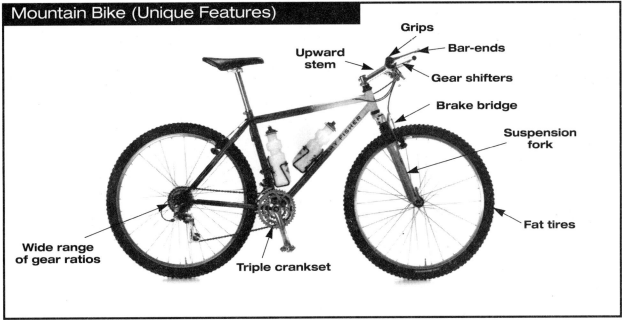

Mountain Bike (Unique Features)

Grips

Bar-ends

Upward stem

Gear shifters

Brake bridge

Suspension fork

Fat tires

Wide range of gear ratios

Triple crankset

moderate rails-to-trails riding on level grades doesn't need suspension the way a guy who lives to speed down mountainsides at 40 miles an hour does. The most popular cushioning system involves suspension built into the fork. (A fork connects the front wheel to the bike's frame.) Suspension forks compress vertically under the force of a hard impact, softening a blow that would otherwise be taken mostly by your hands and arms. Fully suspended models have frames that suspend the rear wheel, too. These don't come cheap: They cost 33 to 100 percent more than a bike with a front suspension. Are the bucks worth the benefit? Your call.

Choose your material. Road and mountain bike frames can be built with different materials, each of which has its advantages and drawbacks. The oldest and most familiar is steel alloy (usually steel mixed with other metals such as chromium and molybdenum)—"cro-moly" in gearhead lingo. Steel is strong and highly durable, but heavy. The most popular alternative is aluminum, which is lighter and doesn't rust, but stiffer and more jarring than steel. A dream material that combines steel's strength with aluminum's lightness exists in the form of titanium; "ti" remains a dream for many cyclists, however, because it's pricey—$1,500 and up for a complete bike.

Which to choose? There are no clear winners or losers here, says Fred Zahradnik, technical editor for

Bicycling magazine. You'll find high-end bikes made of all these materials except mild steel (the stuff they make department store bikes out of).

What will sway you toward one bike or another are additional factors such as the quality of the braking and drivetrain components (let your bike shop expert be your guide) and, more fundamentally, how well you like the feel of the bike when you ride it. And you will ride it before you buy: Any shop that balks at test rides should not be getting your business.

Skis

There's been an explosion of diversity in ski design recently, which is good because it provides lots of choices for people at all skill levels. But it also makes a trip to your local ski shack more confusing. The basic categories of slalom and giant slalom have now been joined by parabolics, which, compared to regular skis, are much wider at the tip and tail and much narrower in the waist; powder skis, which are shorter and wider than skis designed for harder-packed snow; and all-terrain, or mountain skis, designed to handle both powder and hardpack. If you're in the market, here's how to proceed.

Start with boots. "If the boots don't fit, the rest of your experience won't be pleasant no matter what kind of ski you have," says Mary Jo Tarallo, director of public relations for Ski Industries America in McLean, Virginia. Fitting issues are much the same as for shoes: The heel shouldn't slip, and your digits should fill the toe box but not ride the front of the boot. Wear socks like those you'll wear on the slopes; be sure to fit both feet—and plan on spending 20 minutes in the boots while still in the store, to let irritating pressure points reveal themselves. While you're waiting, ask the salesperson if they have a test platform on which you can simulate the movements you'll make on skis.

Assess local conditions. The type of ski you get depends on the kind of skiing you like to do, how often you plan to do it and, perhaps most important, the type of snow and terrain that prevails in areas where you'll go the most. Individual preferences play a huge role, but here are some general guidelines from Lisa Feinberg Densmore, a former member of the U.S. Ski Team.

• *Giant slalom* is now considered the best all-around ski for both short turns and long turns, powder and hardpack if you're a skilled skier, says Densmore. If you're less skilled and hit the slopes on fewer than a half-dozen occasions a year, consider a less performance-oriented all-terrain ski.

• For taking moguls (bumps) and quick turns on the fall line (the most direct path gravity takes you down a slope), opt for more nimble *slalom* skis.

• For skiers of intermediate or higher skill who want to cruise without working too hard at carving turns, consider *shaped* or *parabolic* skis, whose hourglass shape makes for easy changes of direction.

Run the bases. What's inside a ski doesn't matter as much as what's outside, especially on the bottom, or base. Virtually all bases are made of a plastic material called P-Tex, which comes in three grades, according to how well the material glides over snow. "Beginners are often afraid that a better glide means they'll go too fast, but glide isn't a speed issue, it's a control and ease-of-turning issue," Densmore says. "Get as good a base as you can afford."

Factor in your weight. Skis are rated according to the level of skill they're designed for, but if you weigh more than 200 pounds, you can't go by these ratings. "The heavier you are, the more ski you need," Densmore says. "Buy skis one level up; they'll be stiffer and more responsive." Also, avoid cores made of foam, which will quickly lose their bounce under a heavy person, in favor of layered cores containing

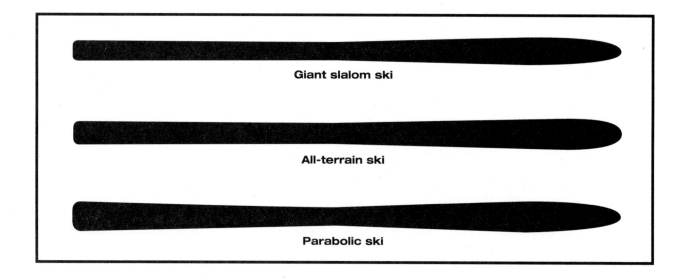

Giant slalom ski

All-terrain ski

Parabolic ski

Getting Gear from Here to There

The major problem with bikes, skis, snowboards, canoes, kayaks and other sporting paraphernalia is where to put them. Not where to *store* them (that's a separate issue whose ramifications need to be hammered out with landlords and/or living companions), but where to put them when you're transporting them from your domicile to wherever funhog heaven is. You could ride, paddle and otherwise self-propel yourself, but for the most part, we're talking about hauling big gear with cars. For that, you'll need a rack.

The first consideration is how often or how far you'll be transporting. For example, if you transport your bike only a few times a season or only drive short distances, you can get by with a rear-mounted rack that clips onto the edges of a hatchback or trunk. These racks, by makers such as Rhode Gear, are inexpensive (usually under $100) but less secure than the major category of "load-carrying systems," the roof rack.

Roof racks are preferable for frequent or long-distance hauling because they're strong, sturdy and extremely secure (they hold gear tightly and also allow you to lock it onto your vehicle), and they evenly distribute weight. Every roof rack consists of two essential elements: bars (usually two) that support whatever you're carrying, and "towers" (typically four), which are structural components that both hold the bars off the roof and affix them to your car. Onto these elements are attached the actual racks that carry your gear. All of this stuff is sold separately.

What you require to make a working system depends entirely on what you're carrying and the make of your vehicle. Some racks, for example, clamp onto your car or van's rain gutter. But if you don't have a rain gutter (and fewer new cars do), you'll need a tower that clips to the door frame or attaches via some other method. One major rack manufacturer, Thule, has more than 200 different "fit kits" for various vehicles.

Thule (pronounced TOO-lee) and Yakima (pronounced YAK-imaw) are the two major manufacturers for versatile carry-anything roof racks. (With some sports, like skiing, additional manufacturers such as Barrecrafter make racks just for that kind of gear.) Both make excellent products with similar prices. "I really can't recommend one over the other without knowing what kind of car you have," says Dan Fleckinger, a sales representative and former manager of the car rack department at Recreational Equipment Incorporated in Conshohocken, Pennsylvania.

If you're in the market for a rack, however, there are a few things you might want to consider before you buy.

• How many cars you'll use. "Thule has a lot of specialty racks for cars like VWs," Fleckinger says. "A specialty rack will fit better, but you won't be able to use it on a different car." Many racks, however, will fit more than one kind of vehicle. Make up your mind which is more important, fit or versatility.

• How long you'll own your car. Load-carrying systems aren't cheap: Figure on paying upwards of $200 to carry just one item, says Fleckinger. That's a hefty investment to a lot of us, and it may not be worth making if you're planning on getting a different car next year.

• How soon you need it. The place you buy from might not have the parts you need, so you can't always walk into the store and just cart off your rack. Shop for your rack at least three weeks before you think you need it, to allow time to order the right components. If you have a new car that just came on the market, call ahead to make sure components are already available.

materials like fiberglass, wood, metal and graphite.

Sweat the details. They can make all the difference.

• Look beyond skin-deep beauty on graphics: Colors should penetrate into the material to prevent inevitable gouges from marring designs.

• Make sure there's metal in the core of giant slalom skis, to ensure superior stability at high speed. Make sure there's little or no metal in slalom or parabolic skis, to ensure livelier performance.

• Look down the length of a ski like you're looking down the barrel of a rifle. If you detect any waves, bumps or irregularities in the finish, choose a different ski.

• To avoid having to fight your way through turns, make sure the metal edges of the tip and tail are rounded off, or "de-tuned," and the base is level with the edges. If the edges are raised above the P-Tex, like rails, the ski will be difficult to turn.

Snowboarding, anyone? They're not skis, but snowboards nevertheless are longish objects you strap your feet into for shushing down hills—except both feet go onto one board. Like mountain biking, snowboarding has quickly become a huge, distinct sport. There are three types of snowboards, but most people use "free-riding" models, which merge the greater lightness and speed of the other types, the freestyle and the Alpine, respectively. There are two types of boots. The first type, soft boots, you lace up, then attach into the board binding. They're flexible, easy to use and most popular. Hard boots, which look like ski boots, provide less flexibility and can demand more skill, says Tarallo.

Canoes

Canoeing seems such an uncomplicated, peaceful pursuit, but any form of self-propulsion has its challenges. A good boat can ease your burden (not to be sniffed at if you happen to be carrying the thing over land) and increase the pleasure you take in your surroundings. Here's what to consider, according to Chuck Weis, editor at large for *Paddler* magazine and chairman of the National Touring and Recreational Paddling Committee of the American Canoe Association.

Chart the waters ahead. Are you heading for turbulent rapids, setting off gear-burdened across vast expanses or launching for an afternoon of lazy paddling in a local recreational area? In answer, the categories of canoes are defined with befitting simplicity.

• *White-water* canoes are highly maneuverable in the interests of dodging boulders and forceful vortexes. If you're deficient in the dodging department, they're also outfitted with flotation bags, which take up room other canoes make available for stowing gear. Much of a white-water model's nimbleness lies in what's called the rocker of the boat—how much the hull curves lengthwise between bow and stern. With a lot of rocker, a white-water canoe has more curvature, less wetted surface and less resistance to side-to-side motion. "It'll turn on a dime and give you nine cents change," says Weis. Which isn't great when you want to paddle in a straight line.

• *Touring* canoes are more straight-ahead vessels and make an excellent all-purpose choice. "You can take them on lakes, rivers—or use them to get serious and take off for a month in the Canadian north," Weis says. Touring canoes are generally more stable than white-water canoes, are longer (17 to 18½ feet) and have higher sides—all of which enable you to load them up with gear or young offspring. The hull has a definite bow and stern, with a fine, narrow line tapering to the front, and a broader line toward the back. This design allows for efficient slicing through water and good tracking—the ability to hold to a straight line.

• *Freestyle and marathon* canoes are more specialized. Freestyle models are designed for the man who delights in the grace and finesse of paddling in still water with minimal strokes—often not even lifting the paddle past the sheen of the surface. There's nothing radical about freestyle canoes, but they're short, leaving little room for gear. They're also lighter,

making them relatively easy to tote around. "They're good for the weekend or after-work paddler," Weis says. Marathon canoes are more hard-core, designed for competition (yes, people even use canoes to race) or any other situation in which you need to go straight fast. They're light, narrow and pointy, with very little rocker—not good to take anyplace you might encounter white water.

• *Multipurpose* canoes, which are what you find in big department stores, are a category altogether lost on seasoned paddlers. Wide, flat and lacking in performance, they're what an old pick-up truck is to a high performance sports car, says Weis. "If you're serious, look for a good canoe shop where you'll find knowledgeable salespeople and hopefully have the opportunity to test-paddle the boats, even if you have to drive a state away to find it," he implores.

Get the hull story. A canoe's performance isn't just about design, but about what the hull is made of, according to Weis.

• *ABS plastic* is the favored material for white-water canoes, because of its batter-resistant combination of strength and flexibility. Polyethylene plastic is a lesser material, but one that's still reasonably strong—and $200 to $300 less expensive.

• *Fiberglass* is well-suited for touring boats because of its strength, durability and low cost relative to Kevlar, which is stronger and lighter. There's no need to spring for Kevlar unless you're planning on doing a lot of portaging. If you get fiberglass, though, make sure it's made in a process called hand layup, as opposed to chopper-gun layup, which produces a heavier, less flexible hull.

• *Aluminum* finds favor only in the realm of the multipurpose boat. "It's at the bottom of the performance scale," Weis says. One problem: It'll stick to rocks that other materials glide over. On the plus side, "it will take a beating," Weis says.

Decide if you want company. Canoes come in either solo or tandem designs—a simple matter of having one seat or two. Tandems are slightly larger and are best for families and stowing large amounts of gear. "Go solo unless you have good reason not to," Weis advises. "Even a lot of couples ultimately find life easier in solo boats."

Kayaks

Kayaks are the fighter planes of the paddler world: sleek, maneuverable, a bit dangerous-looking. They even have a cockpit, which makes you a pilot. The essential differences between kayaks and canoes are obvious to the eye, but when it comes to choosing one, the guiding factors are similar.

Pick your pond. River or open water? Those are the basic choices. White-water, or river, kayaks are short (10 to 13 feet) and have lots of rocker for agile

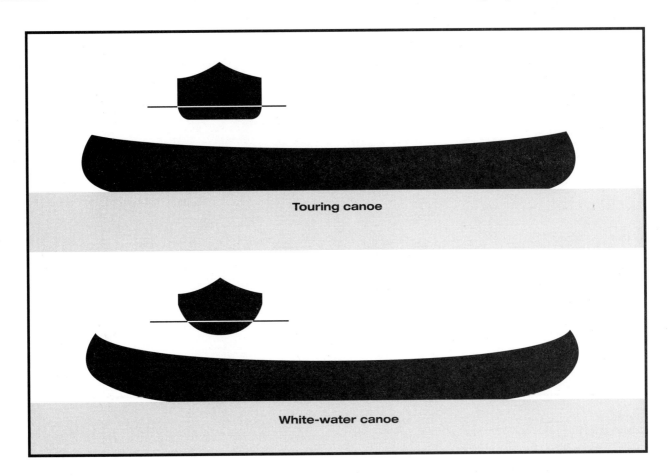

Touring canoe

White-water canoe

turning and darting among rocks. Touring, or sea, kayaks are long (15 to 22 feet), and are more stable for superior tracking over the flat distances of lakes, harbors and oceans, says recreational kayaker Tim Moore, Ph.D., president of Exercise Science Incorporated in Greenbelt, Maryland.

Match construction and function. Most kayaks are made of durable, inexpensive polyurethane, which makes sense for most people. There are two kinds of construction: rotomolding, which produces a thicker, stiffer material, and blow molding, which produces a thinner, more flexible material that needs to be shored up with bracing inside the boat. "Fit is the deciding factor," says Moore. It's not a good fit if your knees, hips or back are smashed against the top or sides of the hull while you sit in the boat (which, for big guys, is often a function of how much the internal bracing of a blow-molded hull gets in the way).

One step up the ladder is fiberglass, which is lighter, faster and the material of choice for more experienced paddlers who get their boats custom fitted. A third, more specialized option is a portable "skin" boat that breaks down so you can pack it to a remote lake or, if transport is an issue, carry it in your trunk.

Backpacks

Backpacking reminds us that the list of true essentials in life is pretty short, since you can strap everything you really need onto your shoulders and walk away from the rest for days, if not weeks. When backpacking, "the big decisions are what size pack you need, based on a realistic appraisal of what you'll be doing, and the type of construction you want," says Jim Gorman, senior editor at *Backpacker* magazine.

Frame your choices. Backpacks come in two basic categories: external frames and internal frames. With externals, the pack is attached to an exposed, H-shaped hard frame. They're best for carrying heavy loads over long distances, not only because of their large capacity, but because of their high center of gravity (much of the load rides above the shoulders), which lets you walk in an upright stance. This makes them bulky and unstable, however, if you're dodging through brush or clambering over rocks.

With internals, flexible stays of aluminum or graphite inside the pack provide structure. Internal packs hug your body closer, ride a bit lower and allow more arm clearance, making them more streamlined and stable when you're hiking in tight spots or rock climbing. However, they force you to lean forward more than externals, which makes it important

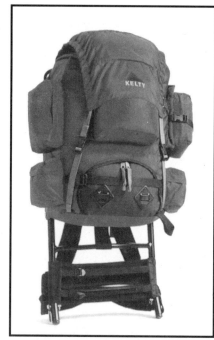
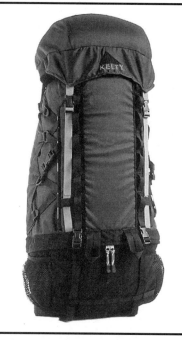
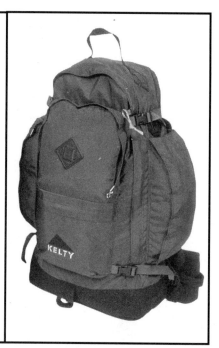

External-frame backpack   Internal-frame backpack   Frameless rucksack

to load cargo for maximum balance.

There's also a third category, the frameless rucksack, which is smaller than full backpacks, but large enough for overnight or weekend adventures.

Do an access assessment. When it comes to stuffing packs, you can either dump everything through an opening in the top (top-loading), or cram your gear into large, zippered compartments (panel-loading). Top loaders are ostensibly drier, since there are fewer openings for rain to get in, and are easy to put things into. Getting things out again, however, can be maddening if the item you need lies buried at the bottom of the pack. Panel loaders boast more convenient access, but there's a premium on zippers that are highly durable and watertight.

Count your capacity. How big a pack you get depends on how much stuff you're willing to haul and how long you'll need it. Here's Gorman's take on how the field breaks down, in cubic inches.

- Above 5,000: "load monster" packs appropriate for hard-core expeditions of many days, perhaps weeks
- 3,501 to 5,000: a standard backpack that will sustain almost any journey lasting a week or less
- 2,500 to 3,500: a light overnight pack ideal for weekend outings
- 2,500 and under: a daypack

Fly-Fishing Gear

Ever since Robert Redford made a movie of *A River Runs through It*, men have been subjected to all manner of self-important poetic tripe on the subject of trout and the means by which we snare them. Let's put all that aside and reconsider the basics here: a man, a river, a rod and something that looks like lunch to a fish. Regarding the places a man's mind wanders to while casting alone in the bubble of a brook: We'll do you a favor and keep those thoughts to ourselves. Instead, here's a brief overview of what you'll need to visit your personal reflective pool, says Dave Decker, owner of The Complete Flyfisher, a fly fishing school in Wise River, Montana.

Get a stick. The kind of rod you buy depends largely on the kind of rivers you'll fish. Smaller rivers (or more crowded ones) call for shorter rods (seven to eight feet) than do bigger rivers, which demand longer rods (nine to ten feet) for longer casts. Beyond that, it's largely a matter of how the rod feels in your hand. Have a salesguy help you pick out a half-dozen models and try them out in the parking lot. One thing to consider before deciding is what the finish on the rod is like: Matte black graphite doesn't reflect the light and spook fish the way a high-gloss polymer epoxy finish might.

Add some string. The line is arguably more important than the rod, because it's the thing you actually cast into the water. (The fly, weighing nearly nothing, trails along for the ride.) Lines come in different weights, depending on the water conditions and the type of beast you're after—they range from 1-weight line, which you might use to hook little, darting trout, to 14-weight line that's more like rope, used to combat marlin and sharks. Beginners seeking a good line for use in a variety of conditions should consider a 5- or 6-weight with a double taper (a narrowing of the line's end for easy casting). You can certainly spend lots on lines in exchange for features like treatments of lubricating chemicals to ease travel through the steel guides on the rod. Do you need the extras? Probably not. Just be sure to get some backing (an extra length of very thin line that's spliced to the main line in case a hooked fish goes on a long run), and tapered leaders (which attach the fly to the line).

Wrap the string on something. Next, you'll need something to spool the line onto the rod. Choice of reel is largely a matter of preference. Be sure to check out the braking mechanism for stopping the line (those using a spring-and-pawl drag are simple and sturdy; those using a disc drag are more adjustable). Whatever you get, make sure all metal parts are anodized as opposed to merely painted, since paint is inclined to chip and rust.

Find some bait. The collector (not to mention the know-it-all) in you may want a bunch of different flies primped in your tackle box. It's also fun—and cost-effective—to make your own flies, a hobby unto itself. But if you really want to catch fish, the best way is to ask at the local tackle shop what artificial bait is biting today and use that.

In-Line Skates

If you remember roller-skating gangs in *The Warriors*, you'll recall that boots with wheels were all the rage 20 years ago, too. The difference today is that the wheels are positioned in a line, one behind the other, creating a bladelike effect that makes the ride more akin to ice-skating. But unlike ice-skating, you can go in-line skating right outside your own door, in driveways, streets and parks, which helps to explain in-line skating's phenomenal popularity.

According to the National Sporting Goods Association, it's the fastest-growing sport in the country. If you're just joining the rush, here are some things to consider.

Narrow the field. The in-line skate market has splintered into several specialty areas, with some models, such as hockey and speed skates, mirroring the ice-skating field. Other categories include recreational skates, used by anyone who values versatility. They're not only for entry-level skaters but are good for those with intermediate skills as well. Fitness skates are similar to recreational models except they have longer frames and bigger wheels for enhanced stability at high speeds. "Aggressive" skates are used for street skating and "vertical" skating done on ramps and half-pipes. Not surprisingly, "recreational and fitness are by far the biggest categories," says Natalie Kurylko, editor of *InLine* magazine, and the ones that make the most sense for most people.

Choose your boot. Since recreational skates are so popular, there's a dizzying abundance of products. Most skate boots are made with injection-molded plastic that holds a removable foam liner. Generally, the frame is bolted to the boot. Some manufacturers, however, make "monocoque" models, in which the boot and frame are molded as one piece. It's a personal decision, Kurylko says: Monocoques are less expensive to produce and tend to be stiffer than two-piece construction. Skates also come with a variety of closure systems. The most common choices are lace-and-buckle combinations and a three-buckle boot. Some people prefer the better fit of lace-and-buckle boots, while others prefer the three-buckle variety because they are easy to get on and off.

Give yourself a brake. With skating, stopping has always been the rub—or should we say the road rash. Standard braking systems require you to lift one foot to apply stopping power, a move that can be hair-raising when you're already struggling to stay upright with both feet on the ground. But now there's another system, known as the ABT braking system by Rollerblade, which allows you to slow with all wheels on terra firma. Before you buy skates, find out whether your brakes are removable (ABT brakes aren't) and if they fit your future skating needs. If you want to play hockey or if your skills advance enough that you don't need ABT brakes, you may need to buy another pair of skates.

Get your bearings. Bearings are the key moving components in skates, and quality is essential for smooth, quiet rolling and overall durability. Oddly, bearings labeled with any variation of the word "precision" (specifically: nonprecision, semi-precision or precision) are of lowest quality and should be avoided. Opt instead for anything given an Annular Bearing Engineering Council (ABEC) rating. Ratings rise in odd numbers from one to nine: Higher numbers signify bearings that roll smoother and faster (and cost more), but are less tolerant of dirt and grit. For most purposes, an ABEC rating of one or three is the best choice for the money, Kurylko says.

Questions and Answers

If you've read the rest of this book (and if you haven't, that's fine with us—feel free to jump around), a few questions may still be nagging at the back of your brain. They may not be the most important questions, but as you walk along, you wonder. And if you find yourself completely satisfied information-wise, well, we still have a few unresolved matters in our minds. We turned to some of the experts we've consulted elsewhere, along with a few other people, research studies and various texts, to come up with answers to the following questions.

My buddy and I started exercising at the same time, but he's made much greater improvements than I have. What gives?

You're a victim of genetic injustice. "It's interesting," says John Duncan, Ph.D., a leading exercise researcher and president of Wellmart, a wellness consulting company also in Denton. Dr. Duncan has made the same observation in studies: "We can give ten people identical exercise prescriptions of running two miles five days a week for six months. Even if all ten people are in the same kind of shape at the start, guess what we find? There's a variation in the results of as much as 60 percent."

Some people are what Dr. Duncan calls high responders to exercise, and some are low responders. The vast majority, however (about 85 percent), respond fairly consistently in a middle range. If you're average, you can expect to see a 15 to 20 percent improvement in cardiovascular fitness over 12 weeks of exercising 30 minutes (at a moderately vigorous pace) three days a week. If you fall short of that, don't lose heart. "The important thing to remember is that for everyone, exercise is dose-related," Dr. Duncan says. "Do more and you get more benefit."

It seems like I add plates for my biceps curls more often than for my leg extensions. Do some parts of the body get strong faster than others?

Yes, indeed (Vagaries of Genetics, Part II), although it's usually the legs that get stronger before the arms, says Wayne Westcott, Ph.D., strength-training consultant to the national YMCA and senior fitness director for the South Shore YMCA in Quincy, Massachusetts. Your overall potential for muscular development depends on the relative length of your muscles and the muscle fiber makeup, which can vary from one part of the body to another.

If you're wondering about the specific potential for developing biceps strength, Dr. Westcott suggests this simple test: Sit with your arm on a table, then bend your elbow 90 degrees and touch your fist to your forehead, like you're posing for Rodin's *The Thinker*. Now contract your biceps and, with your other hand, insert as many fingers as will fit in the crook between your flexed muscle and your forearm. If you can only fit one finger, you have great potential; if you can fit two fingers, you have moderate potential, and if you can fit three fingers, you have minimal potential.

Does bulking up make you less flexible?

"Ah, the muscle-bound theory," sighs Alan Mikesky, Ph.D., director of the Human Performance Lab and associate professor at Indiana University-Purdue University Indianapolis. The pumped-up feeling you get from working out may make you feel like you're becoming a chunk of granite, but in reality, the act of lifting weights—contracting muscles and putting them through a range of motion—stretches muscles, which is good. "As long as you train through a full range of motion, you won't lose flexibility," Dr. Mikesky says. "In fact, you'll gain. Some of the most flexible athletes, aside from gymnasts, are Olympic lifters."

I keep hearing that soreness is bad, but I figure as long as I'm a little sore, I'm on the right track. After all, isn't the idea to push muscles beyond what they're comfortable doing?

There's a fine line to be toed here, says Dr. Westcott. True, "some soreness is good because it means you're making gains," he says. But remember that soreness (and progress) is a function of microscopic muscle damage. You want to break muscles down just enough for them to recover and be stronger by the next workout. If they're overly damaged, recovery won't be complete, and they'll essentially be in worse shape than they were, not better. Stress them again before they're recovered and you'll find it difficult to take them to the next level in stepwise fashion. Soreness and recovery are quite subjective and individual, but as a rule, Dr. Westcott says, being sore the day after a workout is okay. "If you're still sore the second day, though," he says, "you're probably overdoing it."

Will making muscles stronger or bigger boost my sex drive?

Not quite. It's aerobic exercise, rather than muscle-building, that stands to improve your sex drive, if you measure "drive" by either the quantity or quality of sexual experiences, says Roger Crenshaw, M.D., a psychotherapist and sex therapist in private practice in La Jolla, California. In one study, men in their forties who swam regularly had sex more than twice as often as sedentary men their age—seven times a week, as opposed to three times, on average. Another study found that regular exercisers (both men and women) reached orgasm easiest and most often compared to others in a group of 751 volunteers. In this last study, physical condition was deemed an even more important factor in good sex than age.

Some guys tote so much stuff to the gym that they practically carry suitcases. Am I missing something? What's the most perfect way to pack a workout bag so that you have everything you need but not an item more?

Most men overpack, says Owen McKibbin, a former pro beach volleyball player who's now a Los Angeles-based model who has graced the cover of *Men's Health* magazine. McKibbin's profession makes working out essential, but his schedule (with much time spent traveling) demands that he be able to pack light and move quickly.

First, he says, avoid carrying clothes by wearing as much as possible of what you need. "I bring clean underwear, socks and maybe a spare shirt, but I like to wear my workout gear and sweats to the gym," McKibbin says, "and I always wear the same shoes." Beyond that, he packs antiperspirant or deodorant, a bar of soap, a moisturizing lotion such as Polo Sport, a comb, a leave-in hair conditioner that's applied after showering to avoid flyaway hair and a toothbrush, "in case I have a date." And, perhaps most important, McKibbin brings a snack for on-the-go eating, often a small pop-top tin of high-protein tuna or a protein supplement powder that he adds to fruit juice. One

other bit of advice: If you're traveling to warm climes, bring nylon shorts. "You can rinse them in the shower and they'll dry in two hours."

When is it okay to talk to a woman you don't know at the gym?

First, consider how women imagine an attempted pickup progressing: "After I stop laughing, I check for his wedding ring," sneers Liz Neporent, president of Frontline Fitness, a consulting firm that sets up private and corporate gyms in New York City. She continues her distressingly thoughtful and not-too-encouraging response by saying, "Let me tell you when it's definitely not okay." The rules: "Never approach a woman who's in the middle of a set, wears a wedding band, is listening to headphones or scowls at you." Beyond that, however, things become a bit hazy, and it's in the smoke of gender battle that opportunities lie for breaking through defensive frontiers. For example, Neporent says a man shouldn't be encouraged by anything less than flat-out "come here, baby" vibes, but allows that it never hurts for a guy to try. In other words, the essence of the matter, as always, is in the approach. Some of her suggestions:

• Don't make the mistake of thinking that a stock pickup line will work if only it's clever or disarming or sensitive or, for some women, blatantly suggestive enough. Women hate clever, disarming, sensitive or blatantly suggestive lines. And don't bother complimenting a woman on her physique, even if improving it is her reason for being there. Some classic clinkers to avoid: "What exercise do you like for your thighs?" or "If I said you had a beautiful body, would you hold it against me?"

• For an opening line to succeed, it has to sound totally innocent, having nothing whatsoever to do with any sparks of attraction that may or may not—currently or at any point in the foreseeable future—fly. A good gambit is to ask specific questions about specific aspects of a specific routine, such as, "You're able to lift a lot of weight; do you do supersets for your biceps?" If she responds brusquely to such an innocuous question, you've laid so little ego on the line, it doesn't even count as a rejection. If she answers your question, strive only to have a nice conversation.

What should I do when I need to use a machine but some other guy is sitting on it between sets? I always assume he knows the rules about not hogging equipment and is probably taking extremely short rests. But should I allow him to inconvenience me for the sake of his own timing?

"Give him the benefit of the doubt," Neporent advises. "Maybe he's new and doesn't know the ground rules. Or maybe he's just distracted or hasn't noticed that it's become more crowded than when he first arrived. Or maybe he is doing a sophisticated exercise and legitimately isn't finished yet. The main thing is that if you don't ask, you don't know. If you say politely, 'Mind if I work in with you?' you'll usually get a polite answer."

Is it really necessary for me to drink water while I'm working out? Why not just tank up before and after?

Maybe it's not surprising that hydration so often seems a pain. When you're sweating like a pig, you're actually sweating more than a pig: No mammal sweats as much as humans. If you're fully hydrated before a workout, not drinking during exercise isn't going to kill you—unless you're working out in the heat (temperatures in the 70s or higher), or exercising at high intensity or for a long period of time. Then, dehydration might kill you after all. Remember, running at a typical training pace can drain you of two quarts of sweat an hour. To keep up, you need to be taking in more than a quart each hour, says Colonel John Gardner, M.D., professor and physician at the Uniformed Services University of the Health Sciences at Bethesda, Maryland. Dehydration doesn't just make you thirsty, it makes you weak: Muscle strength declines with every percentage point of dehydration. If you're trying to get stronger, what's the point of letting a lack of water sap you? Severe loss of fluids can bring on muscle cramps, headaches, tunnel vision, nausea, diarrhea and, ultimately, heat stroke, which is fatal a third of the time.

I'd like to start a workout program, but I can't afford any exercise equipment right now, much less a gym membership. What are my alternatives?

"I love high tech, but low tech often gets you in better shape," says Neporent. Who needs a $2,000 stationary bike when walking or running will give you a superior aerobic workout with more interesting scenery? For resistance training, good old-fashioned push-ups, crunches and chin-ups will get your muscles in great shape, free of free weights. If you're pushing beyond that point, well, weight is weight. Browse the supermarket aisles for containers that have fat ends and narrow middles (the section where bleaches and cleansers are displayed is a good bet). Dump the contents into something else and fill the container with sand for makeshift dumbbells. For unsophisticated items like jump ropes, don't shell out the $15 to $30 it takes for a high-end model when plastic kid's ropes are available for under $2. "I love my $1.75 jump rope best," Neporent says. "It whips around a lot faster than professional ropes."

Are chores exercise?

Broadly speaking, yes, but naturally it matters what kind of chores you're doing. Here's how some domestic duties favorably compare with various forms of exercise or sports, with calories burned per hour by a 180-pound man noted in parentheses.

Tree pruning (630)=swimming at a slow crawl (630)
Pushing a power mower (486)=biking at 10 mph (486)
Light snow-shoveling (702)=jumping rope (684)
Garden hoeing (576)=playing singles tennis (522)
Sawing by hand (594)=using a rowing machine (558)
Chopping wood (414)=walking at 3.5 mph (432)
House painting (378)=playing volleyball (396)

What's the best way to go about hiring a personal trainer?

You might think that people who say they're personal trainers actually need to have some training themselves, and maybe a paper to prove it, but you'd be wrong. Anybody can call himself a personal trainer. According to a survey by the International Association of Fitness Professionals, 27 percent of those who hang trainer shingles have no formal background in fitness. Here are some lines of inquiry to follow, provided by the association, to find trainers who know their stuff.

Who says? Certification by any of the following six major national groups is a sign of professionalism and dedication.

- The American College of Sports Medicine
- The American Council on Exercise
- The Aerobics and Fitness Association of America
- The International Fitness Institute
- The National Academy of Sports Medicine
- The National Strength and Conditioning Association

Where's the safety net? If something goes wrong, the best trainers know CPR and first-aid, and also insure themselves and their services against personal injury and property loss—something that's particularly important if you'll be training in your own home.

What's your background? Good trainers have been involved in athletics since way back when. They have a longtime passion for fitness that the best of them will have pursued by studying—if not getting a degree in—exercise physiology, kinesiology, anatomy or sports psychology.

How's business? Find out if this is a full-time job; a part-time trainer may not be as committed to you as someone whose livelihood depends on keeping clients satisfied. Ask how many people this person trains a day. A trainer who's in demand isn't necessarily better: You're paying for personal attention, and somebody who's frazzled, distracted or overbooked won't be able to give it to you. Ask for a few references and call them.

How can I make my athletic shoes last longer?

"There's not really that much you can do," says Bob Wischnia, senior editor and resident shoe guru at *Runner's World* magazine. "No matter what, shoes wear out depending on how much you use them, the mechanics of your body, your size and the kind of surface you wear them on." The best bet, Wischnia says, is to buy shoes made with durable materials such as polyurethane midsoles (as opposed to EVA, which is a more cushioned foam, but less durable) and hard carbon outsoles (as opposed to softer rubber). Beyond that, says Wischnia, there are a number of basic ways to avoid shortening the life of your shoes.

- Keep them dry. Getting shoes wet makes the midsoles break down and become brittle.
- Avoid temperature extremes. Shoes kept in cold garages also quickly become brittle in the midsole, and sunlight can turn foam to mush.
- Let function follow form. Using running shoes for basketball or basketball shoes for playing tennis

wears and tears shoes in ways they're not designed to hold up against.

If I'm pressed for time, which is better: taking three-minute rests between two sets, or 30-second rests between three sets?

From a strictly time-management point of view, let's assume you're doing a basic workout with six stations, one set per station. Each station takes a minute to do (assuming ten reps at six seconds per lift). Tacking on an additional set (another ten reps) at each station costs you an additional 6 minutes, and adding a third set is another 6 minutes. Add 30 seconds between each set and you're up to 9 extra minutes. Your total time spent would be 27 minutes.

Now, two sets would only take 12 minutes, but 3 minute rests between those sets would add another 36 minutes to your workout, for a total of 48 minutes. As you can see, it will take an extra 21 minutes if you choose the 2-set, long rest program.

That said, the real answer here depends upon your goals. Remember, longer rests of three to five minutes between bouts of heavy resistance are better for building muscle strength, while shorter rests of 30 to 90 seconds between bouts of moderate resistance are better for building muscle size.

Index

Note: Boldface page references indicate main discussion of topic. *Italic* page references indicate illustrations or boxed text.

A

G

H

Y

Z